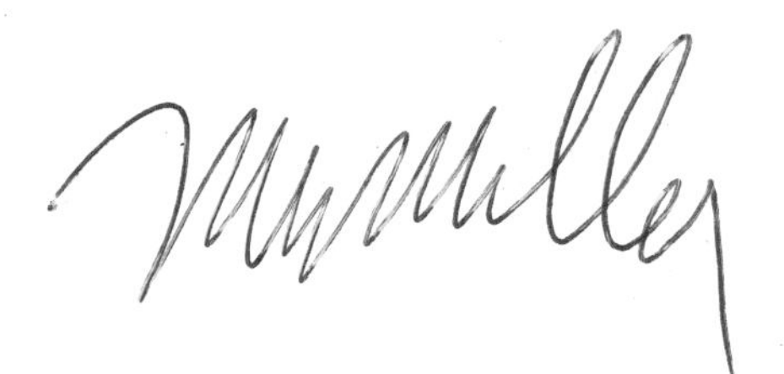

T5-DHH-767

Hydrocarbon Contaminated Soils

Volume IV

Perspectives
Analysis
Human Health and Risk Assessment
Remediation

Edward J. Calabrese
Paul T. Kostecki
Marc Bonazountas

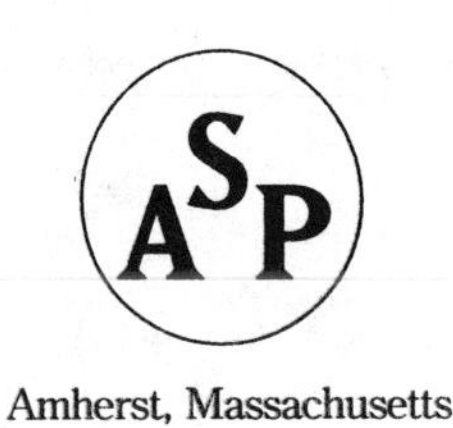

Amherst, Massachusetts

Hydrocarbon contaminated soils/ Edward J. Calabrese, Paul T. Kostecki, Marc Bonazountas, editors
ISBN 1-884940-00-5

Amherst Scientific Publishers
150 Fearing Street, Amherst, Massachusetts 01002

PRINTED IN THE UNITED STATES OF AMERICA

Preface

> "There is limited awareness among the regulators, the petroleum industry, and the public concerning the significance of soil...contamination from petroleum products. Additionally, industry is generally unaware of the potential environmental and financial liabilities they incur should their operations or actions cause contamination."

This statement opened the preface of the proceedings from the first "Environmental and Public Health Effects of Petroleum-Contaminated Soils" conference in 1985. The statement was taken from a state report on petroleum contaminated soils and was described as "where we as a nation stand with respect to addressing the environmental and public health problems associated with petroleum contaminated soils in the 1980s."

It is the 1990s. The industry has matured. We are no longer investigating and characterizing; we are now, not only remediating, but are working to help our companies and customers solve and manage their environmental issues. In the 1990s, we, as a nation, have travelled far from the 1980s along the road to addressing the environmental and public health problems associated with petroleum contaminated soils.

The 1985 and subsequent conferences taught us about the chemistry and fate of petroleum in soil systems, the detection of petroleum contamination by state-of-the-art field measurement techniques, what can be done with petroleum contaminated soils, and possible engineering and remedial action techniques.

Today we seek speed, efficiency, and cost-effective solutions; we are experimenting and using innovative technologies to help us achieve those solutions; and we are fine tuning our efforts by evaluating existing clean-up standards and questioning traditional methods of practice. For example, the papers included in this year's proceedings describe real-time, cost-effective on-site sensors for long term monitoring (Chapter 7) and passive sorbent collection devices for site screening (Chapter 11). Innovative technologies, from immunoassay technology for field screening (Chapter 12), to the Biogenesis[tm] washing process for remediating contaminated soil and sediment (Chapter 24) demonstrate progress accomplishing our work. Utilizing risk assessment as a tool to determine "how clean is clean" shows our ability to examine the standard in search of a better gauge (Chapters 14, 16, and 17).

The evolution of the industry over the past decade is remarkable. Where we once spent countless hours compiling mountains of data in order to characterize a site's contamination, we are now cleaning up this contamination. The developments in data collection and evaluation methodologies and remedial technology, coupled with the experience we've gained over the years and continual changes in the regulatory climate, have greatly improved our capabilities and confidence. The industry has moved to the next level: designing and implementing remedial solutions. And perhaps more importantly, we are committed to analyzing the effectiveness of these solutions - from both a technology and a cost perspective.

The environmental science and engineering community, like many other industries, was swept up in the generous 1980s; getting the work and keeping busy was easy. There was money to be spent. Some even turned customers away. The 1990s can be characterized as a buyer's market, and to succeed we must focus on customer service. We must perform work from a solutions-oriented business perspective, incorporating dollars and sense into what we do every day. The luxury of the 1980s is gone; the reality of the 1990s has set in like every other industry, we are involved in a business, which must be managed with practicality and efficiency, and above all, must serve the customer.

Looking ahead, further technological innovation, better use of risk based techniques, and advances in information technology, accomplished through partnering and teaming across government, industry, and academia, show great promise for our continued progress on the road to solving environmental and public health problems associated with petroleum contaminated soils. And to evolve into the next decade, the industry must continue to focus on our customers, working with them to manage and solve their environmental issues.

Richard G. DeNitto
General Manager
Northeast Region
ABB Environmental Services, Inc.

Rebecca Bozadjian
Manager, Commercial Business Development
ABB Environmental Services, Inc.

Acknowledgments

We wish to thank all the agencies, organizations and companies that sponsored the conference, without their generosity and assistance the conference and this book would not have been possible.

Sponsors

ABB Environmental Services
American Petroleum Institute
Association of American Railroads
ENSR
ETG Environmental
Massachusetts Department of Environmental Protection
Montgomery Watson
Texaco
US Army Corps of Engineers
Woodward-Clyde Consultants and Federal Services

Supporters

Association for the Environmental Health of Soils
Dionex
Envirogen Remediation Services
Health and Welfare Canada
Quantix
RETEC
Roy F. Weston
Tyree Environmental Services
University of Massachusetts Continuing Education
Wastewater Technology Centre, Ontario, Canada
3M

In addition we express our deepest appreciation to the members of the Advisory Committees who volunteered their time to provide guidance and encouragement.

Scientific Advisory Board

Roy Abbate
Dionex Corporation
Keith Angell
Groundwater Technology, Inc.
Michael Arnold
Pennsylvania DER

Christopher Barkan
Association of American Railroads
Bruce Bauman
American Petroleum Institute
Marcos Bonazountas
University of Athens, Greece
Ruddie Clarkson
Montgomery Watson
James Colman
Massachusetts DEP
Michael Conway
United Retek Corporation
John Del Pup
Texaco, Inc.
Richard DiNitto
ABB Environmental Services, Inc.
James Dragun
The Dragun Corporation
Mohamed Elnabarawy
3M
Garth Fort
Monsanto Company
Carol Fussaro
ENSR Consulting and Engineering
Kris Gagnon
Exxon Company, USA
Annette Guiseppi-Elie
Mobil Oil Corporation
Wally Hise
Radian Corporation
Donald Jacobs
Envirogen Remediation Services
Paul Jacobsen
Northeast Utilities
Bruce Jank
Environment Canada
John Lynch
RETEC
Craig McCaffrey
Ohmicron
Frank Peduto
New York DEC
Rod Raphael
Department of Health and Welfare, Canada

Martina Schlauch
Association of American Railroads
Corinne Schultz
Roy F. Weston, Inc.
Leigh Short
Woodward-Clyde Consultants
William Torrey
US EPA Region I
Debby Tremblay
US EPA OUST
Thomas Umbreit
ATSDR
Patrick Vargo
Tyree Organization, Ltd.
Thomas Wysocki
Quantix Systems

Federal Subcommittee Advisory Board

Sidney Allison
Naval Facilities Engineering Command
Greg Grim
US Army Corps of Engineers
Elizabeth Holbrook
Earth Technology
Paul Kavanaugh
RRS-Clemson Technical Center, Inc.
Lynn Kucharski*
Woodward-Clyde Federal Services
Ray Montgomery
US Army Corps of Engineers
Mark Nickelson
Oak Ridge National Laboratory
William Powers
Naval Civil Engineering Lab
Paul Rakowski
Naval Facilities Engineering Command
Edward Smith
US Army Corps of Engineers

* Committee chair

Paul T. Kostecki, Associate Director, Northeast Regional Environmental Public Health Center, School of Public Health, University of Massachusetts at Amherst, received his Ph.D. from the School of Natural Resources at the University of Michigan in 1980. He has been involved with risk assessment and risk management research for contaminated soils for the last eight years, and is coauthor of *Remedial Technologies for Leaking Underground Storage Tanks*, coeditor of *Soils Contaminated by Petroleum Products and Petroleum Contaminated Soils*, Vols. 1, 2 and 3, and of *Hydrocarbon Contaminated Soils*: Vols. 1, 2 and 3; and *Hydrocarbon Contaminated Soils and Groundwater*, Vols 1, 2 and 3, of *Contaminated Soils: Diesel Fuel Contamination; Principles and Practices for Petroleum Contaminated Soils*; and *Risk Assessment and Environmental Fate Methodologies*. Dr. Kostecki's yearly conferences on hydrocarbon contaminated soils draw hundreds of researchers and regulatory scientists to present and discuss state-of-the art solutions to the multidisciplinary problems surrounding this issue. Dr. Kostecki also serves as Managing Director for the International Society of Regulatory Toxicology and Pharmacology's Council for Health and Environmental Safety of Soils (CHESS), as Executive Director of the Association for the Environmental Health of Soils (AEHS), and as Editorial Advisor to the *Journal of Soil Contamination* and *SOILS* magazine.

Edward J. Calabrese is a board certified toxicologist who is professor of toxicology at the University of Massachusetts School of Public Health, Amherst. Dr. Calabrese has researched extensively in the area of host factors affecting susceptibility to pollutants, and is the author of more than 270 papers in scholarly journals, as well as 23 books, including *Principles of Animal Extrapolation; Nutrition and Environmental Health*, Vols 1 and 2: *Ecogenetics: Safe Drinking Water Act: Amendments, Regulations and Standards; Petroleum Contaminated Soils*, Vols, 1, 2 and 3; *Ozone Risk Communications and Management; Hydrocarbon Contaminated Soils*, Vols. 1, 2, and 3; *Hydrocarbon Contaminated Soils and Groundwater*, Vols. 1, 2 and 3; *Multiple Chemical Interactions; Air Toxics and Risk Assessment; Alcohol Interactions with Drugs and Chemicals; Regulating Drinking Water Quality; Biological Effects of Low Level Exposures to Chemicals and Radiation; Contaminated Soils; Diesel Fuel Contamination; Risk Assessment and Environmental Fate Methodologies, and Principles and Practices for Petroleum Contaminated Soils.* He has been a member of the U.S. National Academy of Sciences and NATO Countries Safe Drinking Water Committees, and the Board of Scientific Counselors for the Agency for Toxic Substances and Disease Registry (ATSDR). Dr. Calabrese also serves as Chairman of the International Society of Regulatory Toxicology and Pharmacology's Council for Health and Environmental Safety of Soils (CHESS) and Director of the Northeast Regional Environmental Public Health Center at the University of Massachusetts.

Marc Bonazountas is a civil and environmental scientist, specializing in mathematical modeling of all environmental media and systems: air, soil, water, biota; and global environmental management. He received his engineering degree from the National Technical University in Athens, Greece; his doctorate from the National Technical University of Munich, Germany; his diploma in computer sciences from the Data Processing Institute, Athens; and undertook further studies in water resources systems at the Massachusetts Institute of Technology, and in public policy at Harvard University. He obtained his professorship in 1984 at the National Technical University of Athens, where he is currently engaged in teaching and research related to all environmental media. Prior to joining the university, he was with Rhein-Main-Donau AG in Munich, and Arthur D. Little, Inc., in Cambridge, Massachusetts. He has been involved in numerous U.S. Environmental Protection Agency research and technology projects, and has developed mathematical environmental models, considered today as being standards by the U.S. EPA and other regulatory agencies. Among these models is SESOIL (Seasonal Soil Compartment Model), a theory approved by the U.S. government and various national and international agencies. SESOIL is a standard package for estimating pollution in soil systems from petroleum contaminated sites and other watershed and soil polluting practices. Dr. Bonazountas is a member of CHESS (Council for Health and Environmental Safety of Soils) and a member of the Editorial Board of the *Journal of Soil Contamination.*

Contents

Part I
Perspectives

Part II
Analysis

Part III
Human Health and Risk Assessment

Part IV
Remediation

Hydrocarbon Contaminated Soils

Volume IV

PART I

PERSPECTIVES

CHAPTER 1

Soils Considerations in Navy Risk Assessments

Sheila A. Berglund, P.E., Environmental Programs Directorate, Navy Env' mental Health Center, Norfolk, Virginia

INTRODUCTION

The Comprehensive Environmental Response, Compensation and Liability Act (CERCLA) of 1980, as amended by the Superfund Amendments and Reauthorization Act (SARA) of 1986, provides the regulatory framework for implementing the Department of Defense's Installation Restoration Program. In following the procedural guidelines set forth in the National Contingency Plan, the Department of the Navy conducts studies and investigations at its past hazardous waste disposal sites. A significant part of the process, the risk assessment, is developed during the remedial investigation and feasibility study phase of the program.

Risk assessments are performed to determine if a specific site poses an unacceptable risk to human health or the environment, and thus if remediation is necessary. Risk assessments help in determining how much of a site requires remedial action and to what level it should be cleaned. The risk assessment process is composed of four major steps: data collection and evaluation, exposure assessment, toxicity assessment, and risk characterization. This chapter will briefly discuss each of these steps and address soils issues to be considered during the entire process.

It is important to distinguish between risk assessment and risk management. Risk assessment is the quantitative estimation of the magnitude of health risks and the uncertainties that accompany them. Risk assessment is a scientific process which develops actual risk numbers to be used by risk managers when deciding the best remedial course of action to take on a particular site. Risk management is the ensuing policy judgement of what is an acceptable risk to society. Risk managers combine the information from the risk assessment with other considerations, such as acceptability to the local community, economics, and efficacy and permanence of the remedial alternatives, to reach the remedial decisions necessary to implement an effective clean-up program.

There are many factors which affect the acceptability of the risk posed by a particular site. In addition to addressing the direct and underlying concerns posed by the community surrounding the site, it is the risk manager's responsibility to ensure the scientific merit of the information on which the remedial decisions are made. An understanding of the risk assessment process is essential to meeting the goals of an effective remedial program.

THE SITE CONCEPTUAL MODEL

The site conceptual model is typically developed during the planning stages of the risk assessment. The risk assessor identifies, to the maximum extent practicable, the sources, pathways and receptors located at or near a specific site. Risk to human health or the environment is only possible when all three parameters are present. It is the risk manager's task to eliminate at least one of the three in order to effectively limit or negate the risk posed by the site contaminants.

The risk assessor needs to know the following information to develop the site conceptual model:

- What contaminants are present, including their concentrations at the source and at potential receptors;
- What are the specific sources of contamination at the site;
- How are the contaminants expected to move through the site media; and
- Who are the potential receptors, both human and ecological, including sensitive subpopulations.

THE RISK ASSESSMENT PROCESS

There are four major steps in the risk assessment process. They are data collection and evaluation, the exposure assessment, the toxicity assessment, and risk characterization. Each of these areas will be discussed in detail with particular emphasis placed on the soils considerations involved with each.

Data Collection and Evaluation

The primary purposes of the data collection and evaluation portion of the process are:

- To minimize the possibility of false negative information, in other words, to avoid the situation where the decision based on the risk assessment may not be protective of human health or the environment;
- To determine if the site chemical concentrations are sufficiently different from background concentrations, either naturally occurring or anthropogenic (man-made non-site related causes); and
- To ensure all exposure pathways are identified, examined and characterized.

Data Collection

The Environmental Protection Agency[1] recommends the following course of action when planning for the data collection portion of the process.

Review of Available Site Information

Although most site information in the planning stages of the risk assessment will be incomplete, there are many data sources available to the risk assessor. These include the preliminary assessment and site inspection reports developed prior to the start of the remedial investigation, site historical files and photographs, community relations interviews, and information from agencies not directly responsible for the site such as the Agency for Toxic Substances and Disease Registry or local health departments. For site specific soils information, the risk assessor may turn to the U.S. Department of Agriculture Soil Conservation Service or the U.S. Geologic Survey.

Consider Modeling Parameter Needs

Many risk assessors use computer models to study the fate and transport mechanisms of particular contaminants with respect to potential receptors. Close coordination between the risk assessor, computer modeling staff, and the project planning team is necessary to ensure the required modeling parameters are identified and appropriate data are collected during the on-site field activities. Computer modeling parameters for soils include particle size, dry weight, pH, redox potential, mineral class, organic carbon and clay content, bulk density and soil porosity.

Define Background Sampling Needs

There are two types of background data to be collected; naturally occurring background concentrations of chemicals and anthropogenic background concentrations, those due to human made non-site sources, such as automobiles or industrial activities. Background sampling locations and sample size should be determined in the planning stage using statistics to allow for scientifically valid identification of site related contaminants.

Identify Potential Human Exposures

Potential human exposures may most easily be identified through a review of potentially completed exposure pathways. Using the site conceptual model which is developed during the planning stages, the risk assessor develops a sense of which media at a particular site should be sampled, the probable fate and transport mechanisms for site contaminants, and which specific areas require detailed evaluation. At most sites, contaminated soil is either the primary source of exposure through direct contact or is a media by which other sources become contaminated, for example by the leaching of chemicals into the ground water. The EPA[2-5] has developed a set of guidance documents which deal directly with soil sampling at waste sites. These guidance documents provide information on soil related topics such as the sampling locations, sampling equipment and soil specific issues such as the heterogeneous nature of soils, the designation of hot spots, appropriate depths for sampling, and fate and transport properties.

Develop an Overall Strategy for Sample Collection

The sampling strategy should include the above topics in addition to information important to the on-site field activities. Weather conditions, field screening and analytical capabilities, and costs should be addressed. Most Department of the Navy sites are currently on or are proposed for the National Priorities List (NPL), or have sufficient contamination to be considered for placement on the NPL. The Agency for Toxic Substances and Disease Registry (ATSDR) conducts public health assessments at each NPL site. To increase the compatibility of data used for both the risk assessment and public health assessment, project managers are encouraged to follow the draft guidance set forth in ATSDR's "Environmental Data Needed for Public Health Assessments."[6] A checklist for the environmental data needs for ATSDR's public health assessment pertaining to the soil exposure pathway is provided below.

- Are surface soil results reported separately from subsurface soil results?
- Were surface soil samples taken from zero to three inches?
- Are surface soil results available for before and after removal?
- Are surface soil results available for before and after remediation?
- Is the purpose of each sampling effort described?
- Are exact sample locations, including descriptions and map locations provided?
- Is the depth of sampling points indicated?
- Are samples vertical composites?
- Is the type of sample indicated (grab or composite)?
- Is the sampling scheme for composite samples indicated?
- Is sample analysis information provided (methods, detection limits, concentrations)?
- Is the date of the sample indicated?
- Is the type of soil indicated (sandy, silty, clayey, etc.)?
- Is a description of vegetative cover provided?
- Is land use described?
- Are any special features described?

Define Required Quality Assurance/Quality Control (QA/QC) Measures

The risk assessor should identify the quality requirements of the data to be collected and used in the risk assessment. Sampling methods and analytical protocols must be detailed enough to ensure detection limits, especially sample quantitation limits, are low enough to be useful in comparing site concentrations with health and environmental criteria.

Evaluate the Need for Special Analytical Services

Some site situations will require detection limits lower than the standard analytical services available by the laboratory. In these cases, special services, such as those detailed in the EPA's Contract Laboratory Program[7], should be specified.

Identify Activities During Workplan Development and Data Collection

All of the above data collection areas should be identified as early in the planning process as possible. The risk assessor must be involved during development of the workplans to ensure data collected in the field are adequate to fulfill the needs of the risk assessment.

Data Evaluation

Following data collection, the following activities, as recommended by the EPA[8], should be included in the data evaluation portion of the risk assessment.

Combine Data Available from Site Investigations

Most remedial investigations require several field sampling efforts. The data from each round of sampling must be combined into a single report. Care must be taken to properly identify field procedures and conditions, such as precipitation, temperature and wind speeds/directions. Site maps are particularly important to the risk assessment as they may hold the key to potential receptors in nearby water bodies, recreational areas or housing units.

Evaluate Analytical Methods

Individual attention to analytical methods is necessary even if special analytical services have been specified. Although the EPA's Contract Laboratory Program was established to provide uniform analytical procedures throughout the Superfund Program, it does not ensure consistent quality and reliability of the data resulting from these procedures.

Evaluate Quantitation Limits

The most important quantitation limit for the risk assessor is the sample quantitation limit (SQL). Attention to detail during the data collection planning and sampling stages is necessary to ensure the SQL, which is specific to each individual sample, is below the health and environmental criteria relating to risk, whenever technically feasible. The SQL is also important to identify since, at times, it may be higher than the chemical concentrations detected in other samples from the same site.

Evaluate Qualified and Coded Data

The EPA has established standard qualifiers for use in the Superfund Program.[8] There are two types of qualifiers used: laboratory data qualifiers and validation data qualifiers. There may be two different meanings associated with the same data qualifier depending on when the qualifier was attached to the data. Certain qualified data should not be carried through the quantitative risk assessment.

Evaluate Blanks

Many contaminants found on Superfund sites are also common laboratory artifacts. The use of field and trip blanks, laboratory duplicates and spikes usually allows the data reviewer to separate those contaminants which are related to the site from those which may have been introduced to the sample in the laboratory. It is customary to eliminate sampling data for such common laboratory artifacts as volatile compounds where the detected levels in the site sample are not at least five times the blank concentration. This procedure must take into consideration the possibility of site contaminants at concentrations low enough to fall within the five-fold criteria.

Evaluate Tentatively Identified Compounds

The identification of Tentatively Identified Compounds (TICs) is specific to each laboratory. The number and extent to which TICs are carried through the risk assessment calculations are often a requirement of individual state agencies. The risk assessor must be familiar with the laboratory procedures used to identify TICs and the state regulatory agency requirements regarding TICs.

Compare Site Data with Background

Separate discussions regarding naturally occurring and anthropogenic background concentrations must be included to adequately identify contaminant concentrations directly related to the site.

Identify Chemicals of Potential Concern

The list of chemicals of potential concern should be categorized by each medium. To reduce the total number of chemicals carried through the quantitative risk assessment, indicator chemicals are often chosen. These chemicals should be representative of the total list of chemicals of potential concern which include:

- Those that were positively detected in at least one sample in a given medium with no qualifiers attached or with qualifiers attached that indicate known identities but unknown concentrations;
- Those that were detected at levels significantly above the blank concentrations;
- Those that were detected at levels significantly above the background concentrations;
- Those that were only tentatively identified but may be associated with the site based on historical information; and/or
- Those that are transformation products of chemicals demonstrated to be present.

EXPOSURE ASSESSMENT

The primary purposes of the exposure assessment are:

- To determine who may be exposed and by what pathways;
- To estimate the magnitude of the potential exposures; and
- To determine the average exposure and the reasonable maximum exposure, or the highest exposure that is reasonably expected to occur at a site.

The exposure assessment is performed in the three steps described below.

Characterize Exposure Setting

To characterize the exposure setting, the risk assessment usually addresses two general areas: the physical environment and potentially exposed populations.

Physical Environment

The information in this section should include data on the local climate, including temperature and precipitation; meteorology, including wind speeds and directions; the geologic setting; site and surrounding vegetation, including sensitive habitats; soil type such as sandy, organic, acid or basic; ground water hydrology including depth and direction of flow; and description of surface water, including type, flow rates and salinity.

Potentially Exposed Populations

This section addresses those receptors on or near to the site. The location of current populations with respect to the site should be identified as well as the current and future land uses. Sensitive subpopulations include children, elderly or retired citizens, people who may eat a large amount of locally raised vegetables or locally caught fish or shellfish, and hospital residents.

Identify Exposure Pathways:

The exposure pathway has three requirements: the chemical source or release, the exposure point and the exposure route. The two primary exposure routes for the soils pathway are incidental ingestion and dermal contact. Although not considered a primary pathway, soils may also contribute to the inhalation route via fugitive dust or airborne particles. These routes may be encountered in several exposure scenarios by either adults or children. They are:

- Residential and recreational lifetime exposures to adults;
- Residential and recreational short-term exposures to children; and
- Commercial and industrial occupational exposures to adults.

Quantify Exposure

The EPA[8] provides the following equations for quantifying intakes for the ingestion and dermal contact exposure routes. For ingestion of surface soil, intake may be calculated by:

$$\text{INTAKE} = (\text{CS x IR x CF x FI x EF x ED}) / (\text{BW x AT}) \quad (1)$$

Where:

CS Chemical concentration in soil (mg/kg)
IR Ingestion rate (mg soil/day)
CF Conversion factor (10^{-6} kg/mg)
FI Fraction ingested from contaminated source (unitless)
EF Exposure frequency (days/years)
ED Exposure duration (years)
BW Body weight (kg)
AT Averaging time (days)

For dermal contact with surface soil, intake may be calculated by:

$$\text{INTAKE} = (\text{CS x CF x SA x AF x ABS x EF x ED}) / (\text{BW x AT}) \quad (2)$$

Where:

CS	Chemical concentration in soil (mg/kg)
CF	Conversion factor (10^{-6} kg/mg)
SA	Skin surface area available for contact (cm^2/event)
AF	Soil to skin adherence factor (mg/cm^2)
ABS	Absorption factor (unitless)
EF	Exposure frequency (events/years)
ED	Exposure duration (years)
BW	Body weight (kg)
AT	Averaging time (days)

The EPA[8] has developed standard default exposure factors which must be used to calculate the average and reasonable maximum exposure for each exposure scenario. Table 1.1 provides the standard defaults for the exposure routes and potential receptors for the soils pathways.

Table 1.1. Standard default exposure factors (soil).

STANDARD DEFAULT EXPOSURE FACTORS (SOIL)				
Land Use	**Daily Intake Rate**	**Exposure Frequency**	**Exposure Duration**	**Body Weight**
Residential Recreational	200mg-child 100mg-adult	350 days/yr	6 years 24 years	15 kg-child 70 kg-adult
Industrial Commercial	50 mg	250 days/yr	25 years	70 kg

TOXICITY ASSESSMENT

The following quote summarizes the importance of studying the toxicological properties of chemicals.

"ALL SUBSTANCES ARE POISONS.
THERE IS NONE WHICH IS NOT A POISON.
THE RIGHT DOSE DIFFERENTIATES A POISON AND A REMEDY."
- Paracelsus (1493 - 1541)

The toxicity assessment is performed to determine what adverse health effects a compound may potentially cause in humans and at what doses. To make this determination, multiple adverse effects or endpoints are considered; they include cancer and acute and chronic noncarcinogenic effects such as reproductive or neurologic effects or changes in body weight. The EPA[8] recommends the following actions for completing the toxicity assessment.

Gather Toxicity Information

There are two primary sources of toxicity data, both from the EPA: they are the Integrated Risk Information System (IRIS) and the Health Effects Assessment Summary Tables (HEAST).

Identify Exposure Periods

The exposure periods are the same as the exposure frequencies and durations identified in the exposure assessment.

Determine Toxicity Values for Noncarcinogens

Toxicity values for noncarcinogens are typically derived from experimentation which results in the development of a dose-response curve similar to Figure 1.1. The various effects levels are noted in Figure 1.1. and are combined with uncertainty factors and modifying factors to establish the reference doses and reference concentrations.

Determine Toxicity Values for Carcinogens

A carcinogen is defined as a chemical which causes an increased incidence of tumors above background in an exposed population. Carcinogens are classified according to the level of testing information available for a specific compound. The toxicity values for carcinogens are known as slope factors which are defined as the plausible upper bound probability of excess lifetime risk of cancer; slope factors are expressed in units of risk per (mg/kg-day).

Summarize Toxicity Information

This section typically includes summary information from each of the above areas. In some cases, toxicity information may be presented in groups by affected organ or adverse effect. The risk assessor must coordinate closely with a knowledgeable toxicologist to develop this type of summary section.

RISK CHARACTERIZATION

Risk characterization is the final step in the risk assessment. The EPA[8] recommends the following steps in combining the information from the data collection and evaluation, exposure assessment and toxicity assessment.

- Review outputs from toxicity and exposure assessments;
- Quantify risks from individual chemicals;
- Quantify risks from multiple chemicals;
- Combine risks across exposure pathways;

- Assess and present uncertainty;
- Consider site-specific human studies; and
- Summarize risks.

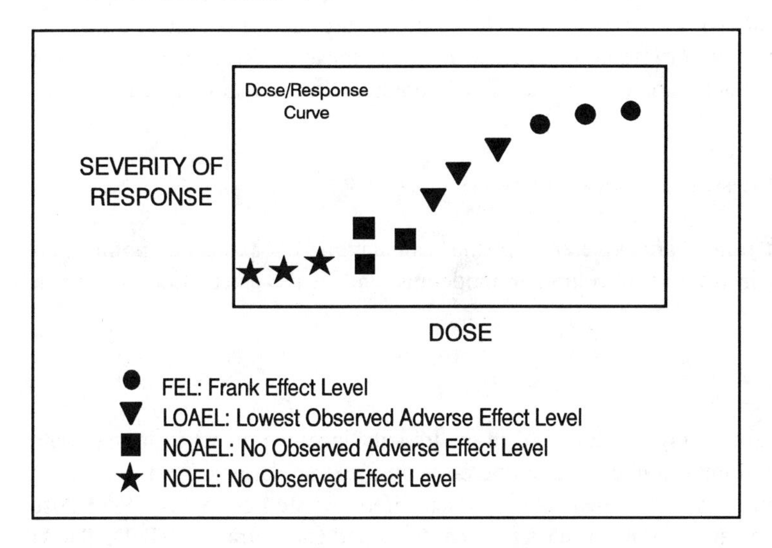

Figure 1.1.

Combining Risks

The result of risk characterization is often a single risk number expressed as a probability (e.g., 4×10^{-6}) for carcinogens and as a hazard index or ratio (e.g., 1.2) for noncarcinogens. The EPA, in a memorandum[9] distributed to each regional office, states: "Regarding exposure and risk characterization, it is Agency policy to present information on the range of exposures derived from exposure scenarios and on the use of multiple risk descriptors (i.e., central tendency, high end of individual risk, population risk, important subgroups, if known) consistent with terminology in the attached Appendix and Agency guidelines." Additional EPA guidance[10] for exposure assessment reiterates that "Several statistical estimators of exposure should be identified, e.g., the 50th, 90th, or 95th percentiles. The distribution should reflect exposures, not just concentrations." Both of these discussions conclude that it is more appropriate to summarize risk as a range of values and not a single point estimate.

Assessing Uncertainty

When combining information, identification of the uncertainties associated with sampling data or standard values used is key to a complete risk assessment. The following information indicates potential sources of uncertainty from each step in the risk assessment process.

Data Collection and Evaluation

With respect to false negatives, there may be concerns that the sampling is not representative, analytical detection limits are above concentrations of concern, or laboratory spike recoveries are low. False positives may be present if sampling blanks are contaminated or laboratory spike recoveries are biased high.

Exposure Assessment

Uncertainties are inherent in the calculation of exposure point concentrations, in the use of computer modeling, and in the calculation of human intakes.

Toxicity Assessment

Uncertainty may be identified in the toxicity information when human data is based on animal studies, when route-to-route extrapolations are used, when lifetime values are founded on less-than-lifetime studies, when low dose concentrations are present, when reference doses and concentrations (RfDs/RfCs) are not statistically derived, and when the mechanism of toxicity is not taken into consideration.

Risk Characterization

The above uncertainties are compounded in the risk characterization with the assumption of risk additivity for carcinogens and dose additivity for noncarcinogens, and when there is a lack of chemical-specific or route-specific reference toxicity values.

SUMMARY

Throughout the risk assessment process it is important to remember that risk assessment involves the use of many health protective assumptions. As a traditionally conservative practice, risk assessments do not predict actual harm that will occur, but rather the potential risk to a hypothetical receptor. In most cases, risk assessments are used as a regulatory decision-making tool to assist the risk manager in choosing an appropriate remedial alternative. The assumptions used in the risk assessment will set a precedent for development of cleanup levels which, in the end, determine the cost of site remediation.

REFERENCES

1. U.S. Environmental Protection Agency, *Risk Assessment Guidance for Superfund, Human Health Evaluation Part A*; OSWER Directive

9285.701A, Office of Solid Waste and Emergency Response, Washington, DC, 1989.

2. U.S. Environmental Protection Agency, *Test Methods for Evaluating Solid Waste (SW-846): Physical/Chemical Methods*, Office of Solid Waste, Washington, DC, 1986.
3. U.S. Environmental Protection Agency, *Field Manual for Grid Sampling of PCB Spill Sites to Verify Cleanups*, EPA/560/5-86/017, Office of Toxic Substances, Washington, DC, 1986.
4. U.S. Environmental Protection Agency, *A Compendium of Superfund Field Operations Methods*, EPA/540/P-87/001, OSWER Directive 9355.0-14, Office of Emergency and Remedial Response, Washing-ton, DC, 1987.
5. U.S. Environmental Protection Agency, *Soil Sampling Quality Assurance Guide*, (Review Draft), Environmental Monitoring Support Laboratory, Las Vegas, NV, 1989.
6. Agency for Toxic Substances and Disease Registry, *Environmental Data Needed for Public Health Assessments*, Federal Register, 58, 12306, 1993.
7. U.S. Environmental Protection Agency, *User's Guide to the Contract Laboratory Program*, Office of Emergency and Remedial Response, Washington, DC, 1988.
8. U.S. Environmental Protection Agency, *Risk Assessment Guidance for Superfund, Human Health Evaluation Part A*; OSWER Directive 9285.701A, Office of Solid Waste and Emergency Response, Washington, DC, 1989.
9. Deputy Administrator, U.S. Environmental Protection Agency, memorandum, "Guidance on Risk Characterization for Risk Managers and Risk Assessors," February 26, 1992.
10. U.S. Environmental Protection Agency, *Guidelines for Exposure Assessment*, Federal Register, 57, 22888, 1992.

CHAPTER 2

Demonstration of the Steam Injection and Vacuum Extraction (SIVE) Technology for Removal of JP-5 Jet Fuel in Soil

Deh Bin Chan, S. Laura Yeh, and Adolph Bialecki, Naval Facilities Service Center, Port Hueneme, California

INTRODUCTION

For several years, the United States Navy has been engaged in the advanced development of specialized techniques for the remediation of subsurface environments contaminated with hazardous materials and wastes such as chlorinated organic solvents, petroleum liquid products, polychlorinated biphenyls (PCBs), heavy metals, and other organic wastes. Recent studies indicate that application of Steam Injection and Vacuum Extraction (SIVE) as a method of remediating volatile and petroleum liquids contaminated soil holds great promise for efficient and cost effective *in-situ* contaminant treatment. Preliminary data shows that steam injection enhances free product mobility and ease of contaminant extraction. The Naval Facilities Engineering Service Center (NFESC) has been jointly tasked by the Naval Facilities Engineering Command (NAVFACENGCOM) and the Environmental Protection Agency/Risk Reduction Engineering Laboratory (EPA/RREL) to further pursue the advanced development and demonstration of SIVE technology.

In this project, the SIVE technology will be particularly applied to remove and recover JP-5 jet fuel in the subsurface soil media. JP-5 is a turbine fuel developed for military use and is used by the U.S. Navy. The fuel is clean burning, is generally a straight run petroleum distillate (little blending occurs), and has a low volatility to reduce the chance of fires on board ships. On a gas chromatographic trace, n-alkanes are the dominant peaks with the branched alkanes, alkenes, aromatic hydrocarbons, and other compounds appearing as small peaks. Generally, fresh JP-5 consists of hydrocarbons which elute from n-C_{10} to n-C_{19} with a maximum near n-C_{13}. Additional properties specified in MIL-T-5624L include a maximum aromatic content of 25% by volume, a maximum olefin content of 5%, and a maximum sulfur content of 0.40% by weight. The viscosity of the Lemoore JP-5 was measured in the laboratory as 1.33 cp at 24°C and has a specific gravity of 0.81.

In late 1987, a leak was discovered in a 16-inch diameter aluminum underground JP-5 aviation fuel transfer pipeline at the Naval Air Station, Lemoore (NASL). The pipeline runs between tank 245 and a refueling island adjacent to runway 32R. The leak caused subsurface contamination of an area later identified as Installation Restoration Site 17 (Figure 2.1). The pipeline

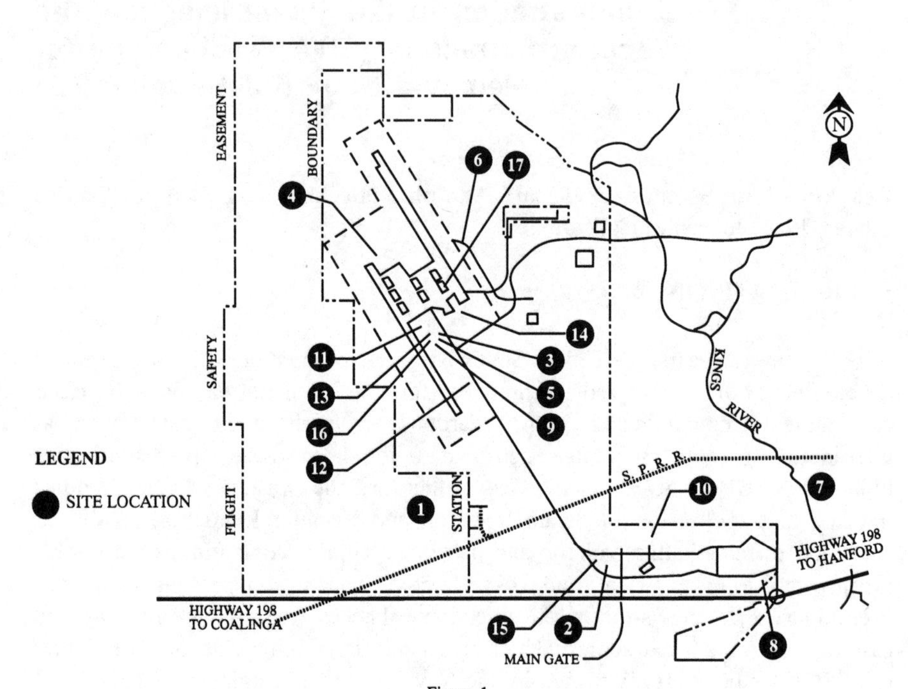

Figure 1
NAVAL AIR STATION, LEMORE, CALIFORNIA
SITES POSSIBLY CONTAMINATED WITH HAZARDOUS WASTE:

SITE 1 LANDFILL
Solvents, Paints, Waste Oils

SITE 2 PESTICIDE RINSE AREA, BLDG. 725
Pesticides, Herbicides

SITE 3 PESTICIDE RINSE AREA, BLDG. 50
Pesticides

SITE 4 OLD FIRE TRAINING AREA
JP-4 and JP-5 Fuels

SITE 5 FIREFIGHTING SCHOOL
Fuels, Solvents, Heavy Metals, andIndustrial Treatment Sludge Poads

SITE 6 OPERATIONS AREA OPEN DITCH
Heavy Metals, Solvents, Paints, Pesticides

SITE 7 HOUSING AREA open ditch
Solvents, Paints, Thinners, Battery Shop Waste, Sanitary Waste

SITE 8 HOUSING AREA SLUDGE DRYING BEDS
Sanitary Sewege, Heavy Metals

*SITE 9 INDUSTRIAL TREATMENT SLUDGE PONDS

*Sludge ponds are now included as part of Site 5.

SITE 10 PESTICIDE APPLICATION LANDING STRIP
Pesticides

SITE 11 TRANSFORMER OIL SPILL BLDG. 3
Waste Oil (PCB)

SITE 12 TRANSFORMER OIL SPILL BLDG. 468
Waste Oil (PCB)

SITE 13 TRANSFORMER STORAGE AREA BLDG. 50
Waste Oil (PCB)

SITE 14 JET ENGINE TEST CELL
JP-5 Fuel Solvents

SITE 15 FRANKLIN AVENUE PESTICIDE RINSE AREA, BLDG. 756
Pesticides

SITE 16 SLUDGE BEDS, BLDG 65
Municipal Wastewater Treatment Sludge

SITE 17 JP-5 PIPELINE FUEL LEAK
JP-5 Fuel

Figure 2.1. Naval Air Station, Lemoore, California. Sites possibly contaminated with hazardous waste.

connects a 120,000 gallon fuel storage tank to a series of refueling islands adjacent to the runway. When in full use, the flow rate through the pipeline can reach over two million gallons per day. The fuel line is buried approximately three feet below grade and is partially covered with asphalt, except at the leak point, where the absence of asphalt apparently led to corrosion of the pipe. Initial removal of fuel saturated soil adjacent to the site of the leak, resulted in an excavation collection pit approximately 14 feet deep. The JP-5 fuel which accumulated in this pit was pumped into a storage tank for disposal. The excavation depth was subsequently increased to 17 feet and later to almost 21 feet. The fuel recovery rate during this period was approximately 40-200 gallons per day. The total fuel recovered from this effort was on the order of 100,000 gallons. An unknown quantity of contaminant (estimated at 200,000-300,000 gallons) still exists on the site.

Under NFESC, the investigations related to the contamination at NASL Site 17 comprise an initial site assessment, SIVE treatability studies both in the laboratory and the field, and design of the SIVE technology demonstration system. The following tasks will be performed in conjunction with the SIVE technology demonstration:

1. Survey of existing monitoring well integrity; redrilling or new well drilling; soil and sediment sampling;
2. SIVE system design and equipment layout;
3. Site preparation;
4. Equipment installation and testing;
5. Technology demonstration.

Data collected from the SIVE technology demonstration will be utilized to develop a remediation plan for Site 17 and for full-scale SIVE system design and implementation in FY95.

SIVE TECHNOLOGY AND APPLICATION SITE CONSIDERATIONS

SIVE Technology

A typical environmental release results in disconnected pools of contaminant in the soil. Application of the SIVE process to this spill consists of steam injection wells around the contaminated soil and vacuum extraction wells within this region. Steam is injected both above and below the water table, if necessary. Groundwater, product and air (including volatiles) are pumped from the extraction wells. The soil is heated as the steam condenses until it reaches steam temperature, creating a steam zone. This steam zone grows toward the extraction wells and pushes much of the contamination ahead of it. In the steam zone, the residual contamination is volatilized at the elevated temperature and swept toward the extraction wells. After steam breaks through at the extraction wells, the injection continues or can be cycled with air injection to continue volatilization and recovery of residual compounds, e.g. JP-5. The recovered fluids are condensed and cooled to ambient conditions. Standard technologies are used to separate the product from water and to treat contaminated air and water. The success of the process for *in-situ* remediation is due to several mechanisms: steam displacement of mobile fluids from the pore space, boiling of high vapor pressure nonaqueous phase liquids, enhanced evaporation rates of low vapor pressure nonaqueous phase liquids, and desorption of contaminants from solid surfaces.

The SIVE process is a thermal enhancement to pump-and-treat and soil vapor extraction, which are conducted simultaneously with the injection of steam. The major benefits of this enhancement are the drastically reduced volumes of contaminated fluid to be handled on the surface, order of magnitude decreases in the time for remediation, applicability to source contamination (*in-situ*) both above and below the water table, and potential for recycling recovered product. The disruption of surface activities is often limited to system installation. Operating the system requires space for equipment, but does not interfere with other activities. The process is feasible to any depth and may be applied underneath structures.

Application Site Considerations

Over one dozen hazardous waste sites were reviewed for the applicability of the combined steam injection and vacuum extraction process. The purpose of the review was to select the one site most amenable to a field demonstration of the technology. Criteria used in evaluating these sites were grouped into two categories: primary and secondary. The primary criteria are necessary conditions for the demonstration and the secondary criteria are issues of practicality. The three primary criteria are:

1. **Type of contaminant.** The range of contaminants for which the process is applicable is yet to be determined. Therefore, only contaminants with proven laboratory success or desirable thermodynamic properties were considered for the demonstration. Laboratory success has been achieved with gasoline, diesel, JP-5, and volatile organic compounds. Thermodynamic properties considered, with desirable properties in parentheses, included boiling point (<100°C), specific gravity (< 1.0), vapor pressure (> 0.12 psi), viscosity (< 2.0 cp), and solubility in water (< 200 mg/l). Potential for modeling the process was also evaluated. A wide-ranging mixture of compounds was considered undesirable. Finally, highly toxic and carcinogenic compounds were avoided for the field demonstration.
2. **Concentration of Contaminant.** The minimum total concentration considered was ten parts per million (ppm). This cutoff was selected to allow for an observable reduction in concentration during the

demonstration. A 99% removal of the contaminant would leave a residual of 0.1 ppm and yield large analytical uncertainties. The optimum concentration of the contaminant was dependent on its type. For example, a concentration of 1,000 ppm for gasoline and 10,000 ppm for diesel was desirable. For compounds denser than water a maximum total concentration was applied, dependent on the particular compound. The maximum concentration represented a value beyond which a bank of separate phase contaminant may form in front of the condensation front and potentially sink through the water. A maximum concentration of 200 ppm for trichloroethylene was typical.

3. **Confining Medium Beneath Zone of Contamination.** The vertical movement of steam, condensate, and contaminant must be controlled to prevent the spreading of the contaminant. This is partially achieved by applying a large horizontal pressure gradient to the flow, but also by naturally occurring horizontal barriers. These barriers can take three forms. A continuous low permeability confining bed such as a clay layer prevents downward migration of all contaminants. For compounds lighter than water and with a low solubility, the water table may inhibit downward movement. Finally, for compounds with boiling points below that of water, a continuous high permeability strata may be filled with steam prior to the injection of steam into the overlying contaminated zone.

The secondary criteria are design considerations which could be compensated for if they are not met. The secondary criteria are:

1. **Defined perimeter of contamination**. The area of contamination must be well-defined to prevent the spreading of contaminants into clean areas.
2. **Relative Site Size**. A small site, less than 1/4 of an acre, could be completely remediated by the demonstration.
3. **Site Accessibility**. The demonstration site is preferably away from buildings, structures, underground utilities, and human intrusion and has adequate work space on the surface.
4. **Adequate Depth of Contamination**. A minimum depth of ten feet is preferable.
5. **Proximity to Existing Facilities**. On-site water treatment plants or steam supplies could be utilized.

Selection of NAS Lemoore, CA.

This site was selected because it satisfied most of the criteria set forth for the demonstration. The JP-5 jet fuel is in high concentrations at significant depth. The water table can act as a barrier to vertical migration of the fuel. The site is very open and accessible. An industrial waste treatment plant on-site could be utilized to process the extracted water. A laboratory study of samples recovered from the site was extremely promising.

JP-5 CONTAMINATION SITE

NAS Lemoore, CA

The Naval Air Station Lemoore (NASL) is approximately seven miles west of the City of Lemoore, CA. Lemoore is midway between Los Angeles and San Francisco, in the central portion of the San Joaquin Valley. As described previously, in December 1987 a leak in a 16-inch diameter aluminum pipe carrying JP-5 jet fuel was discovered at the site. The fuel line is buried approximately three feet below grade. An initial study of the site indicated an areal extent of approximately four acres for Total Petroleum Hydrocarbon (TPH) concentrations in excess of 100 ppm. Floating fuel was observed in five of twelve borings. The vertical extent of the contamination appears to be confined primarily to a silt/sand unit near the water table. The water table is located at a depth of approximately 16 feet. The site is located in an open space between a paved area and a taxiway for jets.

Site Characterization

Five monitoring wells were installed and developed in June 1988. The locations of these monitoring wells and other soil borings are shown in Figure 2.2. Boring log data indicates the site area consists of a silty-clay unit to a depth of approximately ten feet. Underlying the silty-clay unit is a thin, brownish silty-sand approximately 1.5 to 2.5 feet in thickness over much of the area. A relatively thick, fine grained, grayish-brown sand was found in several borings and exceeded ten feet in thickness. This sand may represent a buried steam channel deposit. A clay layer was encountered underneath the stream channel. The depth to groundwater was measured to be 14 to 16 feet below ground surface in June 1988. The groundwater flow appeared to be toward the north-northeast with a gradient of approximately 0.07%.

Soil samples from borings B-1 through B-12 were analyzed for TPH. Results of the analyses are presented in Figure 2. TPH in excess of 1,000 milligrams per kilogram (mg/kg) were detected in samples from five borings. The maximum TPH concentration (89,200 mg/kg) was found at a depth of 16 feet in boring B-1. This sample represents free product floating on the water table. The shallowest sample with a TPH concentration above 10 mg/kg was recovered at 15 feet at a concentration of 3,580 mg/kg in boring B-8. The deepest samples with a concentration above 10 mg/kg were at 25 feet in borings B-1 (1,100 mg/kg), B-10 (9,680 mg/kg), and B-12 (744 mg/kg). The areal extent of JP-5 contamination was estimated to be four acres for TPH concentrations in excess of 100 mg/kg. The vertical extent of JP-5 contamination appeared to be confined primarily to a silt/sand unit near the water table.

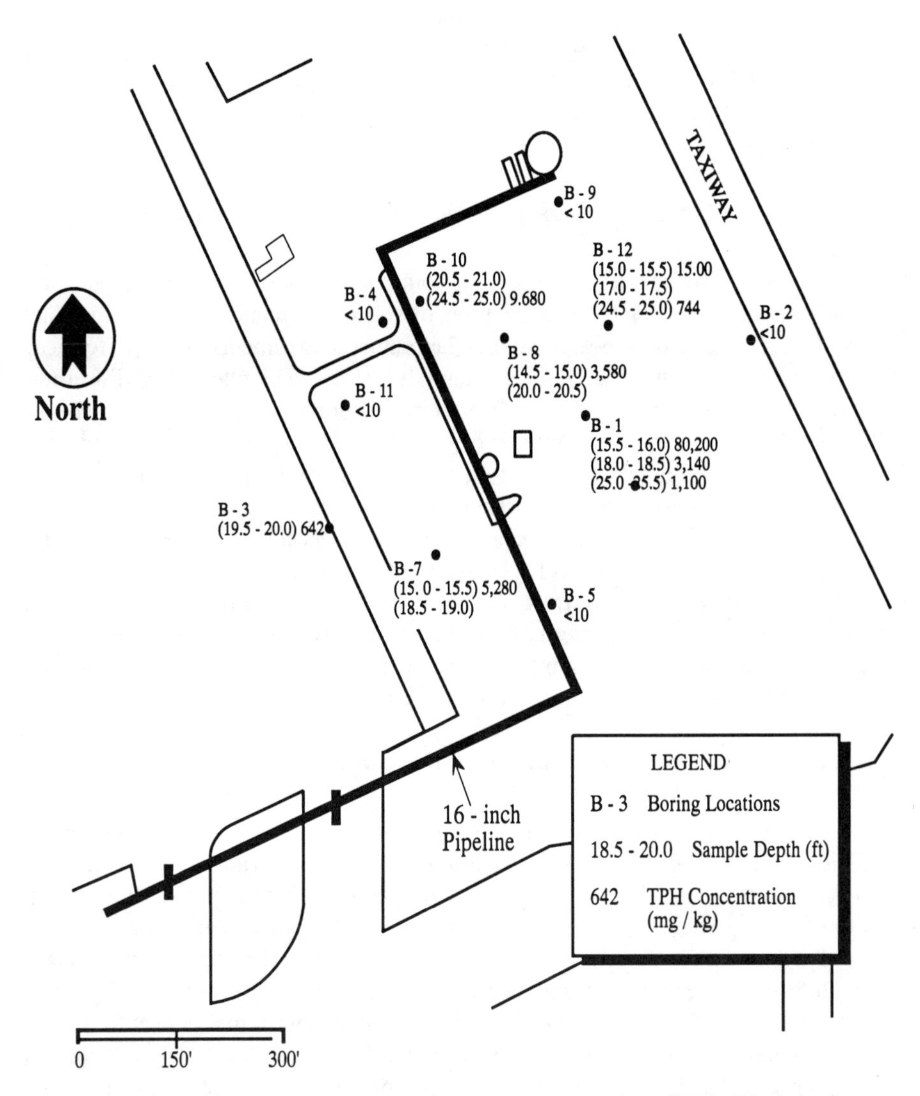

Figure 2.2. TPH concentrations in soil samples (duplicated from ERM - West, Inc.)

Groundwater samples from monitoring wells MW-1, MW-2, and MW-3 were collected and analyzed for TPH and BTEX. No detectable levels of TPH (< 0.5 mg/l) or BTEX (< 0.5 micrograms per liter) were present in the groundwater. Free product jet fuel was observed in the monitoring wells but the thickness was not measured.

METHODS: LABORATORY TREATABILITY STUDIES

To assess the effectiveness of the combined steam injection and vacuum extraction process for *in-situ* remediation of soil contaminated with JP-5 jet fuel at NAS Lemoore, two one-dimensional laboratory experiments were performed. These experiments were used to evaluate the levels and rates of hydrocarbon removal from the Lemoore soil under specific laboratory conditions. In general, it is concluded that excellent removal of the hydrocarbon can be achieved with cycling of the combined process of steam injection and vacuum extraction.

Two samples were prepared using a dry, fine sand and free product jet fuel (JP-5) recovered from the NAS Lemoore site and subjected to steam and vacuum in a one-dimensional experiment. The procedure was varied slightly in each run to aid in estimating the effort required to attain specific cleanup levels. Chemical analyses were performed on the soil before and after the total process and also on liquid effluent samples collected during the steam phase and during the vacuum phase. The results illustrate the effectiveness of the removal process.

Description of the One-Dimensional Experiments

The soil samples were taken from sandy soil and excavated near the region of high fuel concentrations. In the initial site characterization, the maximum concentration of fuel discovered in the field was 89,200 parts per million (ppm). In the first experiment, free product JP-5 recovered from a monitoring well was mixed with the sand to a level of about 100,000 ppm. The total sample weight was 205 grams. For the second experiment, 82 grams of the sand were mixed with 4.1 grams of the fuel to yield a spiked sample with a fuel concentration of approximately 49,000 ppm. The precise contamination level was not known since the excavated sand used in the sample preparation already contained fuel at a level of about 1,100 ppm.

Prior to each run, the spiked sample was packed into a cylindrical stainless steel holder of 1.5-inch inner diameter and a 8.5-inch length and surrounded by unspiked sand from the site. Approximately one inch of Ottawa sand (10-28 mesh) was packed on either end of the unspiked Lemoore sand, and screens were placed between the Ottawa sand and the end plates. A schematic of the initial distribution of sands and fuel in each experiment is shown in Figure 2.3. Once packed, the holder was wrapped with a thin ceramic tape. Two heater tapes were then applied along the length of the holder and covered the entire radial surface area as illustrated in Figure 2.3. The heater tapes were used to maintain adiabatic conditions at the surface during steaming. A thermocouple was placed

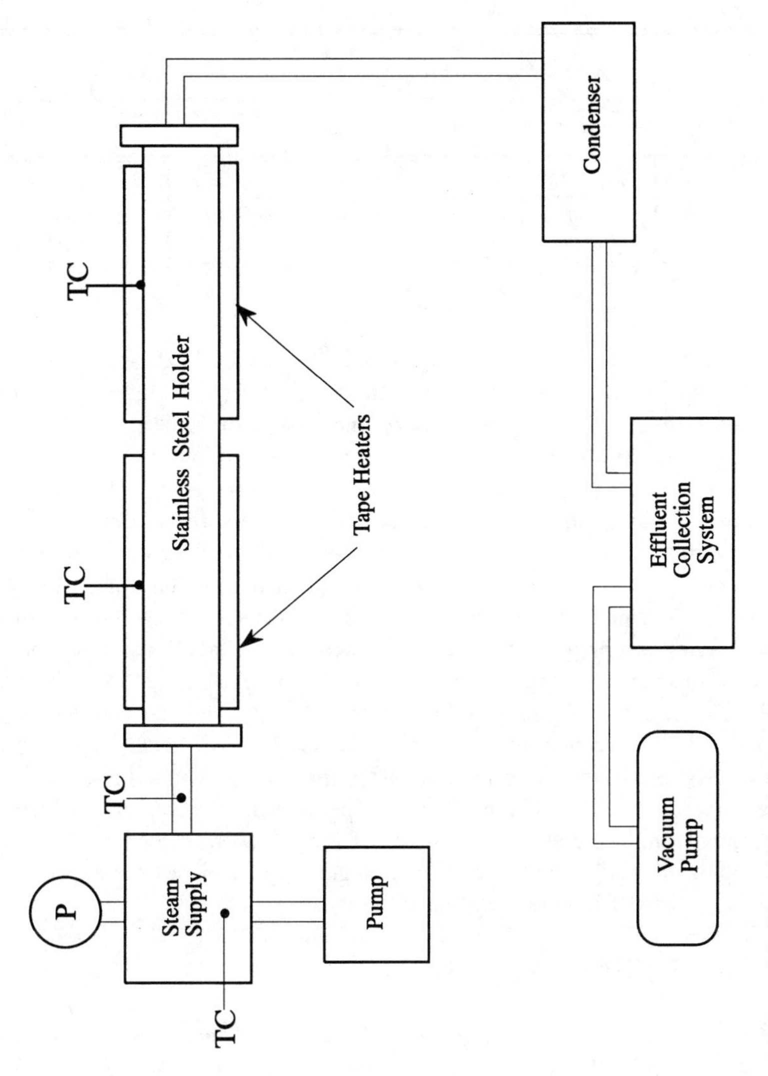

Figure 2.3. Experimental Apparatus.

underneath the heater tapes to monitor the holder surface temperature. Finally, the apparatus was placed in a one-inch thick ceramic blanket. The end plates were covered with additional insulation.

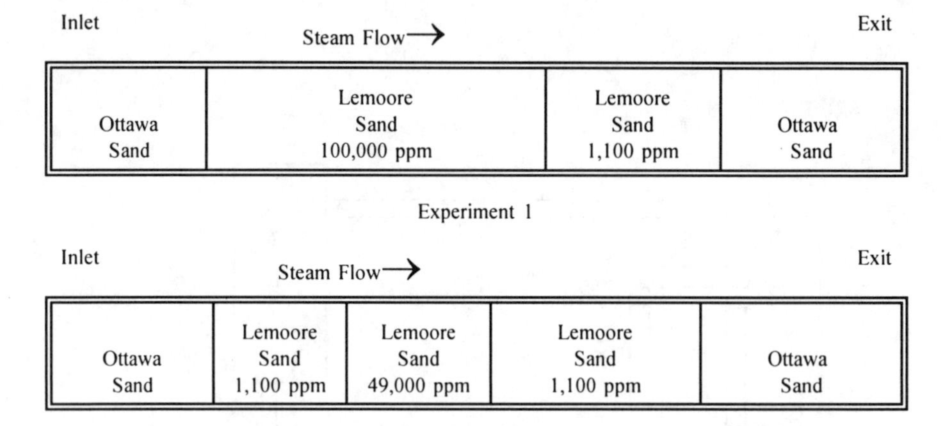

A constant displacement pump supplied deionized, deaerated water at ambient temperature to the steam generator as illustrated in Figure 2.3. Before steam injection, the temperature inside the generator and at the exit were monitored to determine when steady state steam conditions were reached and injection could begin. During injection, the heater tapes were turned on sequentially as the steam front propagated through the core. A flexible 1/8-inch teflon exit line run through an ice bath served as the condenser. The effluent was collected in 40-ml vials. The vials were sealed immediately after filling and refrigerated. A small head space was left in the vials to ensure no loss of free product during capping. After steam breakthrough, the steam injection was continued for varying lengths of time before termination. After the steam injection, a vacuum was applied for a period of time and the condensate was collected. In the second experiment a second cycle of steam injection and vacuum extraction was performed to determine the potential increase in fuel recovery. At the termination of the experiments, the sample holder was disassembled and representative samples of the soil were placed in 40-ml vials and refrigerated. All samples subjected to chemical analyses were transported to a state certified laboratory within 48 hours.

Experimental Results

In the first experiment, the initial flow rate of steam injected was 0.8 ml/min and after 47 minutes the rate was reduced to 0.4 ml/min. Steam breakthrough occurred after approximately 90 minutes of steam injection. Injection continued for another 90 minutes at 0.4 ml/min after which the injection rate was increased to 0.6 ml/min and continued for 90 minutes more. The steam injection was then terminated and the inlet to the apparatus was closed. A vacuum of 28 in Hg was then applied for 60 minutes during which the sample cooled to nearly ambient temperature. Figure 2.4 is a graph showing the water and free product fuel collected in the 40-ml vials. A large slug of pushed fuel appeared in the first vial and was collected before steam was observed in the effluent tubing. The next three liquid samples consisted of condensed vapor effluent. The appearance of the free product fuel shows that part of the pure fuel in the soil sample was being evaporated into the steam vapor. The water in these samples was also saturated with the fuel at a level greater than 100 ppm. The final sample shown was the condensate collected during vacuum extraction. No free product appeared but the concentration of fuel in the condensate was again greater than 100 ppm.

The total amount of fuel recovered was greater than the fuel mixed with the Lemoore sand indicating a high fuel concentration existed in the soil prior to the spiking. Representative soil samples were analyzed for total petroleum hydrocarbons according to EPA Method Modified 8015 by a certified laboratory. The results of the chemical analyses are presented in Table 2.1. The concentration of fuel in the spiked sample prepared in the laboratory was based on a mass balance and was not determined by an analytical method.

The purpose of the second experiment was to determine the effectiveness of cycling the steam injection/vacuum extraction process. In the first cycle the steam was injected at a constant rate of 0.5 ml/min. Steam was observed at the exit after approximately 90 minutes.

Table 2.1. TPH Concentrations in the Soils of Experiment One.

Sample	Pre-Process TPH Conc. (mg/kg)	Post-Process TPH Conc. (mg/kg)
Lemoore Sand (Spiked)	100,000	1,000
Lemoore Sand (Unspiked)	1,100	NA

Injection continued at this rate for an additional 90 minutes before termination. A vacuum of 5 in Hg was then applied and the inlet was left open to allow ambient air to flow through the sample. This first vacuum cycle lasted 60 minutes. Steam injection was then restarted at a flow rate of 0.75 ml/min and after 45 minutes, steam was observed at the exit. Injection continued for another 15 minutes. The second cycle of vacuum at 5 in Hg with an open inlet for 50 minutes before the experiment was terminated.

Figure 2.5 is a graph of the water and free product fuel collected during experiment two. The concentration of fuel in the water is also indicated. The measurement of separate phase fuel was performed volumetrically. The fuel concentration in the water was determined by EPA Method Modified 8015 and was performed by a state certified laboratory. A 3.3-ml slug of fuel pushed ahead of the steam condensation front was collected in the first vial. The second sample consisted of vapor effluent which was condensed outside the apparatus. The concentration of fuel in the water of the second sample was much higher than that of the first sample. This indicates that the solubility of the evaporated fuel was higher than that of the fuel dissolved into the bank of condensate pushed ahead of the steam front. Separate phase fuel appeared in the vapors condensed during the first cycle of vacuum extraction. This did not occur in the first experiment, probably because of the longer period of steam injection. The second cycle of steam injection served to reheat the sample to steam conditions and only a small concentration of fuel was measured in the effluent. The second cycle of vacuum extraction yielded separate phase fuel in the condensed vapors. Based on the weight of the soil sample, the 0.3 ml of fuel recovered during the second vacuum interval lowered the concentration of fuel in the soil sample by 975 ppm. The same trend for fuel concentration in the water samples was detected in the first experiment, but problems in the calibration at the certified laboratory prevent the reporting of accurate absolute values.

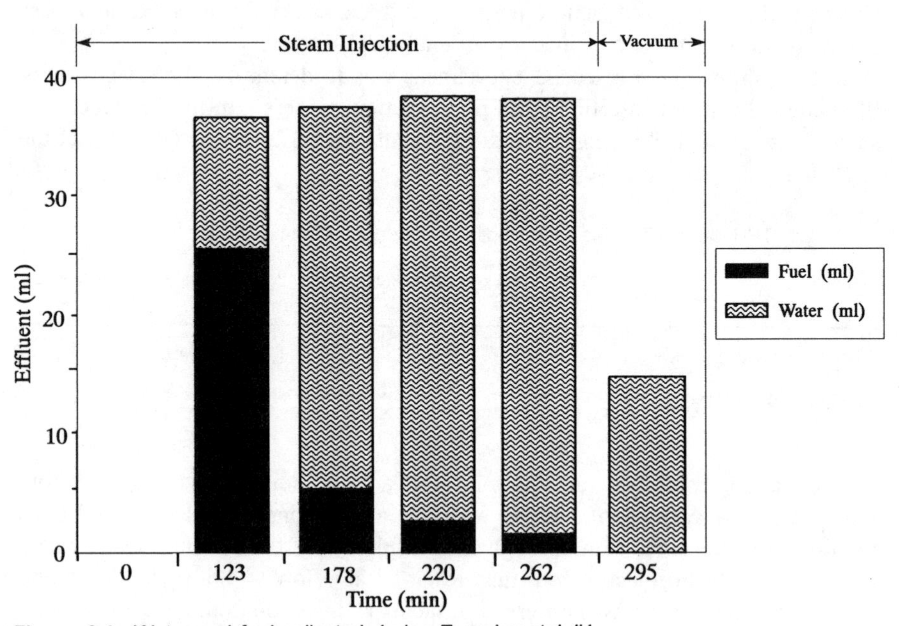

Figure 2.4. Water and fuel collected during Experimental #1.

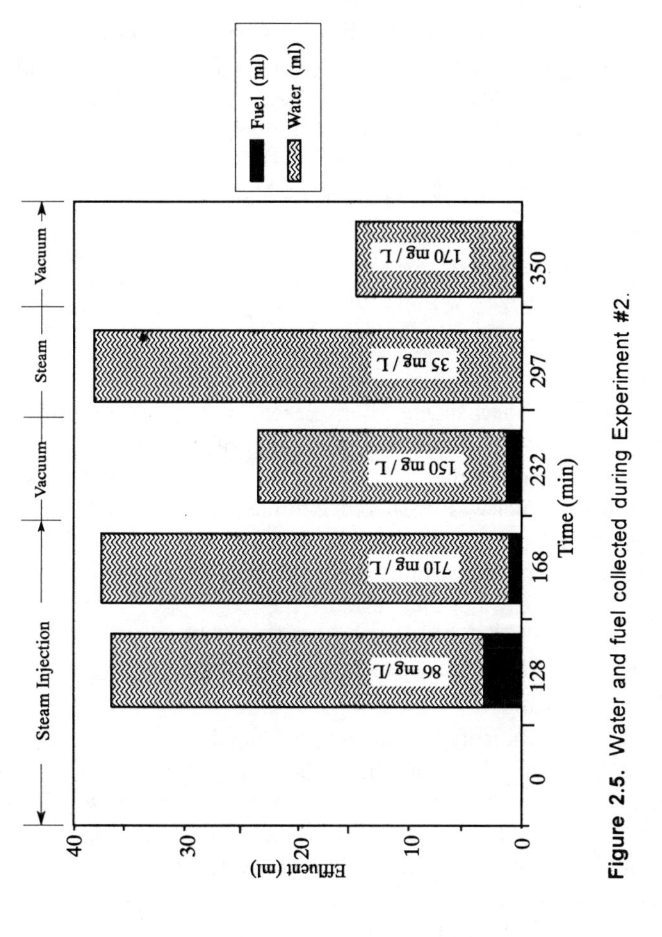

Figure 2.5. Water and fuel collected during Experiment #2.

Representative samples of the soil before and after processing were analyzed for TPH according to EPA Method Modified 8015 by a certified laboratory. The results of the chemical analyses are presented in Table 2.2. The concentration of fuel in the spiked sample prepared in the laboratory is based on a mass balance and was not determined by an analytical method. As shown, the concentration of fuel in the spiked sample was reduced by 99.9%. An overall mass balance can be performed on the second experiment assuming the samples analyzed were truly representative. The total amount of fuel recovered (5.2 ml) was greater than the amount of fuel mixed with the Lemoore sand (5.0 ml). The amount of fuel recovered minus the spiked fuel and the fuel remaining in the soil indicates that the original concentration of fuel in the unspiked sample was 600 ppm. This number compares reasonably with the value of 1,100 ppm determined for a sample of the unspiked sand used in the experiments.

Table 2.2. TPH concentrations in the soils of Experiment Two.

Sample	Pre-Process TPH Conc. (mg/kg)	Post-Process TPH Conc. (mg/kg)
Lemoore Sand (Spiked)	49,000	59
Lemoore Sand (Unspiked)	1,100	140

The predominant mechanisms of displacement of jet fuel by steam injection and vacuum extraction are evident in the results of these two experiments. For large concentrations a separate phase bank of fuel was pushed by the steam condensation front. Fuel was dissolved into the water bank which precedes the steam condensation front. Fuel remaining in the steam zone was evaporated into the steam vapor. Under vacuum, the matrix cools and gives up energy to vaporize the interstitial water and residual fuel.

Conclusions

From these experiments, it can be concluded that cyclic steam injection combined with vacuum extraction should be an effective remediation technique for this site. The second cycle of the process was shown to be particularly effective in lowering the residual hydrocarbon content in the soil. Further reductions would be expected with additional cycles.

DESIGN OF SIVE TECHNOLOGY DEMONSTRATION SYSTEM

Introduction

The purpose of the design of the demonstration plant is to provide sufficient technical descriptions of the various components and plant layout to allow a contractor to construct and assemble the system. The design of the demonstration plant is based on the results from project process modeling, prior field tests, and experience from other projects. The operational specifications of the entire system, the layout of different functional units, the performance specifications of each unit, the design of steam injection and vacuum extraction wells, and the process monitoring borings and devices are included in the design. The design is in accordance with relevant standards, codes and regulations issued by EPA, ASME, ASTM, and local regulatory agents.

The demonstration plant consists of three portions. The first portion includes all the equipment, pipeline, devices above the surface. The function of this portion is to provide steam with desired thermodynamic properties and to treat the effluent extracted or pumped from the extraction wells. The second portion, which interfaces the above-surface equipment to the soil to be treated, includes injection wells, extraction wells, and submersible pumps installed in the extraction wells. The third portion is the temperature and process monitoring system. The temperature monitoring system is physically independent of the injection and extraction system. Process monitoring interfaces with the above-ground equipment to provide information on equipment performance, and mass and energy fluxes. The monitoring system provides crucial information for the operator to control, to steer, and to optimize the SIVE process. Because of the heterogeneities of the soil and the complexity of the SIVE process, the importance of a temperature monitoring system can never be overemphasized. To achieve high sweeping efficiency, the growth of the steam zone must be monitored closely. The injection rate and vacuum extraction rate at each well should be adjusted accordingly to control the growth of the steam zone as much as possible. Since temperature varies dramatically in the vicinity of steam condensation front, temperature logging becomes the most effective way to monitor the growth of the steam zone.

Each portion may include one or more functional units. The specifications of each functional unit are given later in this chapter. The details of each individual functional unit are to be determined by the contractor based on availability, cost, and experience. This flexibility allows the contractor to assemble the plant in the most cost and time effective manner.

The Principles of the SIVE System

The basic function of the plant is to provide the steam required by SIVE and to process the effluents from extraction wells, to provide information to assess the performance of SIVE, and to meet the regulatory requirements of the disposal of the waste water, extracted air, and the recovered jet fuel. Figure 2.6 is an overall flow diagram of the plant. The flow diagram can be divided into three parts. The first part is the steam generator unit that converts water to steam at desired pressure and rate. The second part is a vapor extraction and processing system in which the steam and jet fuel vapor are extracted, cooled, measured, and treated. This system includes the treatment of the hydrocarbon-laden air removed from the subsurface and above-ground equipment. The third is the process liquid treatment system. This system separates, measures, and provides for convenient site disposal of the water and liquid JP-5 pumped from the extraction wells or condensed during vapor cooling.

The steam generator unit is comprised of a water treatment system, a water pump, and a boiler. Since dry steam is required, a water treatment device is included to soften the supplied water to prevent the boiler from being fouled. A water meter is installed in this line to provide a measure of the cumulative steam injected. Blowdown of the boiler and disposal of the boiler waste water will be necessary. A water pump is used to provide sufficient steam pressure. After the water pump, the pressurized water can directly enter the boiler or run through a heat exchanger where the water is preheated prior to entering the boiler. The dry steam from the boiler goes to the two injection wells. The steam temperature, pressure and flowrate are measured and recorded at each injection well head. The boiler pressure and feedwater cumulative volume are monitored and logged manually. The vapor processing line includes a tube-shell heat exchanger, an air-cooled exchanger #1, a separator/pump unit, a separation/-metering unit #1 and carbon canisters (or other comparable air treatment systems such as thermal oxidation). The vapor extracted from the extraction wells is a mixture of air, steam, and jet fuel vapor. Before steam breakthrough, the mixture is mostly air and the concentrations water vapor and jet fuel vapor are relatively low (on the order of 10,000 ppm). After steam breakthrough, the concentrations of steam and jet fuel vapor in the mixture increase significantly because of the elevated temperature. Jet fuel concentrations are expected to be as high as 300,000 ppm in the hot gas. Once the hot vapor mixture is brought to the surface and enters the vapor line, it is cooled in two heat exchangers, where the steam and much of the jet fuel vapor condense to form two separate liquid phases.

In the first tube-in-shell heat exchanger, the water in the shell side from steam generator unit, is preheated before entering the boiler. The water then passes to an air-cooled heat exchanger where it is cooled to ambient air temperature. Under desired operational conditions, the first tube/shell heat exchanger will not be able to remove enough heat from the vapor stream. Also, the boiler is not always operated simultaneously with the vacuum extraction. When the boiler is down, the tube-shell heat exchanger would not function unless the cooling was discarded. Thus, the second air cooled heat exchanger, sized to remove all the above-ambient heat in the extracted gases, is required. The first tube-in-shell feed-water pre-heater is optional, but would lower boiler fuel costs.

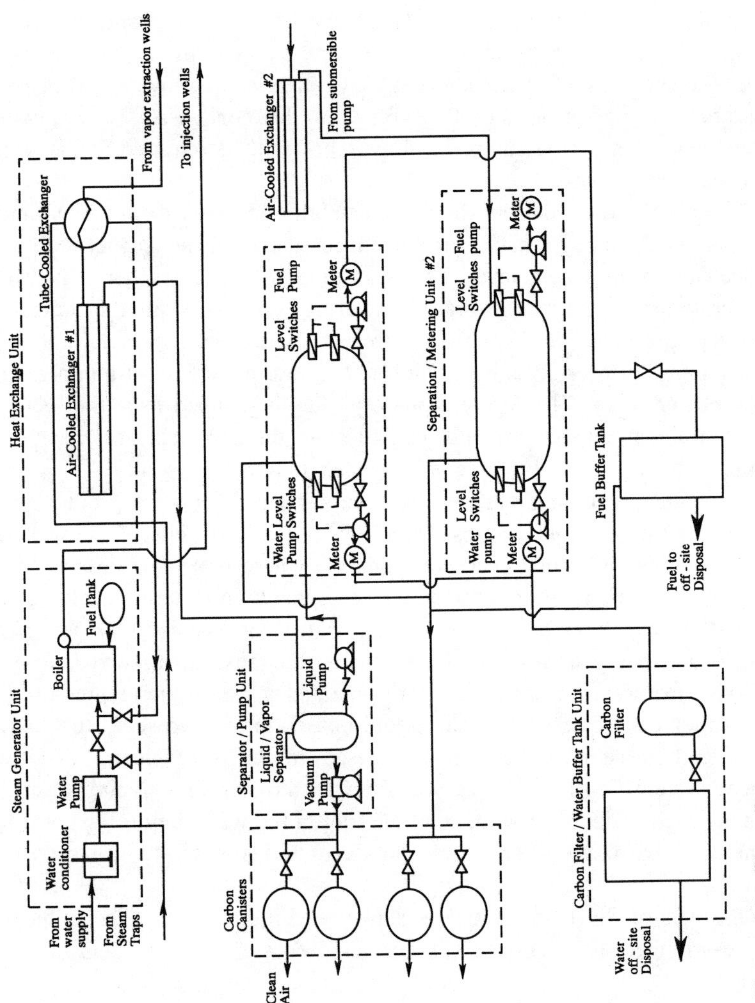

Figure 2.6. Flow diagram.

When the vapor stream leaves the heat exchange unit, the temperature of the stream is near ambient temperature (about 60°F). Liquid phase water and fuel appear in the stream and mix with the remaining gas phase (essentially air), in which the concentrations of water and fuel vapors are near saturation values. The stream is then led to a separator/pump unit where the separation of vapor phase and the liquid phase occurs in a closed cyclone separation vessel. The vapor phase is pulled from the top of the cyclone separator through a pipe to a vacuum pump. The liquid phases of water and jet fuel flow from the bottom of the vessel, into a sump from which they are pumped by a liquid pump. If feasible, the sump should be made of a clear material to allow visual inspection of the phase composition and flow rates of the condensate. To avoid the complete emptying of the sump, level switches will be required in the sump to control the liquid pump.

The vapors expelled from the vacuum pump go to a set of carbon canisters (or thermal oxidation system) where the concentration of the jet fuel in the vapor is reduced to an allowable level for discharging to the atmosphere. The liquid phases are pumped into a separation/metering unit #1, which is operated at atmospheric pressure. In this unit, the free product of jet fuel is separated from the water phase. After separation, both phases are metered and pumped to two separate buffer tanks. The separate phase jet fuel is pumped from the fuel buffer tank to a trailer mounted tank and trucked from the site. The water is pumped from the water buffer tank to the waste water treatment system.

The water processing system also receives water and free product jet fuel delivered by submersible pumps from the extraction wells. The water/fuel stream passes an air cooled heat exchanger #2 where its temperature is lowered to about 60°F. Then the stream enters the separation/metering unit #2 which operates the same way as unit #1. The water and the jet fuel are metered separately and pumped to the two separate buffer tanks mentioned before.

Both separation/metering units are operated at atmospheric pressure. The jet fuel vapor that escapes from the liquid phases in the two separators is led to a set of carbon canisters and then released to the atmosphere. The water treatment system consists of a carbon filter (and/or an air stripping tower with air treatment) to reduce the amount of the fuel in the water before disposal to the pipeline leading to the evaporation ponds of the site waste water treatment system.

A sketch of the plant layout is shown in Figure 2.7. The units of the plant are arranged along a driveway for easy access.

System Specifications

The specifications for each primary component of the plant are listed below:

Boiler

Maximum steam generator capacity*	5,000 lb/hr (2,270 kg/hr)
Maximum steam pressure at well head	20 psig
Steam quality	1.0

*The injection rates of WI-1 and WI-2 were estimated from process modeling to be 2,440 lb/hr and 864 lb/hr. A multiplicative factor of 1.5 is assumed to allow adequate performance if the injectivity of the wells are higher than those inferred from pumping tests of adjacent extraction wells.

Vapor Treatment System

Maximum steam recovery rate	660 scf/min
Maximum vapor mixture recovery rate*	1,300 scf/min

*The maximum vapor recovery occurs after steam breakthrough. The data given here are based on the mass recovery rate of steam to be 0.3 of the injection rate and the volume ratio between recovered steam and air to be one.

Water Treatment System

Maximum water & fuel recovery rate*	240 gallon/min
Maximum water supply required	10 gallon/min
Electrical power supply required	67 kW
Explosion proof level of electric devices (NEC)	Class I, Group C

*The maximum rates of water and fuel recovered by submersible pumps occur before steam breakthrough. After steam breakthrough, steam occupies certain portion of permeable layers previously saturated with water. Thus, the water recovery rates decrease.

Injection and Extraction Wells

A total eight extraction wells and two injection wells are involved in the demonstration project. The well locations are shown in the Figure 2.7. Three extraction wells, WE-2, WE-4, and WE-7 are already constructed. The existing geological data indicate that there is a clay layer below the permeable layers containing the jet fuel. The clay layer acts as a lower boundary of the flow domain. The well bore penetrating into the clay is not useful. Therefore, during the boring of the remaining seven wells, if the bottom clay layer appears shallower than 30 feet, the depth of that well should be changed to three feet below the clay layer or 30 feet whichever is shallower.

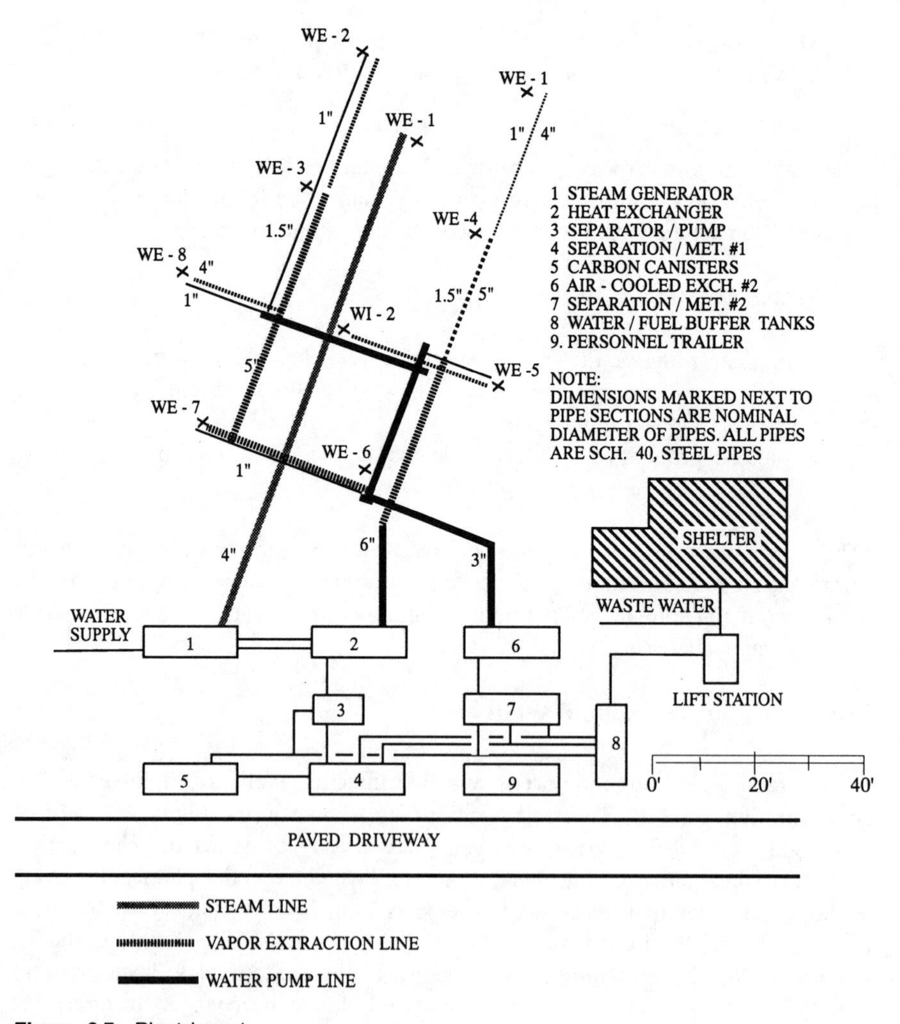

Figure 2.7. Plant layout.

The depths of all of the seven wells are designed to be 30 feet, but are subject to change depending on the depth to the top of the bottom clay layer. There are two injection wells in the demonstration project, WI-1 and WI-2. Their designs are identical and shown in Figure 2.8. The injection wells can be converted to extraction wells during the time steam is purposely turned off. Since the soil around the injection wells are dewatered, there is no need to pump water from the well bores when the injection wells are altered to run vapor extraction. Thus, there are no submersible pumps installed in the injection wells.

The structures of all the extraction wells are identical as shown in Figure 2.9. The final depth of each well may vary depending on the depth of the bottom clay layer at the well site. A submersible pump is installed in each extraction well to pump groundwater during vacuum. When air in a vadose zone is extracted from a well, because of the pressure drop at the well bore, a water cone will be formed in the vicinity of the well bore. The raised water level will block some area of air flow and reduce air flow rate. To overcome this problem, submersible pumps are used to pump water out so that the water level in the well can remain unchanged. Either an electrical or pneumatic pump can be used. The pump rate should be adjustable.

Instrumentation

Besides the pressure, temperature and flow rate measurement mentioned above for each individual functional unit, during steam injection and vapor extraction process, the following measurement should be carried out on the well sites: steam pressure, temperature and flow rate at each injection well; the vapor temperature, vacuum pressure and flow rate at each extraction well head. The information of the ongoing process is very important for the optimization of the process. Since the demonstration plan is not a permanent installation, chart-recording-type instruments are recommended.

Temperature Monitoring System

Subsurface temperatures are monitored by the placement of subsurface thermocouples. To allow for the possibility of continuous temperature logging, the fixed thermocouples will be attached to the outside of a bottom sealed, two inch diameter, 30 foot long, schedule 40 carbon steel pipe, inserted into a bore-hole, and grouted in place, as shown in Figure 2.10. The thermocouples will be copper-constantane, in sealed stainless steel sheaths, attached to 24 gauge, teflon-coated wire, extending to above ground. The coded wires will extend five feet beyond ground level, finished with compatible plugs for quick attachment to a thermocouple output display unit, and housed in a weather-proof enclosure.

The temperature observation wells are to be placed as shown in Figure 2.11. In addition, temperature observation wells are to be placed in each injection and recovery well in the gravel pack. Thus, the total number of temperature monitoring wells is 19. The locations of these wells were chosen to provide de-

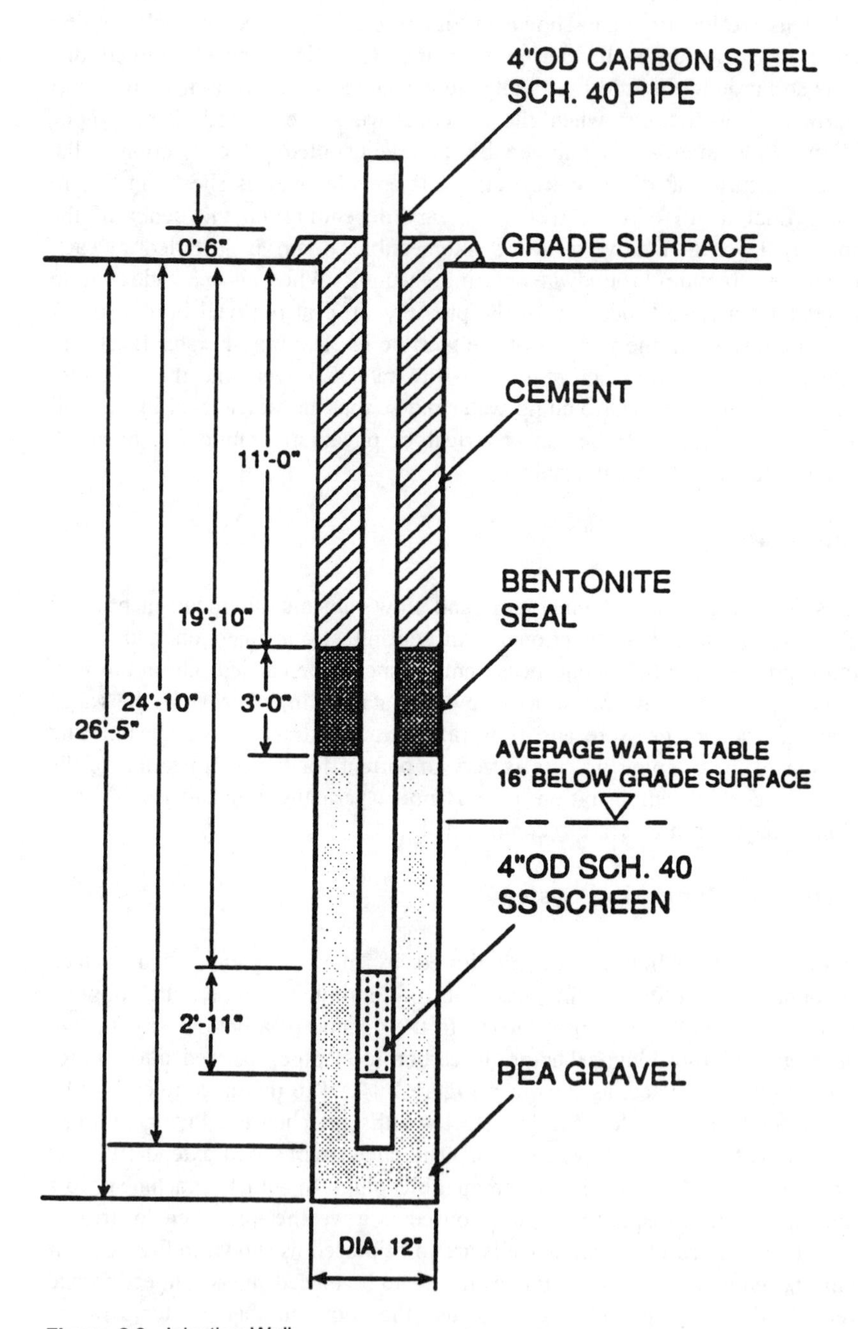

Figure 2.8. Injection Well.

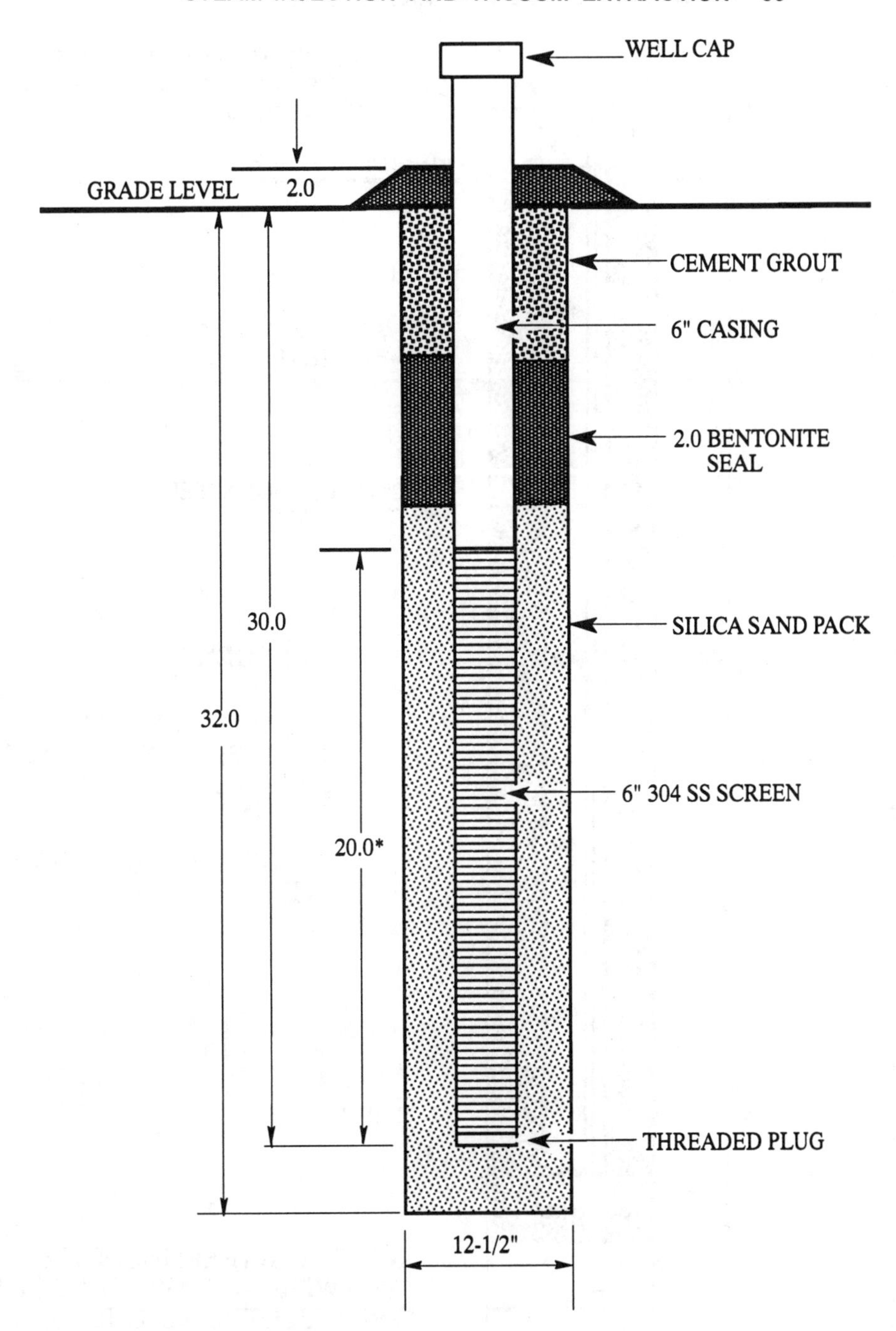

Figure 2.9. Extraction Well.

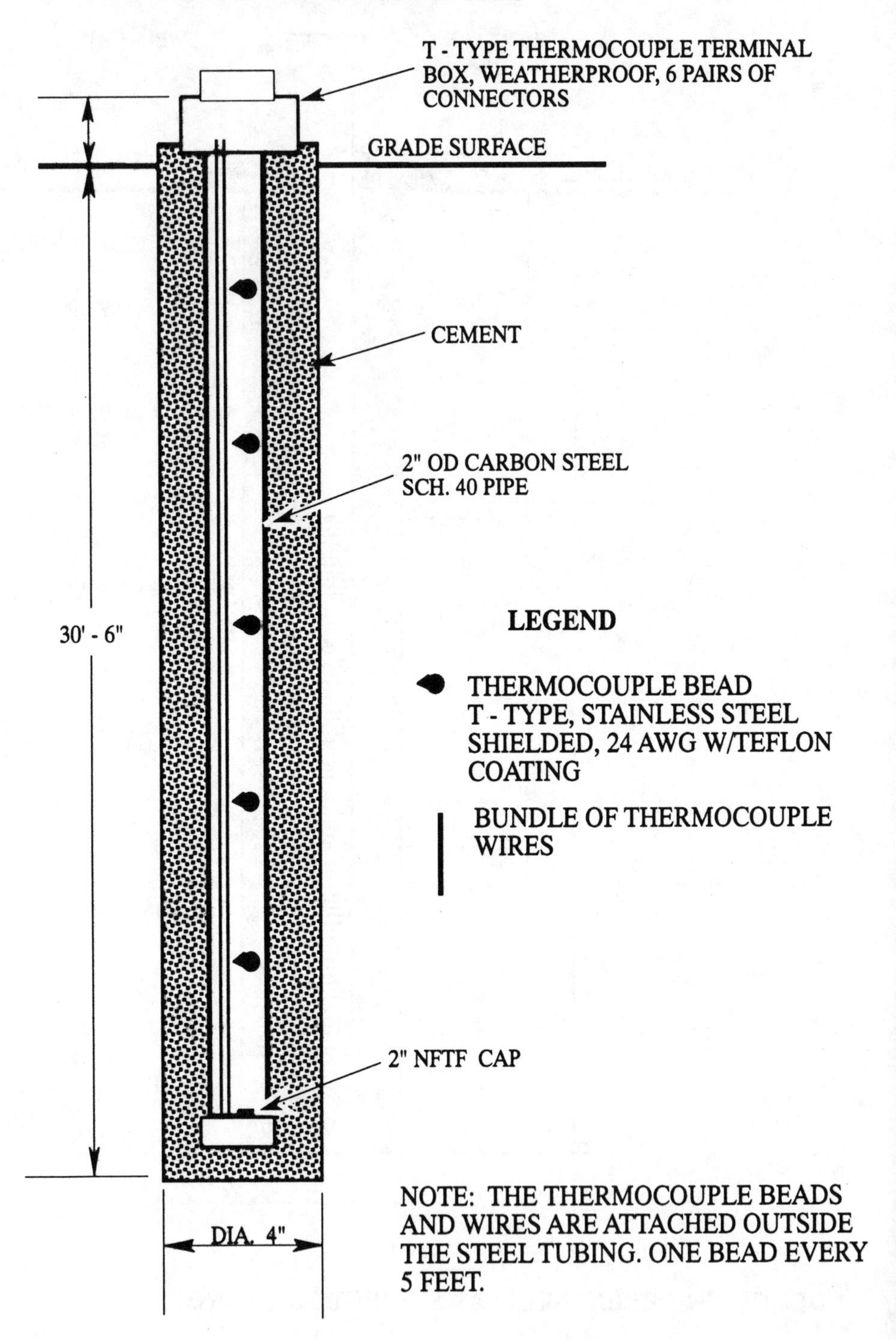

Figure 2.10. Temperature Well.

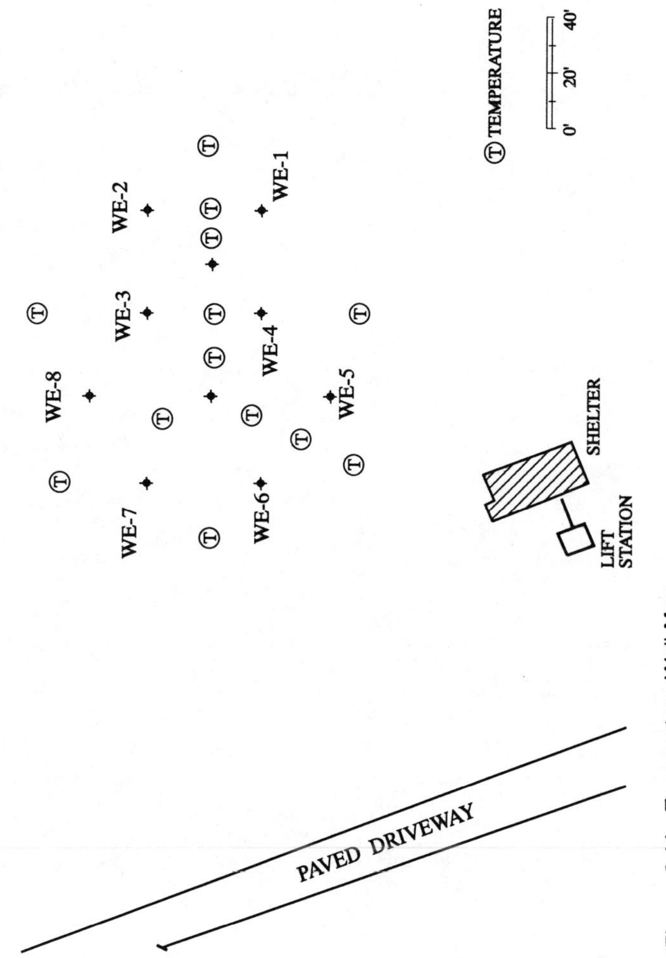

Figure 2.11. Temperature Well Map.

tailed maps of the soil thermal field and information on well-bore dynamics. This placement will facilitate the collection of enough temperature data to allow for process operation optimization and a more precise assessment of the applicability of this process to the remediation of the entire site or other similar sites.

ACKNOWLEDGEMENTS

This project is jointly supported by the Naval Facilities Engineering Command and the U.S. Environmental Protection Agency Risk Reduction Engineering Laboratory (EPA/RREL). Special thanks is extended to Drs. Harry Bostian and Paul de Percin for their technical and financial support. Also, NFESC would like to thank Drs. Kent Udell, Bo Steward, and Zeng-guang Yuan of Udell Technologies, Inc. for their laboratory work and the SIVE system design.

CHAPTER 3

In-Situ Remediation of Low Volatility Fuels

Jeffrey A. Kittel, Robert E. Hinchee, and **Thomas C. Zwick,** Battelle, Columbus, Ohio
Ronald E. Hoeppel, Naval Civil Engineering Laboratory, Port Hueneme, California
Richard J. Watts, Department of Civil and Environmental Engineering, Washington State University, Pullman, Washington

INTRODUCTION

This chapter summarizes data collected at four U.S. Navy and Marine Corps bases to evaluate bioventing technology efficacy in removing low volatility fuels from subsurface soils and the groundwater table. These sites have soil contamination attributed to spills or leaks of fuels having low vapor pressures and very low water solubilities, such as JP-5 jet fuel, diesel fuel, #6 fuel oil (bunker fuel), waste oil, and lubricants. The major contaminant studied is JP-5 jet fuel, a kerosene distillate fraction similar to commercial jet fuel A. Although most of the data were obtained in the field, laboratory treatability studies are included to clarify field information.

Low volatility fuels, unlike gasoline grade fuels, are not removed effectively by soil venting. However, most fuel constituents can be biodegraded under aerobic conditions. The most serious limitations to efficient and complete *in-situ* bioremediation of these fuels and other petroleum hydrocarbons appear to be:

- difficulty aerating contaminated subsurface soils,[1] and
- poor accessibility of the soil microorganisms to the hydrophobic contaminants.[2]

Aeration of the subsurface is difficult because it takes over three times more oxygen, by weight, than hydrocarbon contaminant to promote complete degradation.[3] Thus, use of groundwater as an oxygen carrier becomes impractical because of the poor solubility of oxygen in water. Hydrogen peroxide can provide half its weight as oxygen but it can be toxic or readily degraded by soil microorganisms.[4-6]

Water soluble fuel contaminants are rarely toxic to microorganisms because of the low concentrations found in groundwater. This is especially true for low volatility fuels, which lack significant quantities of the more soluble aromatic compounds found in gasoline. The major components of low volatility fuels are immiscible in water, and thus they remain inaccessible to microorganisms until they have been solubilized or emulsified in the aqueous phase. Emulsification by biosurfactants or synthetic surfactants can be a time limiting process for *in-situ* bioreclamation because of the poor interaction of surfactants with the nonaqueous contaminant phase.[7,8]

Bioventing

In practice, bioventing uses many engineering techniques common to soil venting technology. Both remediation methods are air driven systems that primarily deal with contamination that resides in the vadose zone soils above the water table. Both techniques can be effective for remediating fuel contamination because insoluble fuel hydrocarbons reside at and above the low groundwater level. However, soil venting cannot cost effectively remediate soils contaminated with organic compounds having low vapor pressures. By comparison, bioventing should treat all organic compounds capable of biodegrading under aerobic conditions. The desired purpose of bioventing is to promote *in-situ* aerobic biodegradation rather than to vent fuel vapors to ground surface collection or treatment systems. Oxygen can be transported rapidly through water unsaturated soils, including many with low water permeability (e.g., silts) when low positive or negative pressures are exerted on subsurface soil pores as a result of soil gas extraction and/or air injection. Rapid transport is enabled by the fact that gas diffusion rates are several thousand times those of water and air contains about 25 thousand times more molecular oxygen than aerated water. Vapor transfer through the soil profile, even if not surface vented, should also increase the surface area in fuel contaminated soil pores that can be wetted and colonized by hydrocarbon degrading microorganisms.[9]

Respirometry provides a popular method for measuring aerobic biodegradation rates in soils. This laboratory technique precisely monitors increases in carbon dioxide and/or decreases in oxygen gas levels that result from complete aerobic biodegradation. Using these data, approximate microbial kinetics can be determined. However, soil disturbance or large soil sample variability can often result in laboratory data with little practical value. *In-situ* field respirometry can be used to measure degradation rates in undisturbed, large areas of soil. The technique most often involves measurement of oxygen gas depletion rates following air injection or shutdown of a bioventing system, once atmospheric oxygen concentrations are achieved around soil gas monitoring points. Oxygen depletion rate generally is a more accurate measure of biodegradation rate than carbon dioxide formation, because carbon dioxide can be bound in the soil as carbonates/bicarbonates and is used by many microorganisms as a carbon source for normal microbial biomass production.[10]

Bioslurping

At many contaminated sites, petroleum contamination is present both in the vadose zone and in the capillary fringe as free product. Regulatory guidelines generally require that free product recovery take precedence over other remediation technologies, and conventional wisdom has been to complete free product removal activities prior to initiating vadose zone remediation.

"Bioslurping" is a new dynamic technology that teams vacuum assisted free product recovery with bioventing to simultaneously recover free product and remediate the vadose zone. Bioslurping is a vacuum enhanced free phase petroleum (free product) recovery technology. Unlike other free product recovery (FPR) technologies, bioslurping systems treat two separate geologic media simultaneously. The systems are designed to extract free phase fuel from the water table and to aerate vadose zone soils through soil gas vapor extraction. The bioslurper system withdraws groundwater, free product, and soil gas in the same process stream. Groundwater is separated from the free product and is treated (when required) and discharged. Free product is recovered and can be recycled. Soil gas vapor is treated (when required) and discharged.

Bioslurper systems are designed to minimize environmental discharges of groundwater and soil gas. As done in bioventing, bioslurper systems extract soil gas at a low rate to reduce volatilization of contaminants. In most instances, volatile discharges can be kept below treatment action levels. The slurping action of a bioslurper system greatly reduces the volume of groundwater that must be extracted with the free product when compared to conventional FPR systems. High FPR efficiencies are achieved with pressure induced gradient rather than by the hydraulically induced gradient used by many FPR systems.

FUEL CONTAMINATION SITES

Four U.S. Navy sites were evaluated for bioventing efficiency: Fallon Naval Air Station (NAS) in western Nevada, Patuxent River NAS in southern Maryland, Kaneohe Bay Marine Corps Air Station (MCAS) on Oahu in Hawaii, and Twentynine Palms Marine Corps Air Ground Combat Center (MCAGCC) in southern California. At the first three sites, free fuel has reached groundwater, resulting primarily in a horizontal subsurface plume. At Twentynine Palms, because of very deep groundwater and sandy soils, the plumes are primarily vertical.

Fallon, Nevada

The Fallon NAS site is located in the high desert, with periodically cold winters and hot summers. The plume being remediated appears to be contaminated solely by rather fresh JP-5 jet fuel from a previously leaking supply pipeline. The subsurface soil consists of mixed fluvial and lacustrine deposits in gradational layers of silt, sand, and clay. The soil profile consists of 2.4 to

3.0 meters of silt with sandy-silt interlayers, underlain by 0.6 to 1.2 meters of silty to clean sand and a thick clay stratum, respectively. The shallow aquifer zone is in the sand layer, and the underlying clay acts as an aquitard. The horizontal fuel plume is confined to the sand layer and lower 0.6 meter of the overlying silt layer. The 0.4-hectare bioventing system is constructed within the 2.8- to 3.2-hectare hydrocarbon plume (Figure 3.1). Ambient temperatures in the contaminant zone fluctuate between 12 and 18°C. The groundwater is alkaline and basic (pH 8.9) and of brackish salinity (23 mmho/cm conductivity). Arsenic is a natural contaminant, with concentrations as high as 4 mg/L.

Initial feasibility studies, including soil *in-situ* respiration testing, were conducted in the summer of 1990; the bioslurping system was designed and constructed mainly during late 1991. The system was started up initially in November 1991 but was not run full time until January 1993.

Patuxent River, Maryland

The Patuxent River NAS site is situated in upland forested terrain close to the Chesapeake Bay. Contamination is predominantly aged JP-5 jet fuel, but less aged gasoline grade fuel was observed in parts of the hydrocarbon contaminated soil. The subsurface consists predominantly of mixed fine to coarse fluvial sand, with some thin, discontinuous interbeds of silt and clay that formed in an ice age backwater salt marsh. In some areas thin peat strata exist. The water table and free fuel lie generally at depths of 4.3 to 5.5 meters with an extensive clay layer at depths of 6.7 to 7.6 meters serving as the shallow aquifer aquitard. In general, the fuel does not contact the peat layers except near where fuel seeps from a steep embankment along a creek. The groundwater is slightly acidic and is low in dissolved solids (150 mg/L) and salinity (<0.5 mmho/cm, conductivity); temperatures fluctuate between 15° and 20°C. Groundwater and fuel migration patterns are strongly affected by soil fill deposited in shallow canyons that existed prior to underground tank construction.

Vent wells and monitoring points were installed in three phases from the summer of 1987 to the fall of 1990 over an area of about 28 hectares. The contaminant plumes, originating from several sources, cover an area of about 12 hectares. Extensive laboratory and field treatability and feasibility studies were conducted during the well installation period. Laboratory studies included evaluation of synthetic surfactants, JP-5 soil venting rates, biodegradation rates of individual hydrocarbons in fuel contaminated soils (radiolabel studies), and fuel degradation rates; microbial characterizations; and large soil column evaluations of different nutrient additions and aeration techniques. Field studies included comparative analyses of soil gas and groundwater data, other geophysical evaluations, tracer studies, and geochemical evaluations. *In-situ* respirometry was conducted during the summer of 1990. A bioventing system has not yet been planned for this site.

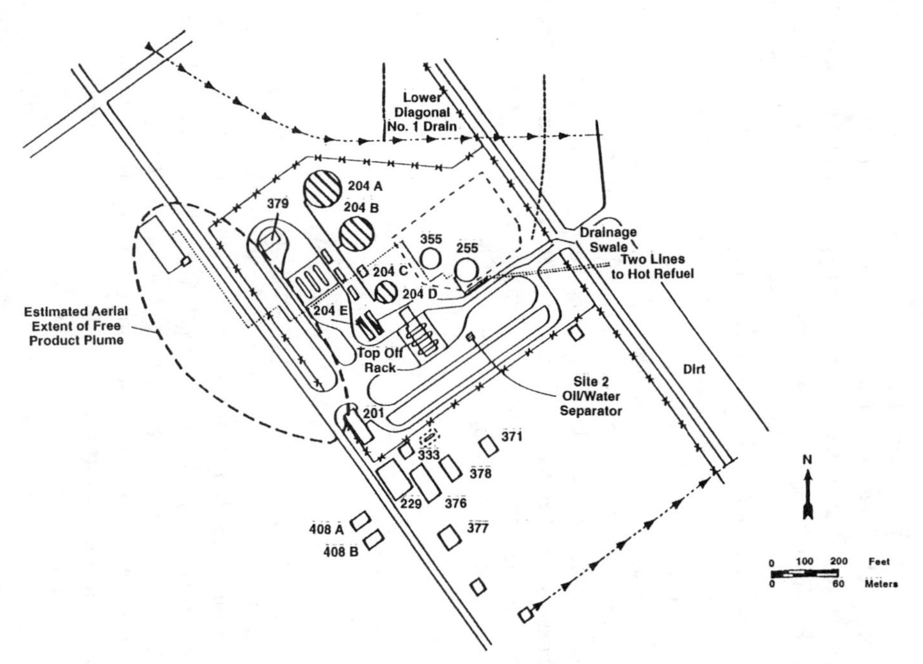

Figure 3.1 Estimated aerial extent of JP-5 free product plume west of Fallon NAS new fuel farm. Bioslurper System will treat an approximate 0.4-hectare plot within plume.

Kaneohe Bay, Hawaii

The Kaneohe Bay MCAS site is located on the Mokapu peninsula surrounded by embayments in a tropical setting with very uniform seasonal temperatures. The contaminant plume is JP-5 jet fuel and it covers nearly two hectares around a previously leaking, very large aboveground tank. The subsurface soil profile consists of sand, silt, and clay originating from basalts; basic volcanic tuff; and coral limestone. The upper section consists predominantly of silty reddish brown sand 0.3 to 4.5 meters thick. This is underlain by a cohesive sandy clay zone that extends to about six meters below ground surface (BGS), at the groundwater table. Highly permeable sand and silty sand is encountered below the groundwater table to about ten meters BGS, where sandy clay and calcareous fines are encountered as the possible aquitard. The fuel appears to reside both in the low permeability zone above and the high permeability zone just below the water table. The groundwater appears to be fresh and unaffected by tides.

During previous investigations, nearly 100 soil borings were emplaced at the field site to delineate the extent of the free product plume. Soil gas monitoring points were installed in August 1993, and soil samples were collected from three borings for chemical analysis. *In-situ* respirometry was performed following monitoring point installation. Construction of a bioventing system over the entire contaminant plume is scheduled for late 1993, with startup in early 1994.

Twentynine Palms, California

The Twentynine Palms MCAGCC includes numerous small and large spill sites of different types of fuels. The major spills are JP-5 and diesel, but #6 fuel oil, gasoline, and waste oil spills all need to be treated *in-situ.* Approximately 12 sites are planned for bioventing studies. Two of these are detailed field demonstrations at sites contaminated with JP-5 and #6 fuel oil. The remaining approximately ten sites will be used for pilot scale bioventing studies.

The subsurface soils at most spill locations consist of rather uniformly graded fine to medium aeolian sand, with few low permeability interbeds. Because the groundwater table is at 61 to 67 meters, most fuel plumes are vertical. At one location, preliminary data indicate that a mixed fuel plume has reached the saline groundwater. The #6 fuel oil demonstration site shows contamination more than 14 meters deep.

Vent well and monitoring point installations commenced in March 1993. Initiation of pilot bioventing system operation was expected before the end of 1993, with commencement of the field demonstrations in early 1994. Air permeability testing was initiated during the summer of 1993.

METHODS: LABORATORY TREATABILITY STUDIES

Effects of Fuel Concentrations on Biodegradation Rates

The effects of total petroleum hydrocarbon (TPH) concentrations on the microbiological degradation of JP-5 contaminated soils was investigated in sealed 40-mL borosilicate volatile organic analysis (VOA) vials. Soil samples collected from the Patuxent River fuel farm were passed through a No. 4 (475 mm) sieve to remove rocks and to obtain a homogeneous sample. To investigate the effect of concentration, the contaminated soil was mixed with uncontaminated silica sand to provide soil concentrations of 180, 490, 830, and 1,570 mg/kg TPH dry weight soil. Then 15 grams of soil were placed in the 40-mL vials. The vials were closed with Teflon™ septa caps and 20 mL nutrient solution (Restore 375) containing 200 mg/L stabilized hydrogen peroxide (IT Corporation), 400 mg/L ammonium-nitrogen, and 20 mg/L orthophosphate-phosphorus was added to each vial. Each treatment per sampling time was replicated in triplicate and the experiment was run for 120 days on an orbital shaker at 20°C. The ammonium concentrations and pH were kept uniform, and the soil-water dissolved oxygen levels were maintained at greater than 3 mg/L by adding hydrogen peroxide through the Teflon™ septa when necessary. The content of each respective bottle was analyzed for TPH by the EPA Modified 8015 Method with methylene chloride extraction. Heterotrophic bacteria counts were determined by serial dilution and plating on solid media after incubation at 37°C for 36 hours.[11] Other analyses included soil-water dissolved oxygen, pH, ammonia-nitrogen, nitrate-nitrogen, nitrite-nitrogen, and phosphate-phosphorus.

METHODS: FIELD STUDIES

Soil Gas Permeability and Radius of Influence

An estimate of the soil's permeability to fluid flow (k) and a determination of the radius of influence (R_I) of the vent wells provide important factors to consider in bioventing system design. On-site testing gives the most accurate estimate of the soil gas permeability, k. On-site testing also can be used to determine the radius of influence that can be achieved for a given well configuration and its flow rate and air pressure. These data are used to design full-scale systems with regard to spacing the vent wells, sizing the blower equipment, and ensuring that the entire site receives a supply of oxygen rich air to sustain *in-situ* biodegradation.

Soil gas permeability, i.e., a soil's capacity for fluid flow, varies according to grain size, soil uniformity, porosity, and moisture content. The value of k is a physical property of the soil; k does not change with different extraction/injection rates or different pressure levels. Soil gas permeability generally is expressed in the units cm^2 or darcy (1 darcy = 1×10^{-8} cm^2). As with hydraulic conductivity, soil gas permeability may vary by more than one order of magnitude on the same site due to soil variability.

The radius of influence is defined as the maximum distance from the air extraction or injection well where measurable vacuum or pressure (soil gas movement) occurs. R_I, a function of soil properties, also depends on the configuration of the venting well and extraction or injection flow rates, and is altered by soil stratification. At sites with highly permeable soils, pressure monitoring alone may not be adequate to estimate R_I for bioventing. At these sites the lack of resistance to air flow will reduce the injection pressure. It is best to monitor changes in soil gas composition, particularly increases in oxygen concentration at oxygen deficient sites, or to use an inert tracer (i.e., helium) to observe the radius of influence. A detailed description of the air permeability test procedure is presented in Hinchee et al.[12]

In-situ Respiration Testing

The *in-situ* respiration test consists of placing narrowly screened soil gas monitoring points into the unsaturated zone fuel contaminated and uncontaminated soils and venting these soils with air containing an inert tracer gas for a given period of time. The apparatus for the respiration test is illustrated in Figure 3.2. Each site had a cluster of three to four probes placed in the contaminated soil of the test location. A 1 to 3% concentration of inert gas (helium) was added to the air, which was injected for about 20 to 24 hours. The air provides oxygen to the soil, while inert gas measurements provide data on the diffusion of O_2 from the ground surface and the surrounding soil and assure that the soil gas sampling system does not leak. The background control location was placed in an uncontaminated site with air injection to monitor natural background respiration.

Measurements of CO_2 and O_2 concentrations in the soil gas were taken before injection of any air or inert gas. After air and inert gas injection was turned off, CO_2, O_2, and inert gas concentrations were monitored over time. Before a reading was taken, the probe was purged a few times until the CO_2 and O_2 readings were constant. Initial readings were taken every two hours and then progressively over four to eight-hour intervals. The experiment was usually terminated when the O_2 concentration of the soil gas was ~5%. A detailed description of the *in-situ* respiration test procedure is presented in Hinchee et al.[12]

Oxygen utilization and carbon dioxide production rates were used to estimate biodegradation rates, expressed in milligrams of hexane-equivalent/kilograms of soil per day. Inorganic uptake of O_2 was assumed to be negligible. Aerating the soil for 24 hours was assumed to be sufficient to oxidize any ferrous ions.

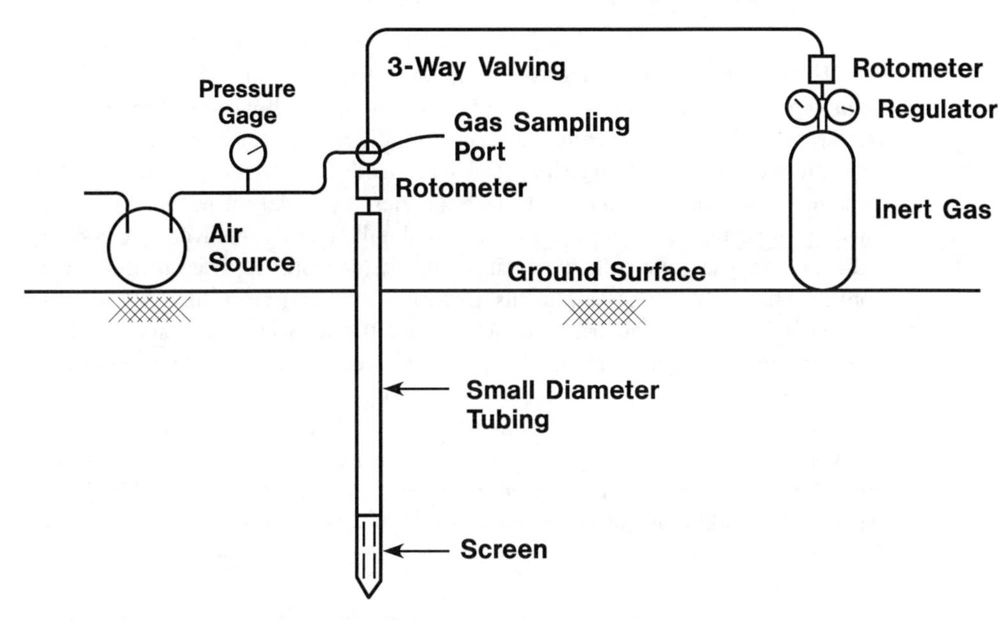

Figure 3.2 *In-situ* Respiration Test Apparatus.

Carbon dioxide production proved to be a less useful measure of biodegradation than did O_2 disappearance. The biodegradation rate in milligrams of hexane-equivalent/kilograms of soil per day based on CO_2 appearance is usually less than can be accounted for by the O_2 disappearance. In the case of the high pH and high alkalinity soils at Fallon NAS, little or no gaseous CO_2 production was measured. This could be due to the formation of carbonates from the gaseous evolution of CO_2 produced by biodegradation.

For the initial *in-situ* respirometry measurements at Fallon, four gas monitoring probes were emplaced to depths of about 1.5 meters in clayey soil contaminated with JP-5; one background gas monitoring probe was emplaced in adjacent uncontaminated soil. Measurements of respiration rates during bioventing at Fallon are conducted using permanent soil gas probes installed in 23 sealed boreholes at three depths (one, two, and three meters) above the water table; two of these probes are located outside the contaminant plume. Three probes at Patuxent River were driven into sand to just above the groundwater table at depths of four to six meters. These served as test, gas control, and background gas sampling probes, respectively. Two permanent soil gas probes were monitored in each of three boreholes at Kaneohe Bay MCAS. Two boreholes were emplaced above the light, nonaqueous phase liquid (LNAPL) plume, and the soil gas probes in each borehole were situated just above the free product layer and just below the upper zone of contamination, respectively. The third borehole was situated outside the LNAPL plume. To date, *in-situ* respiration testing has not been conducted at Twentynine Palms.

Remedial Design: Fallon

The site at Fallon NAS was chosen for a demonstration of the bioslurping technology due to the presence of LNAPL on the shallow water table. The bioslurper technology is unique because it utilizes elements of two separate remedial technologies, **bioventing** and **free product recovery**, to address two separate contaminant media. Both technologies are widely used in some form. Bioslurping combines elements of each to simultaneously recover free product and aerate vadose zone soils, thus enhancing the capabilities of each used alone. Conventional FPR skimmer systems generally are inefficient for FPR because they have little effect on free product outside the recovery well, so efficiency relies on the passive movement of fuel into the recovery well. Dual pump FPR systems increase recovery efficiency by drawing the water table down several feet to create a hydraulic gradient into the well. Although higher recovery rates are achieved, creation and maintenance of the hydraulic gradient can require extraction of large volumes of groundwater that must be treated prior to discharge. In addition, lowering the water table may serve only to trap much of the free product beneath the water table when the water table returns to its normal level.

Bioslurping improves free product recovery efficiency without requiring the extraction of large quantities of groundwater. The bioslurper system pulls a vacuum of 13 to 51 cm of mercury on the recovery well to create a pressure gradient to force movement of fuel into the well. The system is operated to cause negligible drawdown in the aquifer, thus reducing the problem of free product entrapment.

Bioventing of the vadose zone soils is achieved by withdrawing soil gas from the recovery well. The slurping action of the bioslurper system cycles between recovering liquid (free product and/or groundwater) and soil gas. The rate of soil gas extraction is dependent on the recovery rate of liquid from the well system. When free product removal activities are complete, the bioslurper system is easily converted to a conventional bioventing system to complete remediation of the vadose zone soils.

A total of 48 bioventing wells were installed for incorporation into the bioventing system at Fallon NAS (Figure 3.3). Wells were installed to an approximate depth of four m and were constructed of five-cm-diameter Schedule 40 PVC with 2.1m-long, 10 slot well screens. A medium graded sand filter pack was installed across the screened interval. The rest of the annular space was plugged with a wetted bentonite chip plug to near surface followed by a concrete surface seal.

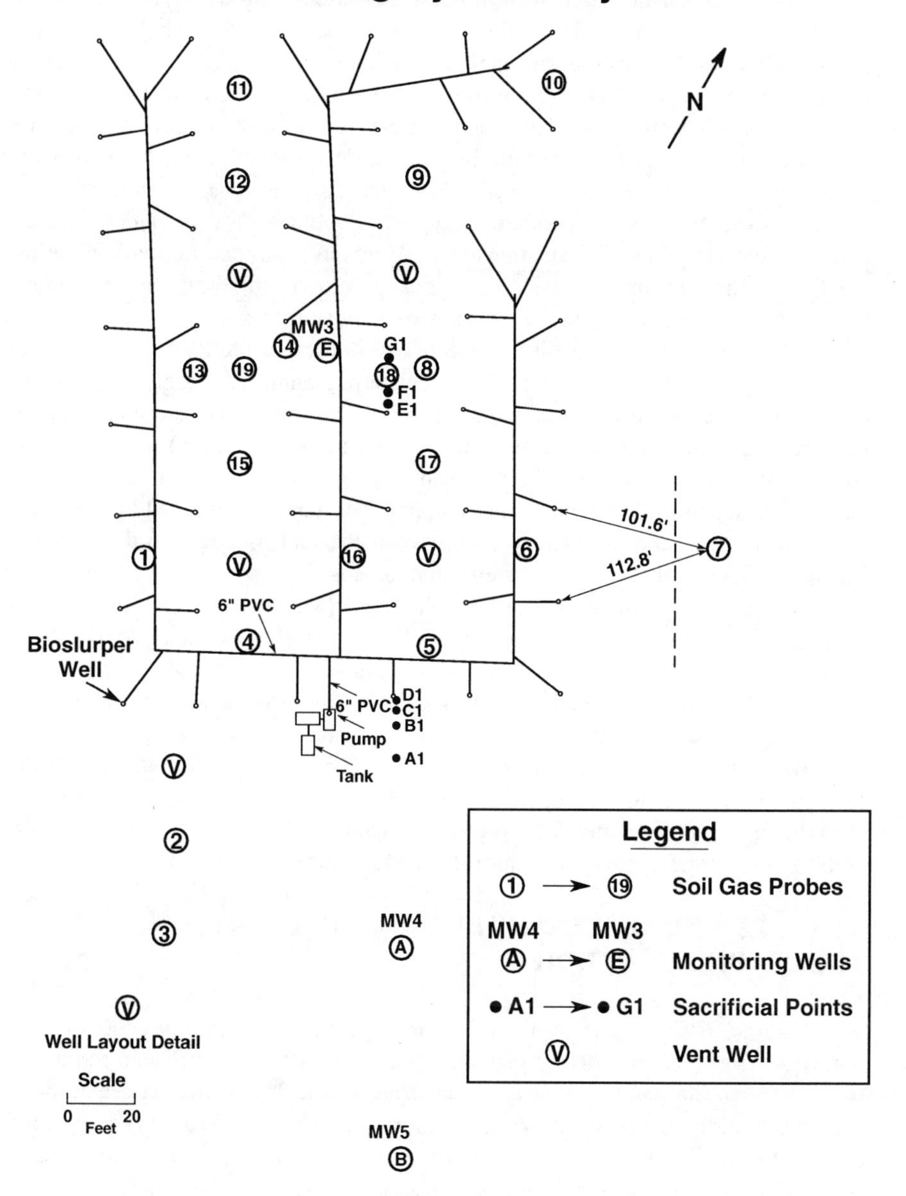

Figure 3.3. Fallon Naval Air Station - Bioventing system layout.

The system is designed to simultaneously vent the soils and skim free product from the water table. To accomplish this, a 2.5 cm diameter PVC suction tube was inserted inside each well through a vacuum-tight well seal. The depth of the tube is adjustable to allow for selective withdrawal of water, free product, and/or soil vapor by placing the suction tube below, at, or above the water table surface, respectively. Each suction tube is tied into a larger diameter (10 cm and 15 cm) PVC pipe manifold. The suction tubes are valved to allow for variable flow adjustment, and an in-line sampling port allows for collection of the process fluids being removed from each well. Each well also has a vacuum release valve at the surface to allow for comparison of free product recovery under vacuum and free product recovery at atmospheric pressure. Under normal operating conditions the vacuum release valve is kept closed to allow for maximum bioventing. Figure 3.4 shows a diagram of a bioslurper well.

All of the bioslurper wells were connected through the PVC manifold to a 10 horsepower dewatering pump. The dewatering pump is capable of pumping water, free phase petroleum, and soil gas from the wells. The liquid discharge from the pump is processed through an oil/water separator (OWS) to separate the aqueous from the petroleum phases. The OWS is connected to a 1,890 L steel tank for collection of free phase petroleum. The tank is equipped with a float switch to shut off the dewatering pump when the tank is nearly full. Figure 5 shows a diagram of the OWS system components.

The aqueous phase discharge from the OWS (Megator Model Meg-S 24.60) is directed to a 529 L PVC tank that also has a float switch for overflow protection. A five horsepower irrigation pump directs the tank water to the Fallon NAS sanitary sewer. The OWS is rated for an aqueous discharge of 15 ppm total petroleum hydrocarbons and can operate at up to 95 L per minute.

The dewatering pump is fitted with a vacuum assembly through which the soil gas is vented to the open atmosphere under permit from the Nevada Department of Environmental Protection. Vapor is discharged through a 3 m high, 5 cm diameter polyvinyl chloride (PVC) stack.

RESULTS AND DISCUSSION OF LABORATORY TREATABILITY STUDIES

Figure 3.6 shows the results of laboratory studies using soil contaminated with JP-5 from Patuxent River that was diluted to different TPH concentrations with clean sterile sand. As seen in the figure, the lower fuel concentrations degraded rapidly, whereas soil concentrations of 830 and 1,570 mg/kg appeared to change negligibly during the four month experiment, despite significant fluctuation in concentration among replicate bottles. In retrospect the total heterotrophic bacterial counts (colony forming units, or CFUs) fluctuated minimally among soil samples having different initial TPH concentrations.

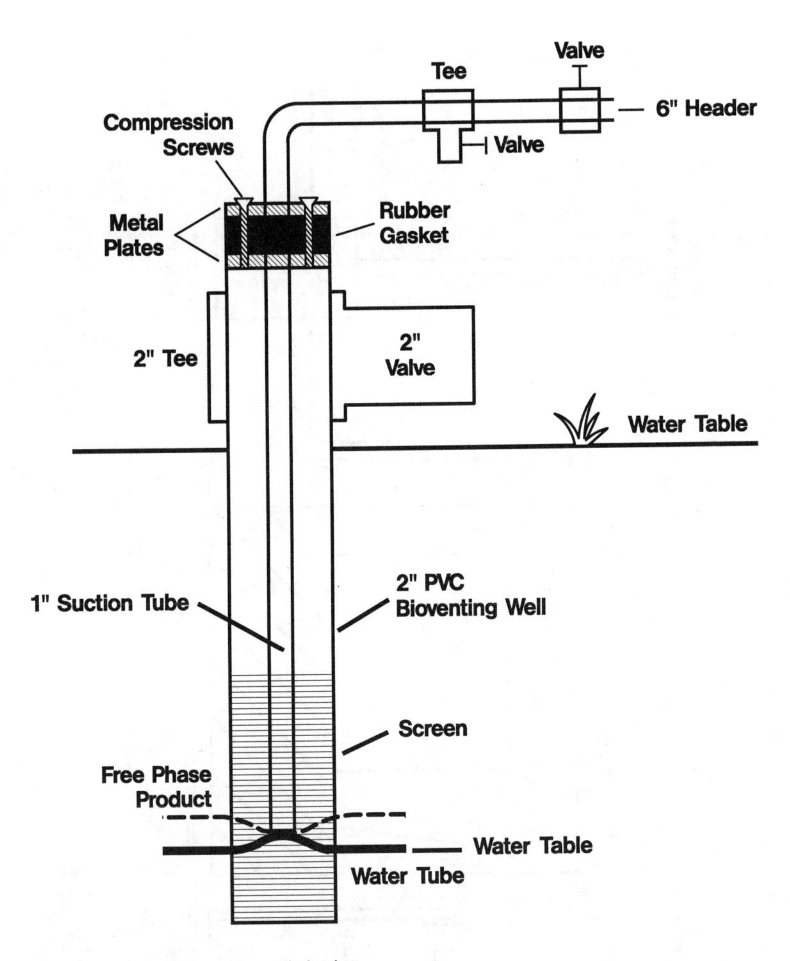

Figure 3.4. Bioslurper well design.

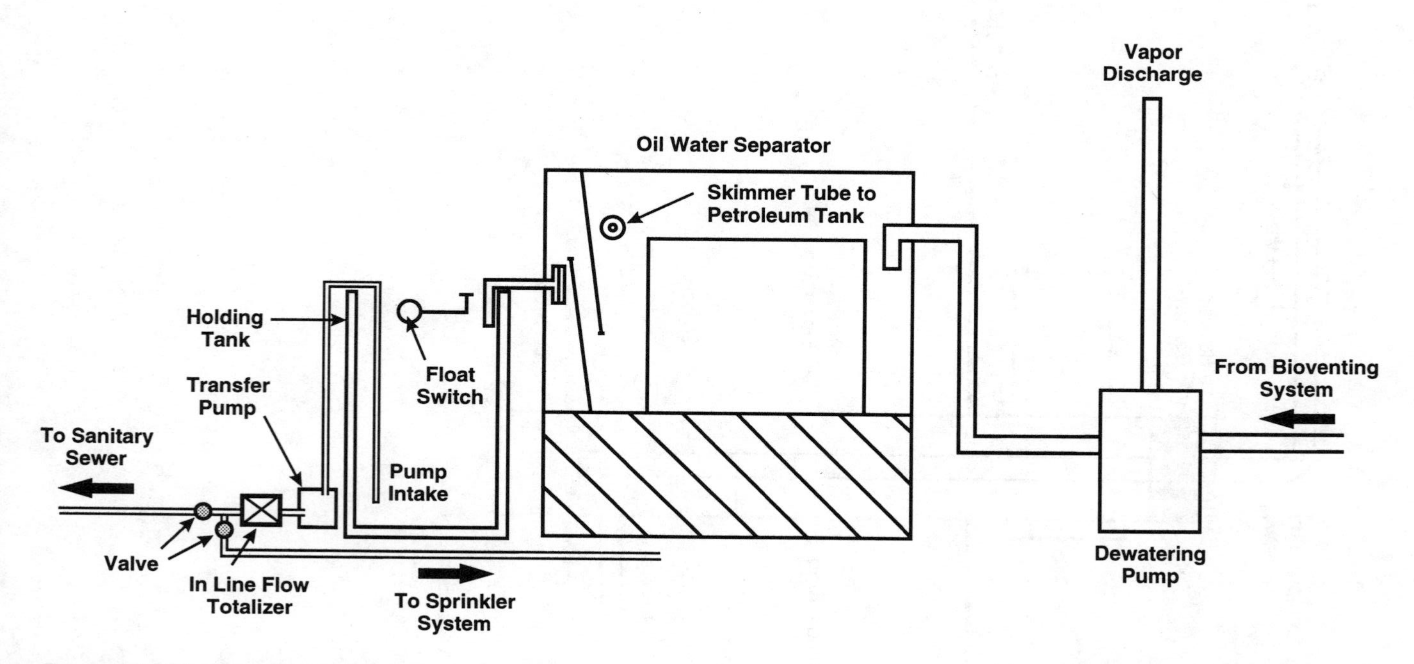

Figure 3.5. Diagram of bioventing system components. (not to scale)

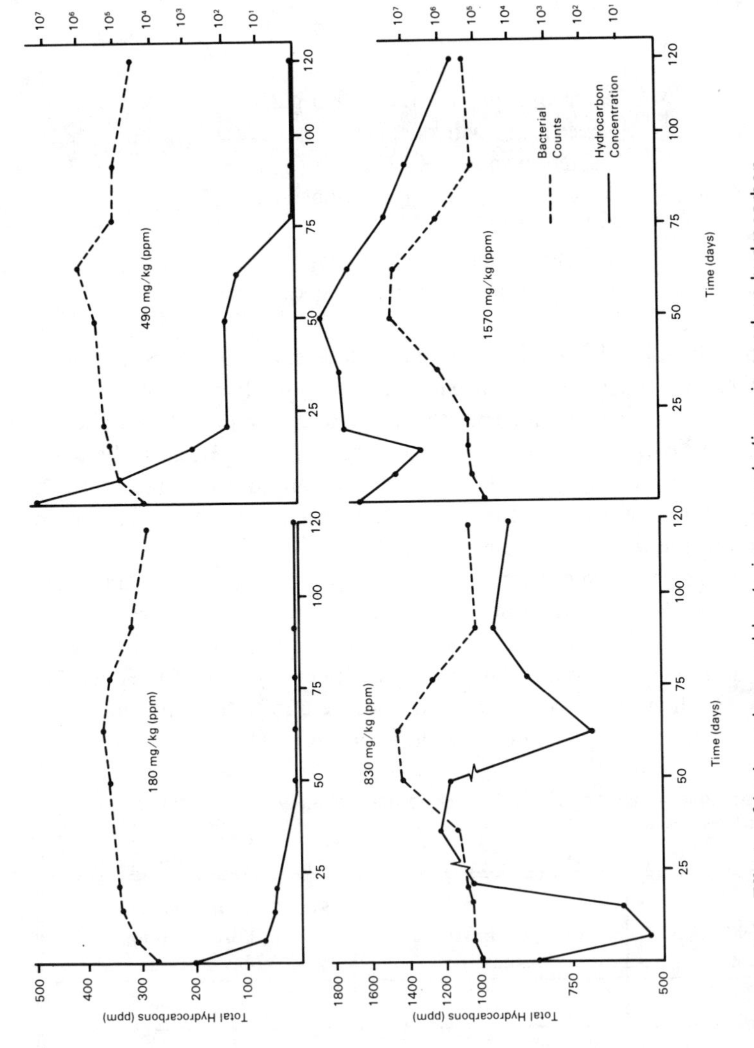

Figure 3.6. Effects of hydrocarbon and bacteria concentrations in sand on hydrocarbon degradation rates.

To evaluate the effect of initial TPH concentration on soil treatment, specific growth rates (Equation 1) and specific substrate utilization rates (Equation 2) were calculated for the logarithmic growth phase at each TPH concentration (triplicate vials of soil):

$$dX/dt=\mu X \quad (1)$$
$$-(dS/dt)/X=kS \quad (2)$$

where

dX/dt	=	microbial growth rate, CFU/g.d
μ	=	specific growth rate, day^{-1}
X	=	bacterial counts, CFU/g
$-(dS/dt)/X$	=	specific substrate utilization rate, (mg/d)/(CFU/g)
k	=	first-order rate constant, day^{-1}
S	=	substrate concentration, mg/kg.

Equation 2 is applied only in continuous flow stirred reactors in which steady state substrate and biomass concentrations are established. In the batch systems used in the experiments, the specific substrate utilization rate may be approximated by normalizing k to the biomass concentration. Because biomass increased during the batch experiments, k was normalized using the mean X during the logarithmic growth phase. Estimated specific substrate utilization rates therefore are reported as $k/X(day^{-1}/CFU/g)$.

Specific growth rates and estimated specific substrate utilization rates for the four initial soil TPH concentrations are listed in Table 3.1. Factorial design analysis of variance (ANOVA) showed that the population means for the four specific growth rates were not significantly different ($\alpha \leq 0.05$). However, ANOVA analysis showed that the estimated specific substrate utilization rates declined as a function of initial TPH concentration ($\alpha \leq 0.05$).

Table 3.1. Logarithmic phase specific growth rates and estimated specific utilization rates for four initial TPH concentrations

TPH Concentration (mg/kg)	Specific Growth Rate (day^{-1})	Specific Estimated Substrate Utilization Rate ($day^{-1}/CFU/g$)
180	0.407	1.03×10^{-6}
490	0.052	5.4×10^{-7}
830	0.093	0
1,570	0.111	0

The concentration effect exhibited by TPH concentrations at or greater than 830 mg/kg in these experiments should not have been limited by dissolved oxygen, pH, or nutrients. The dissolved oxygen concentrations in the soil systems were maintained at ≥ 3 mg/L, and the pH was maintained between 6.5 and 7.0. The concentrations of the two primary nutrient additions, NH_3-N and PO_4-P, decreased negligibly during the 120 day treatment. The results indicate that low degradation rates observed with the higher soil TPH concentrations may be due to surface area and bioavailability phenomena. Bacteria may not be physically capable of degrading significant water immiscible hydrocarbons when present at high concentrations, when the substrate exists as large globules that are poorly accessible to biosurfactants.[13,14]

To evaluate the potential of stimulating the biodegradation of petroleum with TPH concentrations above 830 mg/kg, a vial containing soil contaminated with 2,000 mg/kg TPH was amended with 10 mg/L methanol, mixed with the original soil-water solution. This methanol addition was repeated weekly over the 34 day treatment period. Figure 3.7 shows that the methanol amendment resulted in a significant loss of TPH, amounting to 83% over the experimental period. The specific growth rate and the estimated specific substrate utilization rate for the methanol amended system were 0.87 day^{-1} and 2.28×10^{-5} day^{-1}/(CFU/g), respectively. By factorial ANOVA, these values are significantly greater than the specific growth rates and estimated specific substrate utilization rates for the 830 and 1,570 mg/kg TPH experiments.

Although the results of the experiment with methanol addition were confounded by a lack of decline in bacterial counts over the shorter experimental period and a much higher specific growth rate, the most logical reason for increased hydrocarbon biodegradation rate is the hydrocarbon solubilization effect promoted by a water soluble cosolvent such as methanol. The result would be greater bioavailability of the water immiscible hydrocarbon compounds. Because the experimental vials were continually agitated, the solubilization effect experienced would be much greater than what should be expected in an *in-situ* treatment system, however. Thus these results serve mainly to help define the problem rather than to provide a practical solution.

RESULTS AND DISCUSSION OF FIELD STUDIES

In-situ Respiration Testing

Fallon Naval Air Station, NV

The *in-situ* respiration test at Fallon NAS was performed in the summer of 1990. The observed biodegradation rates ranged from 4.4 to 5.9 mg/kg day as hexane (based on oxygen utilization rates). Carbon dioxide production was not significant during the test.

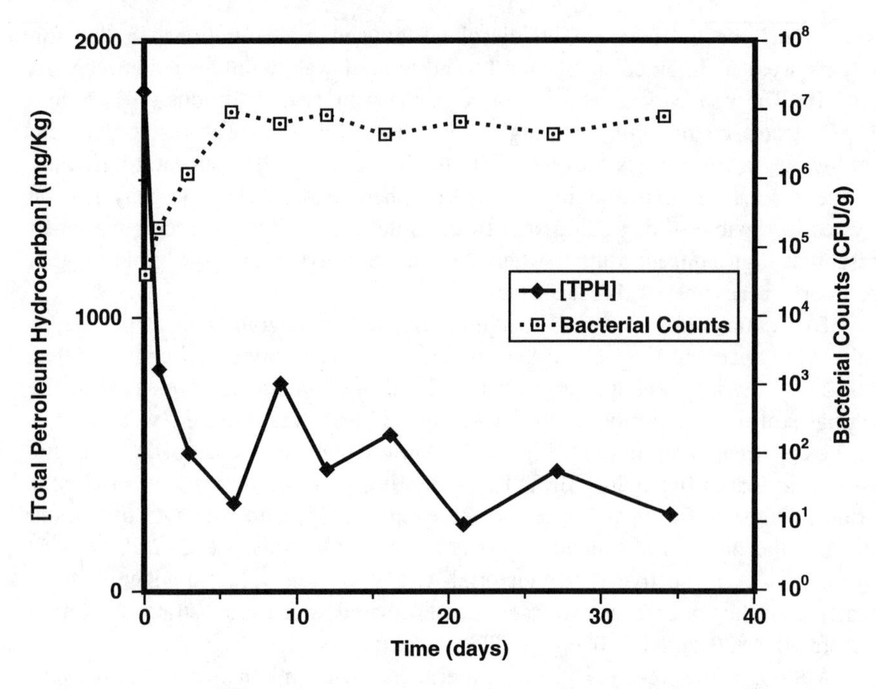

Figure 3.7. Biodegradation and bacterial counts during treatment with methanol Amendment.

Patuxent River Naval Air Station, MD

The *in-situ* respiration test at Patuxent River NAS was performed in the summer of 1990. The observed biodegradation rate was 2.9 mg/kg day as hexane (based on oxygen utilization rate). Carbon dioxide production indicated a biodegradation rate of 1.5 mg/kg day. Detailed descriptions of the respiration tests at Fallon and Patuxent River NAS are described elsewhere.[15]

Kaneohe Bay MCAS, HI

The *in-situ* respiration test at the Kaneohe Bay MCAS was performed in the summer of 1993. Two sequential respiration tests were performed. The first test was performed on August 3, 1993, according to the standard procedure with air injection being performed for 20 hours. Soil gas was sampled for oxygen, carbon dioxide, and hydrocarbon concentrations. Oxygen depletion was extremely rapid, with all monitoring points in the contaminated zone reducing from more than 18% to less than 5% in less than four hours. The helium tracer concentration held constant during the test, indicating that leakage and diffusion were insignificant. Carbon dioxide production was insignificant. The background probe indicated very little oxygen depletion during the test.

Due to a concern that the high chemical oxygen demand at this site might be contributing to oxygen depletion, it was decided to run a second test at the same monitoring points beginning on August 6, 1993. Air and inert tracer (helium 1 to 2%) were injected for an additional 44 hours, and soil gas monitoring was conducted as in the first experiment. Oxygen depletion was slower than in the first experiment, with all monitoring points in the contaminated zone reducing from more than 19% to less than 5% in less than 12 hours. The helium tracer concentration held constant during the test, indicating the leakage and diffusion were insignificant. Carbon dioxide production again was insignificant. The background probe indicated very little oxygen depletion during the test. See Figure 3.8 for *in-situ* respiration data for one monitoring point during each test.

The biodegradation rates observed ranged from 60 to 122 mg/kg day as hexane (based on oxygen utilization rate) for the first test and 22 to 105 mg/kg day for the second test. Carbon dioxide production was insignificant at all points. Table 3.2 presents data for both Kaneohe respiration tests from one soil gas monitoring point. Figure 3.9 presents oxygen utilization rates for all three *in-situ* respiration test sites.

Table 3.2. Kaneohe Bay Marine Corps Air Station - *In-situ* Respiration Data

Kaneohe O_2 Utilization				
Monitoring Point (MP)	Oxygen Utilization Rate (%/hour)		Biodegradation Rate (mg/kg/day)	
Test Date	8/3/93	8/6/93	8/3/93	8/6/93
Background	0.06	0.06	1.2	1.2
MPA (2.3 - 2.6 m)	3.1	1.1	60	22
MPA (1.5 - 1.8 m)	4.1	NS	78	NS
MPB (3.8 - 4.9 m)	6.4	5.5	122	105
MPB (1.8 - 2.4 m)	4	2.8	77	54

NS = No Sample Taken

Air Permeability Testing - Twentynine Palms MCAGCC, CA

At the Twentynine Palms study site, a permeability test was conducted at site 17 Alpha. The test was conducted by injecting air into a single vent well (screened from 19.8 to 0.9 meters) until pressure in the soil gas monitoring points stabilized (approximately 20 minutes). The air injection rate and pressure were approximately 4.5 m^3 min^{-1} and 66 cm of water, respectively. The gasoline powered blower was operated at approximately 1,830 rpm. Soil gas pressures were monitored at all screened intervals of three multi-level screened

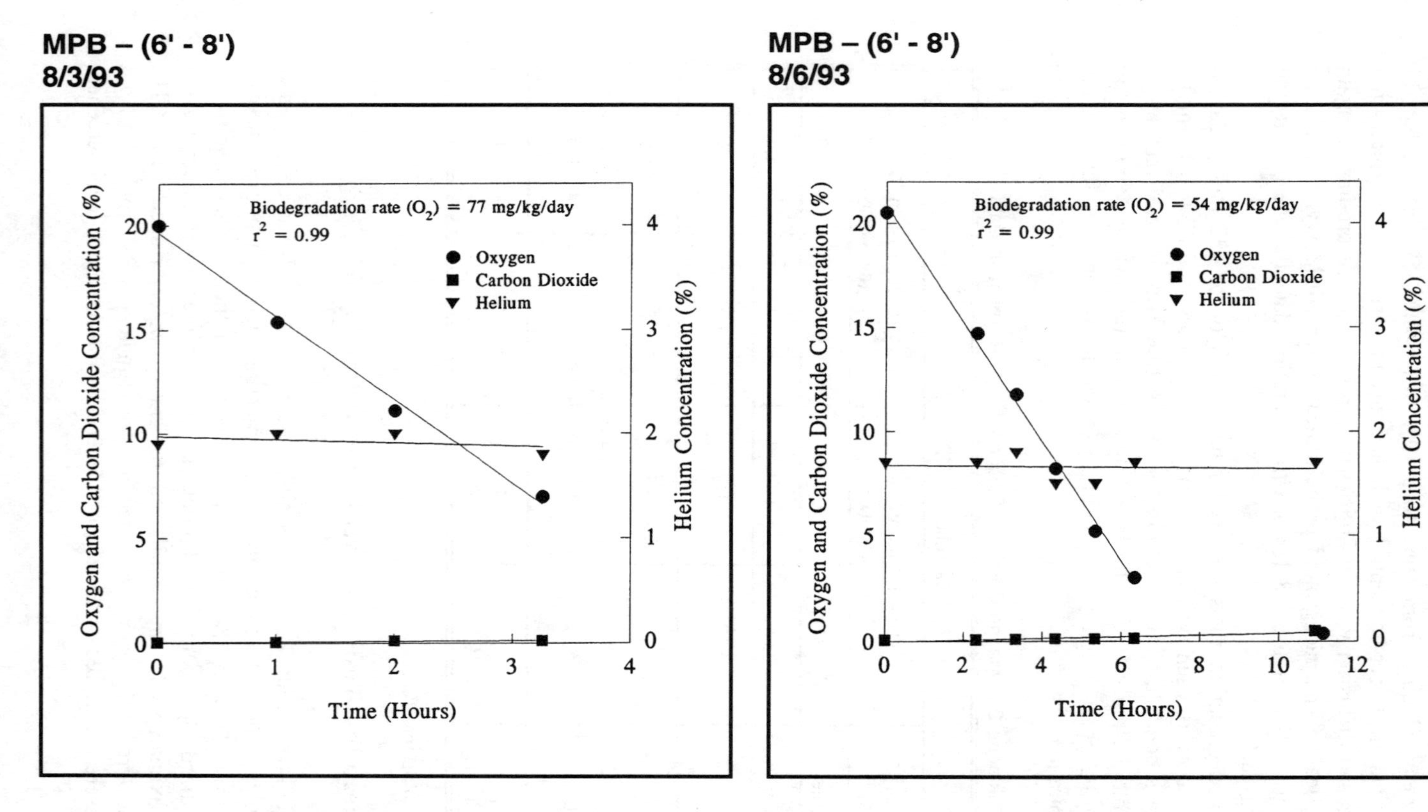

Figure 3.8. Kaneohe Bay Marine Corps Air Station - *In-situ* respiration data.

soil gas monitoring points. Monitoring points (MP) were placed at 55.2 (MP-D), 24.4 (MP-F), and 5.2 (MP-E) meters from the vent well. MP-D is screened at depths of 7.6, 15.2, 22.8, 30.4, 39.5, 48.6, 54.7, and 60.8 meters. MP-E is screened at depths of 1.5, 3.0, 4.6, 6.1, 9.1, 12.2, 15.2, and 18.2 meters. MP-F is screened at depths of 3.0, 6.1, 9.1, 12.2, and 8.2 meters.

The results of the soil gas permeability test conducted at Twentynine Palms have indicated that the radius of influence (R_I) is approximately 49 m. The permeability (K) of the soil was estimated to be approximately 18 darcys, which is typical for medium to coarse sands as observed on the site.

Soil Gas Analysis - Twentynine Palms MCAGCC, CA

Results of soil gas analyses conducted at monitoring points 17A-MP-H and 17A-MP-E are shown in Tables 3.3 and 3.4, respectively. Although total petroleum hydrocarbon (TPH) levels at both sites are similar, with concentrations ranging from 240 to 1,480 ppm, oxygen levels at 17A-MP-H are considerably lower than levels observed at 17-MP-E. Typically, oxygen levels below 5% would indicate that the soils are oxygen deficient and are favorable for remediation by bioventing. The elevated oxygen levels observed at 17-MP-E could suggest that factors other than oxygen concentration are limiting biodegradation in some areas. Other factors that could be limiting biodegradation include moisture deficiency and nutrient deficiency. Future studies will be conducted to identify limiting factors, and bioventing systems will be designed to compensate for site-specific limiting factors (i.e., moisture addition and/or nutrient addition, as appropriate).

Bioslurper System Operation - Fallon NAS, NV

The 0.4-hectare study site at Fallon NAS is located in an open field just downgradient from the JP-5 fuel supply pipeline for the NAS fuel farm (Figure 3.1). The site was selected because of the large LNAPL plume and lack of structures in the vicinity, and to avoid planned construction activities at the *in-situ* respiration test site studied in 1990. Full scale startup of the bioslurper system was initiated in January 1993. Process monitoring includes tracking the mass of hydrocarbons removed in liquid, gaseous, and dissolved form, and monitoring the mass of hydrocarbons remediated via *in-situ* biodegradation. The mass of free phase fuel recovered is measured daily. The OWS aqueous discharge is sampled monthly and is analyzed for TPH. Stack vapor discharge is sampled and analyzed for TPH using field instrumentation daily and is sent

Table 3.3. Soil Gas Data - Twentynine Palms MCAGCC

17A-MP-H						
Depth (m)	June 16, 1993			July 16, 1993		
	O_2 (%)	CO_2 (%)	TPH (ppm)	O_2 (%)	CO_2 (%)	TPH (ppm)
3.0	0	20	280	7	12	580
6.1	0	20	380	0	20	660
9.1	0	19	460	0	18	860
12.2	0.2	18	440	0.5	17	1000
15.2	0.3	18	490	0.9	17	1040
18.2	2	17	470	3	16	960
21.3	3	16	410	3	15	880

Table 3.4. Soil Gas Data - Twentynine Palms MCAGCC

17A-MP-E						
Depth (m)	June 16, 1993			July 16, 1993		
	O_2 (%)	CO_2 (%)	TPH (ppm)	O_2 (%)	CO_2 (%)	TPH (ppm)
1.5	17	2	470	19	0.8	240
3.0	14	4	900	17	3	920
4.6	11	6	1010	13	6	1200
6.1	9	7	720	10	7	1200
9.1	5	11	710	6	11	1440
12.2	6	10	720	6	11	1400
15.2	8	8	720	9	8	1480
18.2	9	7	640	9	8	1340

to a laboratory for analysis quarterly. The TPH concentration in the aqueous effluent has ranged from 50 to 130 ppm. The mass of hydrocarbons emitted from the bioslurper system vapor discharge averages approximately 2.3 kg per day.

The bioslurper system is being operated to maximize fuel recovery while minimizing the volume of groundwater that must be extracted. Average FPR rates have ranged from 25 gallons/day (gpd) to 7 gpd, whereas groundwater extraction rates have ranged from 0.5 to 0.3 gallon per minute (gpm). Figure 3.10 presents the free product and groundwater recovery data for the bioslurper system from full scale startup to date.

The bioslurper test site is located approximately 150 meters from the site where initial *in-situ* respiration testing was conducted. Most soil gas monitoring points within the test site have very low respiration rate measurements, with O_2 concentration of 15 to 19% observed 3 months after soil gas probe emplacement. This contrasts with the respiration rates 18 months earlier at the fuel farm (Figure 9).

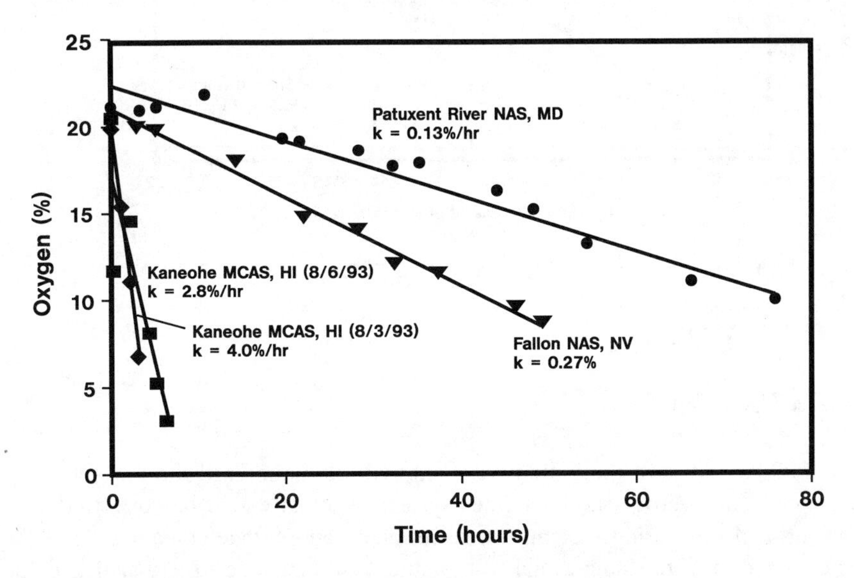

Figure 3.9. Oxygen utilization rates measured at three test sites.

It appears that biodegradation at the test site is being inhibited by some factor other than oxygen deficiency. Free fuel is trapped in a narrow soil zone, confined beneath a silt layer. This excessive fuel concentration could be the major limiting factor. The JP-5 release is very fresh, making it possible that the microbial population has not had time to adapt to the fuel. Corrosion inhibitors in the fuel may also be inhibiting microbial activity. Oxygen-deficient conditions have been observed just 30 meters from the bioslurper study site. A soluble hydrocarbon plume from gasoline contamination may be influencing respiration rates in this area. Bench-scale laboratory studies are ongoing to determine the reason for the observed poor respiration rates at the bioslurper test site, compared to sites displaying oxygen deficiency.

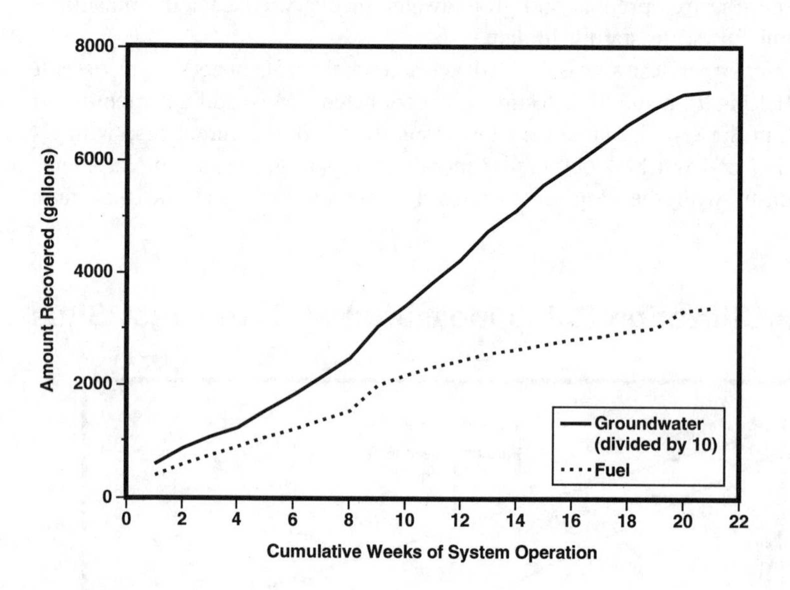

Figure 3.10. Free product recovery data for NAS Fallon.

FUTURE WORK

Fallon NAS, NV

FPR activities at the Fallon NAS site will continue until the fuel recovery rate approaches zero. The bioslurper system eventually will be converted to a conventional bioventing system to treat residual vadose zone contamination. At the completion of the study, final soil samples will be collected and analyzed for post-treatment characterization.

Kaneohe MCAS, HI

A full-scale bioslurper demonstration project is planned for the Kaneohe Bay site. Pretreatment site characterization will be conducted in the winter/spring 1994, and system installation is planned for mid to late 1994.

Twentynine Palms, CA

Site characterization and vent well/monitoring point installations continued through 1993 at Twentynine Palms. Pilot and demonstration scale bioventing projects initiated in late 1993. One area of immediate interest is further investigation of bioventing efficiency utilizing passive aeration, which will involve controlled movement of air into bioventing wells with changes in barometric pressure. Another area of interest is to evaluate the effect of soil moisture biodegradation rates and develop methods for deep irrigation of contaminated soil that is now essentially dry, to enhance fuel bioremediation.

REFERENCES

1. Hinchee, R.E., D.C. Downey, and E.J. Coleman. Enhanced bioreclamation, soil venting and ground-water extraction: A cost-effectiveness and feasibility comparison, in *Petroleum Hydrocarbons and Organic Chemicals in Ground Water Prevention, Detection and Restoration: A Conference and Exposition*, Houston, November 1987.
2. Bury, S.J., and C.A. Miller. Effect of micellar solubilization on biodegradation rates of hydrocarbons. *Environ. Sci. Technol.* 27:104-110, 1993.
3. Hinchee, R.E., and M. Arthur. Bench-scale studies of the soil aeration process for bioremediation of petroleum hydrocarbons. *J. Appl. Biochem. Biotechnol.* 28/29:901-906, 1991.
4. Hinchee, R.E., D.C. Downey, and P.K. Aggarwal. Use of hydrogen peroxide as an oxygen source for *in-situ* biodegradation. Part I. Field studies. *J. Hazard. Mater.* 27:287-299, 1990.
5. Huling, S.G., B.E. Bledsoe, and M.V. White. The feasibility of utilizing hydrogen peroxide as a source of oxygen in bioremediation, in R.E. Hinchee and R.F. Olfenbuttel (Eds.), *In-situ Bioreclamation: Applications and Investigations for Hydrocarbon and Contaminated Site Remediation.* Butterworth-Heinemann, Boston, 1991, 83-102.
6. Morgan, P., and R.J. Watkinson. Factors limiting the supply and efficiency of nutrient and oxygen supplements for the *in-situ* biotreatment of contaminated soil and groundwater. *Water Res.* 26(1):73-78, 1992.
7. Downey, D.C., R.E. Hinchee, M.S. Westray, and J.K. Slaughter. Combined biological and physical treatment of a jet fuel-contaminated aquifer, in *Proceedings, Petroleum Hydrocarbons and Organic Chemicals in Ground Water: Prevention, Detection and Restoration.* National Water Well Association, Dublin, OH, 1988, 627-645.
8. Wilson, J.S. and S.H. Conrad. Is physical displacement of residual hydrocarbons a realistic possibility in aquifer restoration? *Proceedings, Petroleum Hydrocarbons and Organic Chemicals in Groundwater.* National Water Well Association, Dublin, OH, 1984.
9. Hoeppel, R.E., R.E. Hinchee, and M.F. Arthur. Bioventing soils contaminated with petroleum hydrocarbons. *J. Ind. Microbiol.* 8:141-146, 1991.
10. Ong, S.K., R.E. Hinchee, R.E. Hoeppel, and R. Scholze. *In-situ* respirometry for determining aerobic degradation rates, in R.E. Hinchee and R.F.

Olfenbuttel (Eds.), *In-situ Bioreclamation: Applications and Investigations for Hydrocarbon and Contaminated Site Remediation.* Butterworth-Heinemann, Boston, 1991, 541-545.

11. Watts, R.J., P.N. Mcguire, and R.E. Hoeppel. A simple method for conducting laboratory treatability studies for assessing potential for *in-situ* bioremediation. *Biotechnology Techniques.* pp. 385-390, 1993.
12. Hinchee, R.E., S.K. Ong, R.N. Miller, and D.C. Downey. Test Plan and Technical Protocol for a Field Treatability Test for Bioventing. Report to U.S. Air Force Center for Environmental Excellence, Brooks AFB, Texas, 1992.
13. Stucki, G. and M. Alexander. Role of dissolution rate in biodegradation of aromatic compounds. *Appl. Environ. Microbiol.* 53:292-297, 1987.
14. Thomas, J.M., J.R. Yordy, J.A. Amador, and M. Alexander. Rates of dissolution and biodegradation of water-insoluble organic compounds. *Appl. Environ. Microbiol.* 52:290-296, 1986. 15. Hinchee, R.E., S.K. Ong, and R. Hoeppel. A treatability test for bioventing. *84th Annual Meeting and Exhibition, Vancouver, B.C.,* Air & Waste Management Association, 1991, 91-19.4.
15. Hinchee, R.E., D.C. Downey, R.R. DuPont, P.K. Aggarwal, and R.N. Miller. "Enhancing biodegradation of petroleum hydrocarbon through soil venting." J. Hazard Mater. 27:315-325,1991.

CHAPTER 4

Environmental Justice Initiatives Along Louisiana's Mississippi Corridor

William A. Kucharski, P.E., Louisiana Department of Environmental Quality, Baton Rouge, Louisiana

The state of Louisiana is located at the mouth of the Mississippi River, and over 600 miles of the river are located in Louisiana. Between the cities of Baton Rouge and New Orleans, there are approximately 60 land miles and 120 river miles. There are also in excess of 85 major chemical and petro-chemical manufacturing and refining facilities. Over 1.5 million people live and work in the nine parishes (counties) between these two cities. Approximately 600,000 people are minorities representing 40% of the population in the area. Orleans parish, where New Orleans is located, has a 62% minority population. Unemployment for minorities is three times higher than for whites in these parishes (approximately 16.6% versus 5.4%).

I will show you a few slides of the Mississippi corridor from Baton Rouge to New Orleans. There are in excess of 85 major industries along this stretch of the Mississippi. The list of companies reads like a petrochemical patent directory. Dow, DuPont, Allied Signal, La Roche Chemical, Formosa Plastics, Rhone Poulenc, BASF, Shell Chemical, Exxon Chemical, Marathon, Shell, Exxon, Placid Refinery, Ethyl, Vulcan, Ciba Geigy, Kaiser Aluminum, Union Carbide, American Cyanamid and Georgia Gulf. This is not all of the companies and some have more than one plant along this part of the river.

Most of the people residing in the nine river parishes will have a major chemical or petrochemical facility within 10 miles of their home. Many have facilities much closer. The terms "environmental racism", "environmental equity" and "environmental justice" have all been used to describe a condition of disproportionate impact being received by a powerless constituency. If we can all assume that the closer to a facility one lives, the greater the potential threat to their health, then Louisiana can expect to be challenged by these issues.

The Louisiana Department of Environmental Quality (LDEQ) has decided to address this issue directly and not wait until we are forced into action by outside interests. Before a discussion of where a program such as this might be expected to go, it would be appropriate to review the history of the Environmental Justice movement itself.

Attachment 1 is an Environmental Equity Chronology, prepared by Harris, DeVille & Associates, Inc (a Baton Rouge public opinion firm). A brief summary of this history follows. The start of the environmental justice movement can be traced to as early as 1979 when a non-scientific study revealed that all of the city of Houston's solid waste landfills and 75% of their incinerators were located in black neighborhoods. In 1982 in Warren County, North Carolina, residents in this predominately black county protested the state's proposal to locate a PCB landfill there. Over 500 people were finally arrested, including Dr. Benjamin F. Chavis, Jr. current executive director of the NAACP. A 1983 GAO investigation of hazardous waste landfills in the south revealed that three of four permitted facilities were in predominantly black communities. In 1987, the United Church of Christ's Commission on Racial Justice (CRJ) released "Toxic Wastes and Race in the United States--A National Report on the Racial and Socioeconomic Characteristics of Communities with Hazardous Waste Sites". This study concluded that 60% of black and hispanic Americans live in communities with uncontrolled hazardous waste sites (Dr. Chavis has been associated with the CRJ since 1982). To date, I am unaware of any published studies that refute these figures.

If there are such trends in our country, we must ask the question, what can be done? We can obviously be more aware of this data whenever siting/permitting decisions are being made, but what we do for those communities that already have industrial facilities located them. This question is the topic of this chapter. I will describe the steps taken in the development of a pilot environmental justice program in Louisiana.

As one begins a new process, it is usually a good idea to determine where you are starting so that you can look back on the beginning at a later date and be able to identify changes. One way in which this can be done is by conducting attitude surveys. These surveys are becoming more and more common in our society. After 1% of a vote is cast in a national election, our news stations are predicting winners and losers. We are told what most people think and we can get a breakdown of opinion by age, sex, race, income or preference. We sometimes see so many results that we lose sight of how complex and difficult it is to design and implement a good survey.

There are many good survey firms available to anyone that has the necessary dollars. One does not buy the results of a survey. One buys the form, the questions, the technique that will provide unbiased answers. In Baton Rouge, the capital of Louisiana, a prominent attitude survey company is Harris, Deville & Associates. The poll results I am now going to quote are used with their permission. The results are quite interesting and revealing.

The first question asked individuals to define the main problems which keep Louisiana from being a better place to live. Only 5% of the black and white respondents thought that environment/pollution was the cause. This was the only area of agreement. When it came to the other choices, Whites were three times more likely than blacks to blame the politicians, and twice more likely to blame the economy. Blacks, on the other hand, were three times more likely to blame crime and law enforcement, and twice more likely than whites to blame unemployment as the primary cause keeping Louisiana from being a better place to live. This set of questions is important. To me it says that blacks are underemployed and subjected to more crime than whites, while whites blamed more esoteric villains: politicians and the "economy".

There are many other differences between how blacks and whites view the environment and industries. When asked whether or not chemical companies in Louisiana can operate in an environmentally sound manner, 86% of whites said yes to only 66% of the black respondents. Only 8.5% of the whites said no to this question, while 23% of the blacks said that the chemical companies could not operate in an environmentally sound manner. If you think that the high favorable response for that question means things are really pretty good, wait. The same people were asked if chemical companies tell the truth about their environmental impacts. Only 11.5% of whites and 14.1% of the blacks said yes. 77% of the whites and 80% of the blacks said no. Not only were the respondents convinced that the chemical companies did not tell the truth about their environmental impacts, when people were asked whether the companies could be trusted, only 20% of the respondents said yes. (18.8 white, 21.1 black).

Respondents were asked what they thought the cause of cancer was in Louisiana, and 77.8% of the black respondents answered pollution/environment. To this question only 38.8% of whites responded the same way. However, 32.7% of the white respondents answered chemical plants/industry. No black respondent claimed this answer. When the two answers are combined, pollution/environment and chemical plants/industry, over 70% of white respondents blame industrial sources as did almost 78% of blacks. Several slides are shown that will show some of the trends in these, and other opinions related to the environment and industry.

These data were collected for the chemical industry in Louisiana. Whether or not these responses are relevant to any other state or jurisdiction is not important. What is relevant is the fact that the black and white residents of Louisiana have markedly different perceptions of the environment and those things in the environment that may effect them. It may well be the same situation in other states.

It has already been stated that the LDEQ had decided to take on thie environmental justice issue. One of the first efforts that was undertaken occurred in 1992, when the Louisiana Department of Environmental Quality received an unsolicited proposal from a local university. This proposal was designed to determine the attitude of local communities toward "Environmental Equity". As the proposal was reviewed, it became obvious that having only a community view would not be as helpful as being able to compare the views of the industries at the same time on the same issues. When this process was started, I knew very little about the intricacies of good survey preparation. I now wish I had known more.

The survey was put together to draw out attitudes of local residents about the adjacent industries and industries about the environmental justice question. The concentration of major industries along the Mississippi has been shown to you. Interspersed between these companies are located some very old cities, towns and communities. Many of them have primarily minority residents. The resident survey was augmented by an additional set of questions for gauging industrial attitudes. This seemed to be a very simple process. You ask questions, you receive answers and you create great analyses with the results. It did not turn out just that way.

The industry survey was reviewed by the Louisiana Chemical Association (LCA) and with their help, the survey was distributed to approximately 100 chemical companies located along the river. Approximately 64 companies responded. Over 500 individuals were queried in four river parishes. Over 60% of the respondents lived less than two miles from an industrial facility, while 96% lived within ten miles of an industrial facility. So, we have 500 people that live near industrial facilities and we have 64-65 facilities responding to a survey. Our report has not yet been correlated to show which responses were associated with which facilities and vice versa. The questions were not identical and so the answers are not really comparable. In short, we have two surveys that we can not use as we intended.

Some of the results were very interesting however.

In the area of regulations:

1= yes, 5=no	Blacks	Whites	Industry
Are the regs too strict?	4.03	3.86	2.76
Should DEQ enforce more?	1.65	1.74	3.09
Should Industry self regulate?	3.56	3.86	3.63
Should repeat violators be shut down?	1.92	2.05	2.00

Complaints (% answering yes)

Noise	55.7	31.8	37.0
Odors	73.4	53.4	51.9
Local Hires (not enough)	60.2	42.0	38.9
Flaring (at night)	45.3	25.0	14.8
Plumes/smoke	47.0	26.1	11.1

Positive and Negative Aspects of Facilities

% that "agree" or "strongly agree"			
Should residents be compensated?	84.3	77.3	5.6
Should Locals have some voice in Operations?	82.1	75.0	66.7
Is there adequate monitoring?	26.4	52.3	98.1
Is AQ unchanged?	55.5	46.6	24.1
Does the facility threaten human health of the community?	64.4	51.1	5.6
Do the benefits of living next to a facility outweigh the risk?	19.2	47.7	37.0

Does the facility generate needed tax dollars?	38.8	67.0	96.3
Employment opportunities have improved for local communities	22.9	61.4	75.9

As you can see, there are several questions that show some extensive areas of differing perceptions/opinions. For example, facility responders were very strong in the belief that their facilities did not pose human health problems for the surrounding communities (5.6%), while 84% of the black residents and 77% of the white residents answered yes. There are surprises however. The question of the benefits to nearby residents versus the risks showed that industry respondents were closer in their views (37%) to black perceptions (19%) than whites (48%). The question of compensation to people who live close to an industrial facility was clearly one of potential conflict, with only 5.6% of industry responding with a yes, while 82% of the community respondents agreeing that such compensation should be made to nearby residents. When one looks at some of the related data, such as average family income of the respondents, this disparity becomes clearer. Of the community respondents, over 60% had under $15,000 annual family incomes.

This simple survey clearly erased any questions as to whether or not such a program was necessary in my state. It became clear that there was much to do. The next step was to review and interpret the survey and begin to try and establish a program that would be responsive to the problem, whatever that turned out to be. There is nothing simple or non-controversial in this area. LDEQ contacted several minority community leaders as well as the Louisiana Chemical Association (LCA) and Mid Continental Oil and Gas (Mid Continent), the API of the region. We all sat down and attempted to review and analyze the survey results and to begin to discuss what we might do. There was one thing obvious about the survey, there is a major difference about how minority communities and white communities and industry people view the world. The survey, while imperfect and in many ways inadequate, did show that there were many major differences in perception.

Where did everyone agree? We agreed that there were significant problems. This is about the only agreement that we were able to reach. We did not really agree about what the actual problems were, only that there were many. Some of the problems that are most obvious include a real fear by residents for their lives. This is augmented by poverty, unemployment, a lack of education and a lack of hope. The real question that we had to ask ourselves is whether anything, any program could work.

LDEQ began to actively pursue the creation of an Environmental Justice Program in early summer of 1993. After we received the preliminary survey, we contacted EPA Region 6. They had attempted to create an Environmental Justice Program, but the results were not as good as expected. LDEQ therefore asked Region 6 if they would like to help fund a pilot program for Louisiana. The answer was yes, and the grant is presently working itself through the federal process. This grant will make a successful program possible, however, no amount of cooperation or financial support, can guarantee success. Thanks to their support however, the chance to succeed or fail is now possible.

Currently, Louisiana has a community outreach program that is sponsored by local industries. The industry fully funds professional facilitators who work with Citizen Advisory Panels or CAPs. A CAP provides a forum wherein a community and an industry can communicate on equal footing. This became the model for the Louisiana Environmental Justice Program. There are several restrains associated with establishing an Environmental Justice Program. There are also a couple of basic principles that I have painfully discovered. I would be happy to describe them for you.

The first is the awareness that any solution, any program that is established must be responsive to the first rule of politics, namely, **ALL POLITICS ARE LOCAL.** What this means is that you can never make progress or solve the problems of "the state". Success will be local in nature or you will not have success. This is why Louisiana will focus our efforts on local involvement, local commitment and local solutions. The state's program will be the coordination of all of the local efforts.

The second principle is that there is no single leader in the minority community. No one speaks for all of the people. Some of the loudest people speak only for themselves, although you might not learn this until after it is too late. The third principle, and probably the most important, is that if such a controversial program is to have any chance of succeeding, the program must have a bottom up organization. The dictate, the top to bottom flow of ideas and solutions, will not work in my opinion. Fourth, there must be a firm commitment from the industries in the affected areas. Without their support, there is no program.

Having described the basic format, let me go on to describe in more detail what the Environmental Justice Advisory Panels (EJAPs) will be expected to do and how they might be organized. We anticipate having the EJAPs contain several representatives of selected communities from a narrowly defined geographic area. Representatives of senior management (the plant manager will be asked to actively participate) from the local industries must also be part of the process. The industry representative must have the power to commit the company's resources to the process and be willing to do so.

One challenge is how one chooses such communities and the representatives, and how one gets the affected industries to the table. First, however, the Panel locations have to be selected. After the locations have been picked, then the topics that the EJAP will address must be selected. There will have to be basic guidelines and "rules of engagement" for the EJAP meetings. It is my opinion that in order to maintain a focus on solvable problems, one of the rules will have to be a limit of initial topics pursued by the panel. There will be many other rules. The formulation of such rules will be led by the independent facilitator.

The role of the independent, neutral facilitator as well as the role of the regulator in this process, should be discussed. The independent facilitator will be the referee, the guide, the mediator. This is a critical position. While the members of the EJAP will be responsible for progress and for staying on track, the facilitator will be responsible for keeping the communications lines open and maintaining the opportunity for success.

The other important point is that the regulator, in this case the LDEQ, will not be a part of the panel. LDEQ will be represented at the meetings, but it will not be an active participant. This is because the solutions to the problems might include the LDEQ, but the major solutions will be determined between the industries, and the communities. The program will be started and funded by the LDEQ, but the work, the communication and the solutions will be solely their responsibility.

The goals of the EJAPs are very basic: To improve the communication between effected communities and the industries that surround them. This program is not designed to be a big giveaway forum. Neither the industries, the regulators nor the community representatives have expressed such goals. What I believe might happen is that the communities will be able to gain more credibility and more power through an honest association with responsible companies. There are those who do not care for real world solutions. There are those who only want to tap free money sources through this process, and there are those who will never admit that there are any reasons to fear living next to a chemical plant or petroleum refinery. There is much to be done.

In closing, it must be said that this process may not succeed. There may be too many mutually exclusive agendas to find success. This, however, will not be known until we try. Selection of the communities, (three groups will probably be chosen to start the pilot) has already begun. It is expected that the actual selection of the representatives will occur in the fall of 1993. Community organization and training will be assisted by the EPA grant, as will the funding of a full time Environmental Justice Coordinator for the state. It is hoped that we can have the first EJAP up and running by January of 1994. The pilot program is being funded by EPA Region 6 for a year.

APPENDIX A

Environmental Equity Chronology

Harris, DeVille & Associates, Inc April 27, 1992

1979 A non-scientific study of black life in Houston, Texas, reveals that all of the city-owned municipal solid waste landfills and six of the eight garbage incinerators are located in black neighborhoods.

1982 State officials decide to locate a PCB landfill in predominantly black Warren County, North Carolina. Residents rise up in protest. The civil rights arm of a major U.S. Protestant denomination, the United Church of Christ's Commission on Racial Justice (CRJ), becomes involved. Civil disobedience follows, and more than 500 people are arrested, including CRJ's executive director, Rev. Benjamin F. Chavis, Jr. CRJ, which was founded in 1963 in the midst of the civil rights movement, begins to turn its attention to environmental issues.

1983 The General Accounting Office (GAO) launches an investigation of the socio-economic and racial composition of communities surrounding the four major hazardous waste landfills in the South. The GAO report reveals that three of the four landfills were located in predominantly black communities.

1985 The Center for Environment, Commerce and Energy is founded as the first national African American environmental organization.

The National Council of Churches' Eco-Justice Working Group begins focusing on environmental equity issues.

1987 CRJ releases its landmark study, *Toxic Wastes and Race in the United States -- A National Report on the Racial and Socio-Economic Characteristics of Communities with Hazardous Waste Sites.* While presenting the report at the National Press Club in Washington, D.C., Rev. Chavis uses the term "environmental racism" for the first time. Among the major findings:

- Communities with the greatest number of commercial hazardous waste facilities had the highest composition of racial and ethnic residents.
- Although socio-economic status appeared to play an important role in the location of commercial hazardous waste facilities, race still proved to be more significant.
- Three out of every five black and Hispanic Americans live in communities with uncontrolled toxic waste sites.

1990 The Conference on Race and the Incidence of Environmental Hazards is held in January at the University of Michigan. This is the first time that an academic conference on race and the environment is held at which a majority of the presenters (nine of twelve) are people of color.

In September, the organizers of this conference meet with EPA Administrator William K. Reilly and Council on Environmental Quality Chairman Michael R. Deland. The meeting is supposedly the first for an EPA Administrator with a predominantly minority group to discuss environmental equity issues. In response, Administrator Reilly organizes an EPA workgroup to study and report to him on the issues raised at the Michigan conference.

1991 The First National People of Color Environmental Leadership Summit is held in October in Washington, D.C., attracting more than 600 participants and national media coverage. Rev. Chavis and former New Mexico Governor Toney Anaya serve as co-chairmen of the four-day summit. The major theme is that minorities are victims of "environmental racism," and among other things, they make it clear they want to become part of the "lily-white" mainstream environmental movement.

1992 February '92 is a watershed month for the environmental equity movement.

EPA releases a draft report entitled "Environmental Equity: Reducing Risk for all Communities." The report, which was the work of EPA's Environmental Equity Workgroup that was organized by Administrator Reilly in 1990, concludes there is a general lack of data on environmental health effects by race and income. The report also details a list of eight recommendations to EPA, the first of which was for the agency to increase the priority it gives to issues of environmental equity. The release of the draft report attracts considerable national media coverage, and U.S. Rep. Henry Waxman of California chairs a subcommittee hearing on the relationship between race and environmental regulations. In general, environmentalists are critical of the report. The final version of the report is released in June.

At about the same time this was going on in Washington, the Louisiana Advisory Committee of the U.S. Commission on Civil Rights conducts two days of fact finding environmental equity hearings in Baton Rouge. The primary focus of the hearings centers around claims that minority groups are being subjected to a disproportionate share of Louisiana's environmental problems.

1992 (cont) The March/April edition of the *EPA Journal* focuses exclusively on the environmental equity issue.

In May, the Federal Environmental Justice Act of 1992 is introduced in Congress. The purpose of the act, sponsored by Sen. Al Gore of Tennessee and Rep. John Lewis of Georgia, is to assure that areas with the highest concentrations of toxic chemicals are scrutinized to ensure equal protection under the law and non-discriminatory compliance with all applicable environmental, health and safety standards.

In September, the Louisiana Department of Environmental Quality funds a year-long, $40,000 study on environmental equity. Two professors at the LSU Department of Political Science are the principal investigators, and both have limited knowledge of industry.

Also in September, EPA creates a headquarter-level Office of Equity.

In December, the Birmingham, Alabama-based Southern Organizing Committee for Economic and Social Justice holds the Southern Community/Labor Conference for Environmental Justice in New Orleans. More than 2,500 civil rights, environmental and union activists attend, and participants network, share common experiences and try to find ways to become more effective in their fight against environmental racism.

1993 EPA Region 6 forms an Environmental Equity Planning Committee in preparation for an environmental equity conference in June. Industry is grossly underrepresented.

On March 18, EPA conducts a public hearing on the proposed HON rule in Baton Rouge. Among the claims made by those who testify: "Environmental racism is predominant in this area. Plants are on top of poor and minority communities, poisoning them, devaluing their land, etc."

On March 27-28 in Birmingham, the Southern Organizing Committee for Social and Economic Justice holds a follow-up strategy session to December's Environmental Justice Conference. The stated purpose of the session is to outline strategies and develop an action plan.

On March 29, the U.S. Commission on Civil Rights announces it is launching an investigation of EPA's enforcement activities in minority communities. In a March 8 letter to EPA Administrator

1993 (cont) Carol Browner, the commission's acting staff director says the probe is "a preliminary examination of environmental equity issues and civil rights enforcement activities at the EPA."

During the first quarter of the year, inquiries from national media about equity issues become more frequent for Louisiana Chemical Association member companies.

On April 9, Rev. Chavis is selected as the new executive director of the National Association for the Advancement of Color People (NAACP). One of his goals is for the NAACP to become active in environmental issues.

In May, the Louisiana Advisory Council of the U.S. Commission on Civil Rights is scheduled to release its written report on environmental equity issues in Louisiana.

U.S. Rep. John Lewis of Georgia plans to reintroduce the Environmental Justice Act of 1992 once a new sponsor comes forward in the Senate.

CHAPTER 5

Lessons Learned From Installation of an Environmental Horizontal Well

Daniel B. Oakley, HAZWRAP, Science and Technology, Inc.
Mark D. Nickelson, HAZWRAP, Martin Marietta Energy Systems, Inc.
HAZARDOUS WASTE REMEDIAL ACTIONS PROGRAM, Environmental Restoration and Waste Management Programs, Oak Ridge, Tennessee

INTRODUCTION

Williams Air Force Base (AFB) is located 20 miles east of Phoenix, Arizona, in the city of Mesa (Figure 5.1). During September 1989, Williams AFB was added to the Environmental Protection Agency's National Priorities List. The major site at Williams AFB is a Liquid Fuels Storage Area (LFSA) which has been used to store jet fuel since 1942 (Figure 5.2). The LFSA was composed of numerous underground storage tanks and several thousand feet of four inch and six inch diameter delivery pipe. Numerous spills and leaks over the years have resulted in a free product plume on the uppermost unconfined aquifer at approximately 220 ft BLS. The free product plume has been estimated to be between 650,000 and 1,400,000 gal (IT Corp, 1991). The associated dissolved contaminant plume as defined by the 5 ppb benzene line is approximately 1700 ft long by 600 ft wide.

The uppermost unconfined aquifer which contains the contaminant plume extends from approximately 220 to 250 ft Below Land Surface (BLS) and is composed of intermixed clay, silt, and sand (Figure 5.3). Deposits are representative of channel, floodplain, terrace, and alluvial fan deposition (Laney and Hahn 1986). The uppermost aquifer is underlain by a 20 ft. thick clay aquitard. Below the aquitard is a semiconfined aquifer that is several hundred feet thick and is used as an irrigation and drinking water supply.

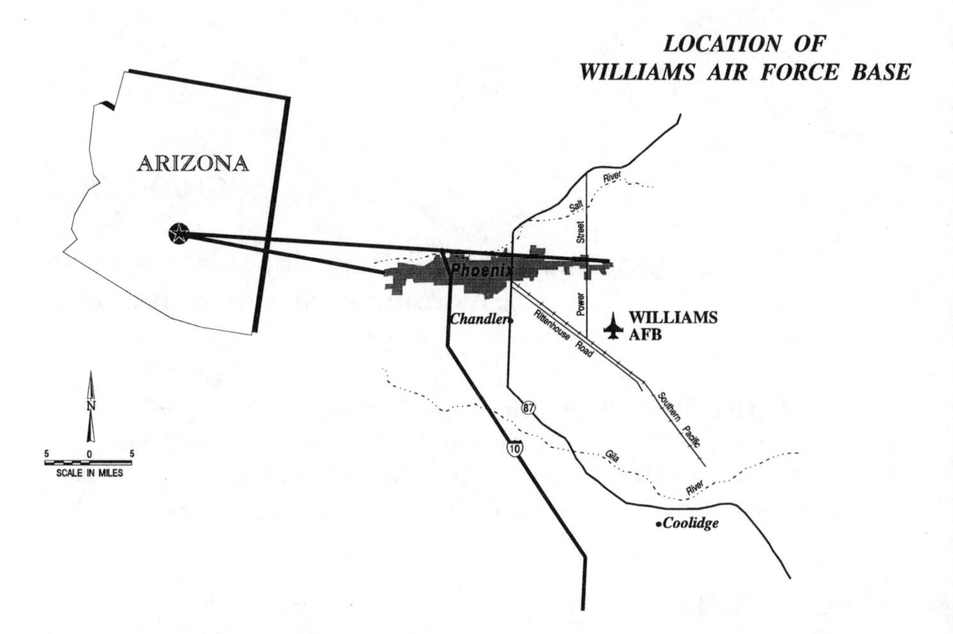

Figure 5.1. Location of Williams Air Force Base.

A Pilot Study/Demonstration Study (PS/DS) began in 1991 to evaluate the effectiveness of horizontal vs. vertical wells for containing and remediating the contaminant plume. As part of this study, the longest, deepest environmental horizontal well was successfully installed during July 1992 after two unsuccessful installation attempts.

DRILLING METHOD

River crossing technology developed for installing utility conduits under rivers was adapted for this well installation. The custom-made rig used for installation included a hydraulically operated, gear-driven feed frame trailer, a control trailer, and a mud tank/mixer trailer. The gear-driven feed frame trailer is raised at one end, and the other end is placed in a mud pit to set the entry angle.

For this installation a nine inch diameter pilot hole was drilled at an initial angle of 20 degrees to the ground surface. A curved section was drilled to make the borehole horizontal. After drilling the 500 ft long horizontal section, the borehole curved upward to an exit location approximately one-half mile from the entrance location. The borehole was then reamed to a 16 or 18 inch diameter, and the well materials were pulled into place from the exit to the entrance location.

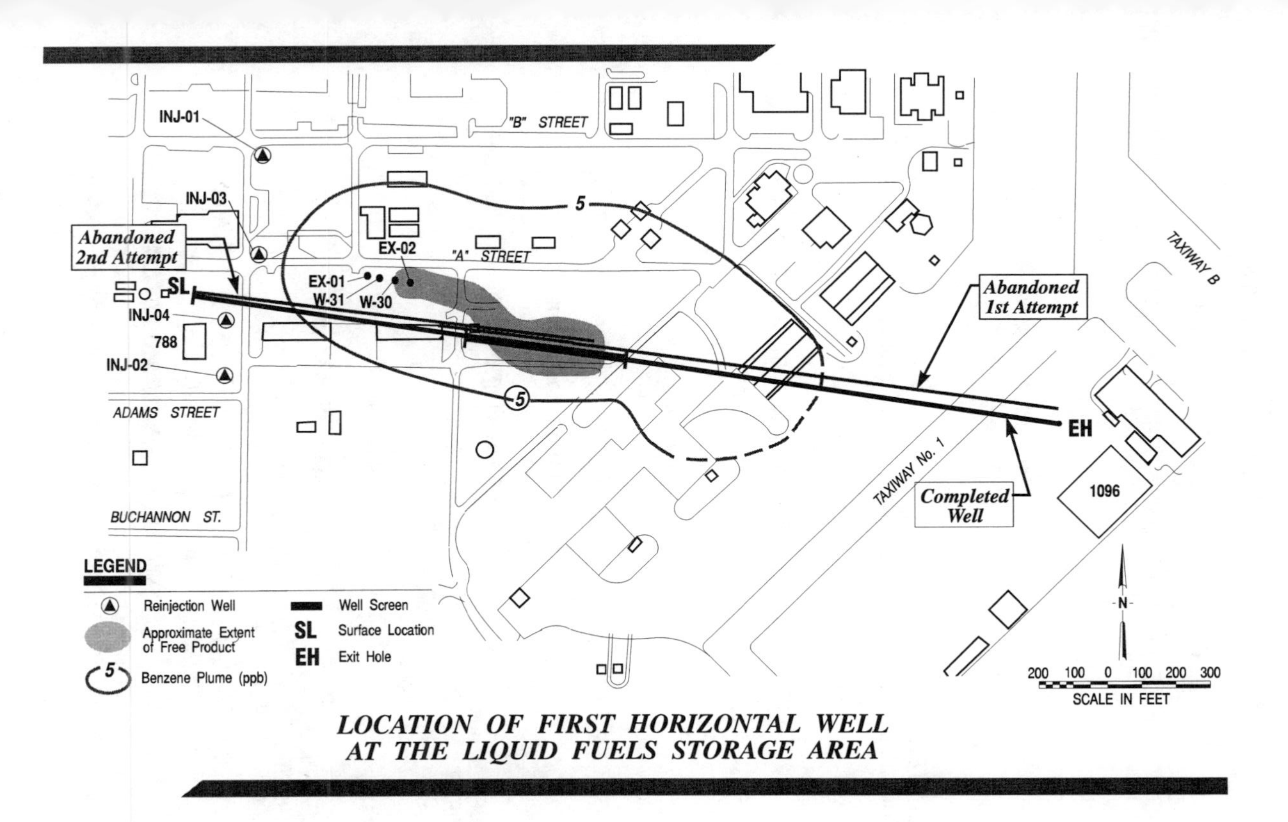

Figure 5.2. Location of First Horizontal Well at the Liquid Fuels Storage Area.

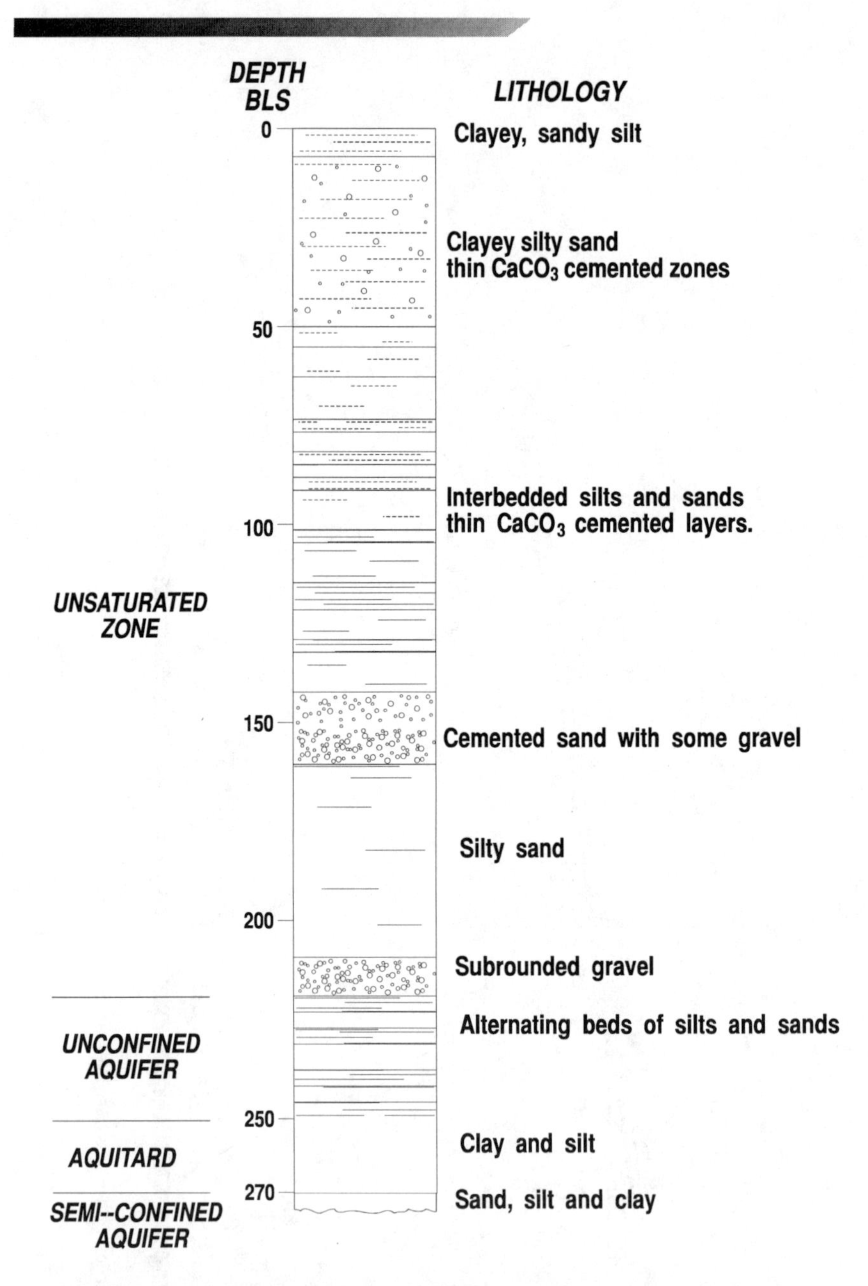

Figure 5.3. Hydrostratigraphic Column of Upper Unit. *Williams Air Force Base.*

During pilot hole drilling, the drill string is steered using a bent subassembly. Increasing the borehole angle up or down, left or right, is achieved by orienting the bent subassembly in the desired direction and jetting while advancing the drill string without rotation. Drilling a straight hole without changing the angle is accomplished by advancing the drill string while rotating and jetting.

A downhole magnetic guidance system, located in the probe directly behind the drill bit, is connected to the surface by wire line and determines the real-time inclination and azimuth of the bent subassembly. Based on this information and the pipe length, trigonometry is used to determine the borehole location. Secondary confirmation of the borehole location is obtained by halting drilling operations every 30 ft (one joint length) and applying an electrical current to the wire loop on the surface, thereby creating a magnetic field of known geometry and intensity over the path of the borehole. The magnetic field is measured at the probe and modeled. The location of the probe is then determined relative to the proposed borehole path.

INSTALLATION ATTEMPT NUMBER 1

Drilling of the first attempt began on April 23, 1993. Workdays were typically 12 hours long. The pilot hole was drilled to 632 ft length, and the curved section was drilled by building angle. At a drilling distance of 837 ft from the surface location (235 ft BLS), the horizontal section began. After drilling 500 ft of horizontal section, angle was again built until the exit angle of 16 degrees was achieved (Figure 4). The pilot hole was successfully completed 1264 ft from the end of the horizontal section (2601 ft from the entrance location). At approximately 150 ft true vertical depth, the secondary confirmation survey (TruTracker®) began to vary considerably from the downhole magnetic tool for depth measurements. During the remaining borehole, TruTracker® located the borehole up to 12 feet below the location measured by the downhole magnetic tool. The azimuth readings were in agreement between the two tools. Because of the discrepancy in borehole depth determined by the two methods, a gyro tool was pulled through the borehole for depth confirmation. The gyro tool indicated the horizontal section was between 232.8 and 234.8 ft BLS. This measurement was within the borehole specification that the horizontal section be between 232.5 and 237.5 ft BLS.

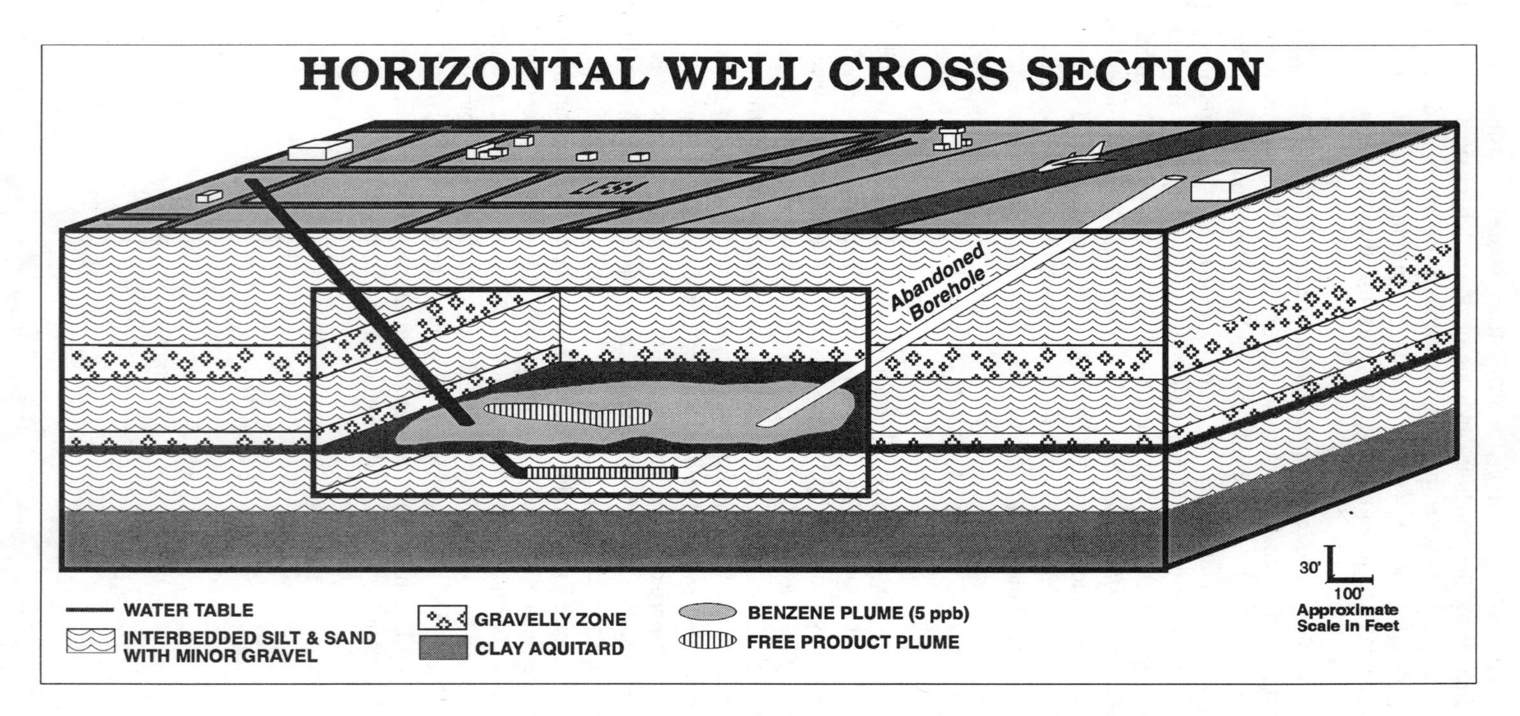

Figure 5.4. Horizontal Well Cross-Section.

The pilot hole was then enlarged by push reaming with a 16 in. diameter bit. During both pilot hole drilling and reaming, a quar-gum based drilling mud, Revert®, was used as the drilling fluid. Revert® was selected because after two to three days it naturally breaks down offering significant advantages over bentonite drilling fluids during well development. During drilling of the initial borehole, it was noted that less solids than expected were generated from the shale shaker and desander because Revert® has no gel strength. Therefore, it did not effectively carry out the sand and gravel from the deep borehole. Because the borehole integrity appeared to be good, installation of the well materials began after reaming.

The original installation method called for installing 870 ft of six inch diameter stainless steel riser followed by 500 ft of six inch diameter prepack stainless steel screen, followed by 1230 ft of six inch diameter high density polyethylene (HDPE) riser. This completion would have allowed two access points to the well. Two tremie pipes were pulled through with the casing so that additional sandpack could be placed around the prepack screen and the risers could be grouted in place. Backfilling would occur from each end of the borehole beginning at the middle of the 500 ft well screen. The well materials and tremie pipes would be attached to a special pulling head which swiveled. This allowed rotation of the drill string without rotating the well materials or tremie pipes.

Borehole reaming was completed on April 29, and 70 ft of casing/tremie pipe were pulled in at the exit hole. Installation of the remaining materials began the following day. Because the crew was welding on each piece of casing/screen and two tremie pipe lines, installation proceeded slowly but steadily until all of the riser, screen, and 620 ft of HDPE was installed. At this point, approximately 14 hours after installation began and 27 hours after reaming was completed, the well materials broke. The tremie pipes were still intact at this time. A second rig was mobilized to the site and set up at the exit hole location. Attempts were made to locate the break, these attempts were not successful. After working the string some more, the swivel assembly failed and all well materials were abandoned downhole.

Several factors could have contributed to the failure including:

- the Revert® drilling mud did not sufficiently clean sand and gravel from the borehole because Revert®, like all polymer muds, has no gel strength to keep sands and gravels in suspension. Therefore, borehole clogging problems occured at the curved section of the borehole in the gravel zone;
- the installation process, which required welding the casing and tremie pipes together, required too much time, and the borehole was left open too long after reaming and collapsed on the well materials;
- the outside diameter of the well materials went from 6 inch stainless steel riser to over 7 inches for the prepack screen, resulting in a funneling effect as the materials were pulled through the borehole with

eventual sediment buildup and sticking around the riser/screen connection;

- the tremie pipes got wrapped around the casing materials downhole, contributing to the sticking problem.

Based on these factors, the well installation was redesigned. A bentonite based drilling mud was chosen in order to maximize borehole stability and enhance solids removal from the borehole. A polymer additive, Mudup, would be used as much as possible in an effort to minimize downhole bentonite while maintaining gel strength. The well materials were changed to 11 inch diameter epoxy coated carbon steel and a custom-made prepack screen with six inch inside diameter and 10.75 in. outside diameter. This provided a 1.7 inch thick sand prepack, thereby eliminating the need for installing sandpack around the screen with tremie pipes. The larger diameter well materials also increased the tensile strength of the installation materials string. The exit hole riser was eliminated to help minimize installation time. Installation time would also be minimized by welding the well together and placing it on rollers prior to installation. This would allow a continuous pullback of the well materials, thereby eliminating the wait for welding during installation.

INSTALLATION ATTEMPT NUMBER 2

Drilling of the second installation attempt began on June 16, 1992. At 575 ft drilling length, the threads on the bottom hole assembly (BHA) stripped and the BHA was lost downhole. The assembly was successfully fished out in two days. The threads were remachined and the old borehole re-entered. The borehole was then drilled to 665 ft when a short occurred in the wireline to the downhole magnetic guidance system. The drill string was tripped out of the borehole and the short was repaired. The borehole was then drilled to 1008 ft, two joints into the horizontal section, before a gyro survey was run to confirm the borehole depth. The tool was pushed downhole inside the drill string with a router truck. After four attempts, the tool was successfully pushed to 680 ft for surveying. When the gyro tool was removed from the drill string, it had broken the wireline to the downhole magnetic guidance system. Attempts to move the drill string at this point were unsuccessful. The drill string apparently became differentially stuck. Differential sticking can occur when the hydrostatic head in the borehole is substantially higher than the hydrostatic head in the formation being drilled. The higher hydrostatic head in the borehole causes water in the drilling mud to be forced into the formation, causing the drill string to become stuck against the borehole wall. This effect is enhanced in curved boreholes like the one being installed at Williams AFB. The drill rig motor mounts were damaged in an attempt to free the drill string. A new rig was mobilized to the site.

We attempted to remove the drill string by using a jarring tool. The jarring tool was attached to the top of the drill string on the feed frame trailer. Acting similar to a rubber band, the jarring tool was pulled back until it released an instantaneous downward force on the drill string. Because our drill string was at a 20 degree angle to ground surface, the force was dampened. If the drill string had been at 90 degrees to ground surface, the entire weight of the drill string would be released downward. The jarring tool was operated for 3 hours before it failed.

An eight inch diameter overwash casing was then brought on site. The overwash casing was drilled over the drill string to a depth of 710 ft before it also became stuck. At this point the drill string was abandoned in place.

In order to prevent future sticking problems caused by letting the drill string sit in the borehole too long, we decided to drill the next attempt on a 24 hour per day schedule with two crews. The drill string would also be kept moving as much as possible in order to reduce the chances of its becoming differentially stuck.

INSTALLATION ATTEMPT NUMBER 3

Drilling of the third installation attempt began on July 6, 1993. After drilling 1411 ft, a short occurred in the wireline to the BHA. Eight drill rods (240 ft) were tripped out and the short was repaired. Drilling began again and another short occurred. After tripping out 12 more rods, the drill string became stuck. Spotting fluid (Pipe Lax Env®) designed to break down the mudcake was added to the borehole. Twenty 55-gal drums of spotting fluid were added to the borehole. An additional barrel was added on the hour for 8 hours. A jarring tool was placed at the top of the drill string and used during the second half of this operation. After nine hours of working the drill string, it finally broke free. All of the drill rod was tripped out of the borehole.

On July 11 the borehole was reentered. In order to further reduce the possibility of sticking, the drilling mud was thickened. After pushing the drill string 902 ft into the old hole, the TruTracker® indicated we were 34 ft right of the old borehole. The drill string was tripped out of the hole to 425 ft. At this point the driller was sure we were in the old hole. At 871 ft, the TruTracker® again indicated we were 30 ft right of the old borehole. At this point we decided there was magnetic interference causing miscalculations by TruTracker®. The TruTracker® data, which was secondary confirmation information, would be ignored. At 2015 ft, the wireline again shorted. We considered drilling out to the exit hole without the steering operating. Because of nearby buildings at the exit hole location, we decided to trip out and fix the short. There were some tight spots while tripping out, but the drill string never became stuck. The short in the wireline was fixed and the borehole re-entered. The pilot hole was then successfully completed to the exit location at a total drilling distance of 2624 ft. A 16 inch diameter reamer bit was added at the exit location and pulled back to the entrance location. Drill pipe was shuttled from the entrance to the exit location and attached to the drill string so a complete string remained in the borehole at all times. After completing the 16 inch diameter pull ream an 18 inch diameter pull ream was performed. Solids removed from the drilling mud during drilling and reaming were approximately five times those removed during attempt No. 1. This experience demonstrates the necessity of having a drilling fluid with gel strength for removing cuttings when drilling deeper installations.

Preparations were then made for the well installation. The well materials had been welded into one continuous run on rollers so they could be pulled into place with minimal delay. A 16 inch diameter reamer bit was followed by a swivel assembly followed by the well materials. The well materials were successfully pulled into place in 5 hours (Figure 5) considerably less time than the first installation attempt which required 14 hours to pull 2000 ft of well materials.

SUMMARY AND CONCLUSIONS

The longest, deepest environmental horizontal well has been installed at Williams AFB in Arizona. Through the three attempts required before successful installation, a wealth of information regarding environmental horizontal well installations has been accumulated. The primary lesson learned is that streamlining and simplifying the installation process should be a major focus of environmental horizontal well design. If sandpack around the well screen is required, prepack screen should be required in order to ensure an adequate sandpack around the screen and minimize the need for installing tremie pipes with the well materials. This procedure is especially important during the well materials installation phase of open hole completions. Minimizing the possibility of borehole collapse can also be achieved by performing 24 hour/day drilling operations—especially important on difficult installations such as long and deep boreholes in unconsolidated sediments.

Additionally, stabilizing and cleaning the borehole through the use of well suited drilling muds is essential to successful completion. For deep completions, quar-gum-based drilling mud does not have the gel strength to adequately carry sand and gravel to the surface. This situation can result in too many solids remaining in the borehole with potential clogging problems during the well materials installation phase.

Another lesson learned is that borehole location systems which locate the BHA through a surface magnetic system such as TruTracker® are unreliable below 150 ft BLS. The downhole magnetic guidance system offers reliable location information up to depths of 235 ft BLS. Therefore, if there is a discrepancy between the two systems, the downhole magnetic guidance system should be trusted.

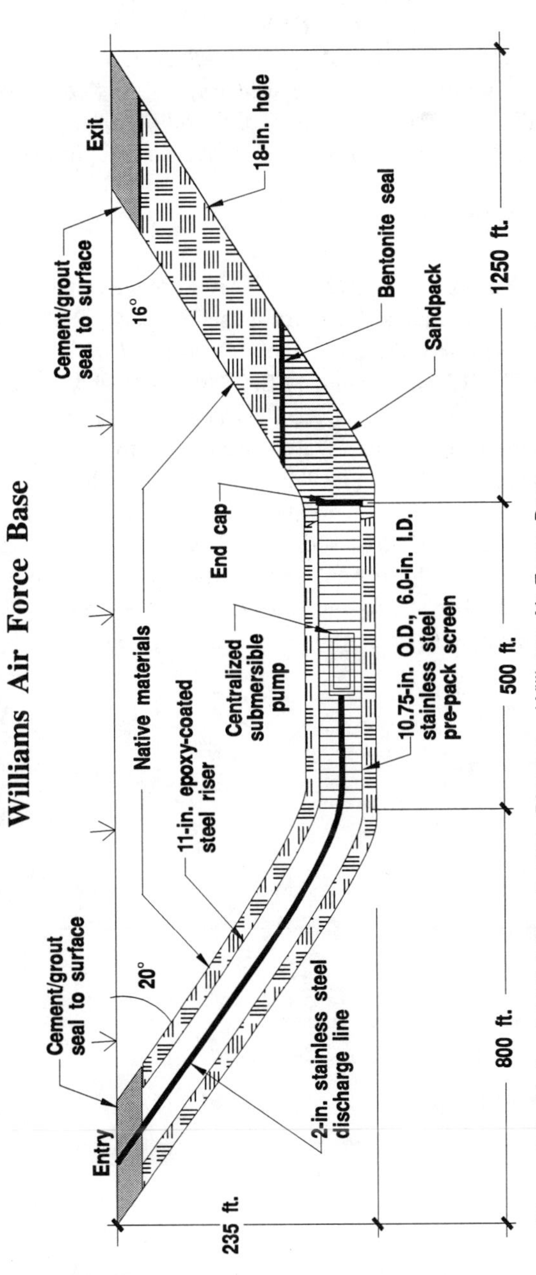

Figure 5.5. Horizontal Well Construction Diagram. *Williams Air Force Base.*

Because environmental horizontal well installations are a new application of existing technologies, there are important lessons learned from each installation. Sharing these lessons learned will advance this important new technology so that costs for future installations can be reduced. This, in turn, will lead to more economic applications of environmental horizontal well technology.

REFERENCES

1. IT Corporation 1992, U.S. Air Force Remedial Investigation/Feasibility Study, Williams Air Force Base, Arizona, Remedial Investigation Report, *Liquid Fuels Storage Area - Operable Unit 2, Vol. 1.*
2. Laney, R.L. and Hahn, M.E. 1986. *Hydrogeology of the Eastern Part of the Salt River Valley Area, Maricopa and Pinard Counties, Arizona*, U.S. Geological Survey, Water-Resources Investigation Report 86-4147.
3. Oakley, D.B. et al., 1992. "The Use of Horizontal Wells in Remediating and Containing a Jet Fuel Plume - Preliminary Findings," presented at Petroleum Hydrocarbons and Organic Chemicals in Ground Water: Prevention, Detection, and Restoration Conference, 1992.
4. CDM Federal Programs, 1993, *U.S. Air Force Demonstration Conceptual Design*, Williams Air Force Base, Arizona.

CHAPTER 6

Navy R&D Program For Site Restoration

William J. Powers, Ph.D, Naval Facilities Engineering Service Center (NFESC), Port Hueneme, California

INTRODUCTION

Unlike the Army and the Air Force, the Navy's Environmental Program is comprised of a network vice a single Center of Excellence. This network provides a major advantage in that it allows the needed expertise to reside close to the customer. Since customer requirements are constantly changing, this structure also allows for rapid contraction and expansion to meet these changing requirements. Therefore, the Navy operates through many non-overlapping organizations with specific missions coordinated at the Systems Command (SYSCOM) level. There are four major SYSCOMS. The Naval Facilities Engineering Command (NAVFAC) is the SYSCOM with cognizance over shore facilities and has major oversight of the Navy's approximately $300-400 million Environmental Program. This program is managed by the Director of Environment, Code 40, at NAVFAC Headquarters located in Alexandria, Virginia. The Naval Facilities Engineering Service Center (NFESC) is NAVFAC's center for technical expertise. NFESC was formed out of the need to consolidate numerous functions.

In March of 1993 the Base Realignment and Closure (BRAC) Committee recommended that the Naval Civil Engineering Laboratory (NCEL) be realigned.[1][2] This was necessary considering that the Navy of the future will be smaller and is already facing a decrease in resources. NAVFAC readily accepted this challenge and was established a new organization on October 1, 1993. This new organization is named the Naval Facilities Engineering Services Center and it consolidates the missions of five organizations into one which offers greater efficiencies through the sharing of expertise in related engineering fields and will further enhance the support provided to the engineering field divisions (EFDs) and naval activities worldwide.[4][5] The new right-sized organization is comprised of approximately 550 engineers, scientists and technical support staff with a budget of approximately $118 million. To date the basic organization and management structure is in place to fully implement the new organization. In addition, a project is underway to build a facility to house the west coast components at the Naval Construction Battalion Center (CBC). The east coast component will be located at the Chesapeake Division of NAVFAC located at the Washington Navy Yard in Washington, D.C. Until the new facility is built, most of the NFESC personnel will remain at their present locations.

ORGANIZATION

Since the Navy of the future will be smaller due to the new force structure projections, many Navy organizations have been restructuring at all levels to meet the decreased requirements.

A. Naval Facilities Engineering Command Headquarters (NAVFAC). NAVFAC Headquarters in Alexandria, Virginia, was recently reorganized by functional areas. The Environmental Director is now Code 40 which oversees the Installation Restoration Program. NAVFAC's mission is to serve as the Navy's expert for facilities, public works, Seabees and environment ashore. Their strategy is to be an environmental leader in all phases of their business and to be a proactive steward of the environment.

B. Engineering Field Divisions (EFDs). NAVFAC works through its five EFDs and two new field activities (FAs), Northwest and Midwest, to provide day to day operational installation restoration and BRAC site closure support to its bases. Figure 6.1, shows the location of NAVFAC Field Divisions and Activities (10). If you need additional information concerning NAVY fuel and hydrocarbon remediation efforts contact Mr. Ted Zagrobelny at NAVFAC Headquarters at (703)325-8175, Mr. Steve Eikenberry, NFESC at (805) 982-1347 or NAVFAC field representatives at:

Midwest Activity -
Mr. Mark Barnes,
Env. Proj. Mgr.
(708)688-4197

Southern Division -
Mr. James Malone
Installation Restoration
(803)743-0602

Northwest Activity
Mr. Patrick Visicek
Operations Div. Head
(206)396-5984

Northern Division -
Mr. Richard Fini
Env. Restoration Branch
(215)595-0567

Pacific Division -
Ms. Darlene Ige
Installation Restoration
(808)471-8410

Atlantic Division -
Ms. Nina Johnson
Installation Restoration
(804)445-6643

Chesapeake Division -
Mr. Frank Peters
Env. Restoration Branch
(202)433-3760

Southwest Division -
Mr. Jim Pawlisch
Env. Div. Dir.
(619)532-1396

Western Division -
Mr. Gerald Katz
Env. Prog. Dir.
(415)244-2501

Figure 6.1. NAVFAC Field Divisions and Activities.

C. Naval Facilities Engineering Service Center (NFESC). NFESC consolidates five major Navy commands including Ocean Engineering and Construction Project Office (FPO-1), Communications/Electronics Facilities Project Office (FPO-2), NAVFAC Chief Engineer Office (FAC-04B), Naval Civil Engineering Laboratory (NCEL), and the Naval Energy and Environmental Support Activity (NEESA) into one center.(6)(7) NFESC is comprised of five major technical departments including Shore Facilities, Ocean Facilities, Energy and Utilities, Amphibious and Expeditionary, and the Environmental Department. The mission of this organization is to "deliver quality, specialized technical products and services, RDT&E, consulting and field engineering in all five technical department areas of responsibility.(8)(9)

ENVIRONMENTAL PRODUCTS AND SERVICES

The Environmental Department located at NFESC Port Hueneme, California, has the capability to provide a full spectrum of research and development testing and evaluation (RDT&E) along with other needed products and services in the areas of air compliance, pollution prevention and installation restoration. This department has approximately 151 scientists and engineers and manages an operating budget of approximately $50 million a year.

A. Air Compliance. In the area of air compliance, responsibilities include managing the Hazardous Air Pollution (HAP) Program, Low Emission Vehicles (LEV) Program, Indoor Air Quality Program, Air Permit Program and hands-on compliance assistance for our customers in the field.

B. Pollution Prevention. Also in the Environmental Department is the Pollution Prevention Program which provides services including best management practices, industrial facilities modernization, hazardous waste minimization, technology transfer, hazardous materials reutilization, solid waste management and oil spill planning for Navy activities.

C. Installation Restoration. The Installation Restoration Program also resides within the Environmental Department. This program is comprised of about 55 scientists, engineers and technicians with a funding of approximately $20-25 million a year. This program provides Navywide support in the areas of quality assurance/quality control (QA/QC), training, remedial action contract (RAC) management, remedial investigations and feasibility studies (RI/FS), technology transfer, and preliminary assessment.

   i. Technology Demonstrations. Fifteen installation restoration technology development projects and demonstrations are currently underway Navywide. The following major installation restoration projects related to chlorinated compounds and fuels and hydrocarbons are summarized below:

a. Chlorinated Compounds. There are approximately 1,790 sites contaminated with chlorinated compounds. PCBs are a contaminant at approximately 900 sites or six percent of all Navy installation restoration (IR) sites. Therefore, NCEL is developing a process for onsite, cost-effective treatment for soils contaminated with PCB. The Base Catalyzed Decomposition Process (BCDP) was developed jointly by NFESC, Battelle Northwest, and the Environmental Protection Agency (EPA). It is being demonstrated at the Navy Public Works Center on Guam. If successful, this research effort will provide a low temperature process which uses an inexpensive nontoxic chemical to achieve decontamination for a fraction of the cost when compared to conventional methods.

b. Hydrocarbons. Petroleum oil and lubricants are contaminants at approximately 4,000 or 30% of Navy IR sites. Therefore, NFESC has seven research projects which address various aspects concerning soil/hydrocarbons remediation. At Naval Air Station (NAS) Lemoore, California, *in-situ* steam injection vacuum extraction (SIVE) technology is being demonstrated for removal of JP-5 in an arid soil matrix. JP-5 is a Navy unique fuel which has lower volatility than other jet fuels and possesses special remediation problems.

In-situ bioventing is being demonstrated at NAS Fallon, Nevada. This project is designed to develop the process further and to obtain detailed cost effectiveness data for using low-level soil venting to promote aerobic biodegradation of low volatility fuels including JP-5. It will also be demonstrated for other Navy fuels such as marine diesel and bunker fuel in subsurface soils.

Many Navy sites require groundwater remediation where fuel contamination has occurred such is the case at CBC Port Hueneme, California, where NFESC is demonstrating underground fuel pump and treat technologies. This system uses existing wells in conjunction with a granular activated carbon (GAC) vapor extraction system and a gasoline generator. An enclosed spray aeration system at the site is being evaluated for performance and ability to remove BTEX and TPH from the groundwater. This system is designed for interim corrective actions at the site and is expected to reduce cleanup time by 50%. Anaerobic degradation a more innovative technology is being demonstrated at the Naval Weapons Stations, Seal Beach, CA for remediating a gasoline spill. This demonstration is being performed by NFESC and the Orange County Water Board. The objective of this demonstration is to investigate *in-situ* anaerobic degradation of gasoline hydrocarbons by use of indigenous microorganisms. As far as is known this is only one of four on-site anaerobic degradation study in the nation. If adequately demonstrated this technology will have numerous applications within DOD and the private sector. Information generated from this limited study will be used in the design of a full-scale anaerobic biodegradation treatment system.

The Navy has hundreds of miles of piping systems that carry a variety of fuels. NFESC is working on developing leak detection systems for high capacity fuel lines; utilizing a vadose zone fuel detection technology for leaks in these systems. These early warning systems will enable quick response and will minimize environmental damage and cleanup costs.

The Navy has some of the world's largest bulk fuel storage tanks. These large tanks are located at the Red Hill underground storage tank facilities on Oahu. This facility consists of a bank of 20 bulk tanks each containing 12 and one half million gallons of fuel. The Red Hill facility supports the fleet and industrial complex at Pearl Harbor. The tanks were field constructed during the 1940s. This tank farm was originally designed to stop up to one years supply of fuel for the entire Pacific sheet. Each tank is approximately 250 feet deep and 100 feet wide and are linked by an underground tunnel cut out of the surrounding lava rock. This project is designed to develop and demonstrate an improved system for level measurement and hydrostatic measurement for accurately inventorying fuel stored in these large bulk tanks.

In an effort to expedite the commercialization of new environmental restoration technologies for remediating soil contaminated with hydrocarbons the Department of Defense and the Navy opened a 3.8 acre site for demonstrating efficient cleanup technologies. The site is located at Port Hoeneme, CA and will be managed by NFESC in cooperation with the CBC Environmental Department. At this site engineers will initially conduct a demonstration of *ex-situ* bioremediation technologies similar to a Heap Pile Bioreactor for remediating fuels using soil removed from a tank farm. In the future *in-situ* technologies will also be demonstrated. The National Test site can also be used by private companies to test, evaluate and demonstrate new remediation technologies. The Navy in conjunction with state and federal regulators will be using the data generated at the National Test Site to develop procedures to certify hydrocarbon remediation technologies for use at similar sites across the country.

The Navy, like industry, has the difficult and costly task of remediating and cleaning up its past disposal sites. Many past methods of disposal are no longer allowed by federal and state regulations and many alternatives which in the past were standard practice have proven to be extremely costly both environmentally and economically. Realizing this, the Navy intends to continue to provide research, development and demonstration of new alternatives that can provide less costly and more environmentally acceptable solutions.

IV. REFERENCES

1. News Release, SECDEF Public Affairs Office, March 12, 1993.
2. 1993 List of Military Installations Inside the United States for Closure and Realignment, March 12, 1993.
3. News Release, Naval Civil Engineering Laboratory, Public Affairs Office, March 12, 1993.
4. Naval Facilities Engineering Command, Products and Services Transition Team Briefing, May 26, 1993.
5. Naval Facilities Engineering Center Analysis of Production Organization Structure, Products and Services Transition Team, March 30, 1993.
6. Naval Energy and Environmental Support Activity, Organization Chart, April 30, 1993.
7. Naval Civil Engineering Laboratory Staffing Chart, June 1993.
8. NAVFAC Points of Contact, Environmental Technology Exchange, 1993.
9. Naval Facilities Engineering Service Center, Command Briefing, July 1993.
10. Navy Environmental Technology Xchange.

PART II

ANALYSIS

CHAPTER 7

Detecting Hydrocarbons in Contaminated Soil Using a Fiber Optic Chemical Sensor Based on Fluorescence Modification

Richard P. de Filippi, Ariano Technologies, Inc., Charlestown, MA

REAL TIME MONITORING OF HYDROCARBON CONTAMINANTS IN THE ENVIRONMENT

On Site Real Time Monitoring Needs

Monitoring of contaminated soil and groundwater is required during site assessment, remediation, and post-closure. During a site assessment, the chemical constituents are identified and their concentrations are usually determined by sampling and laboratory analysis. Sophisticated instruments such as GC-MS are used for many organics, including volatile hydrocarbons. Once the chemical species have been identified, however, simpler sensors which are specific for certain constituents or classes of constituents could be used, not only to complete the mapping of contamination during assessment, but to track the progress of remediation and to monitor the site post-closure as well.

Particularly for long term monitoring, on-site sensors can be of great benefit. Off site analyses are expensive, and are often a major cost in a remediation project. Off site analyses cannot be real time, and thus there is a time lag between the sampling event and the analytical result, sometimes making control of the remediation process problematic. Such time lags also cause delays in warning of the appearance of post-closure contamination. Also, off site analyses mean that representative samples must be taken and preserved. In the case of certain analytes, such as volatile organics, representative samples are very difficult to produce and maintain.[1] Because of these drawbacks of off site analyses, on site real time analyses are preferred, even with some sacrifice in specificity or sensitivity. This chapter describes an instrument employing a fiber optic chemical sensor for on site real time analysis of volatile hydrocarbons.

Hydrocarbons Among the Most Common Environmental Contaminants

Chemical contaminants in soil and groundwater at industrial and government sites are quite varied, including a wide range of fuels, solvents, metals, and radioactive materials. In an early study of the Superfund program, EPA reported the most common chemicals found at contaminated sites.[2] High on the list of contaminants present at National Priority List (NPL) Superfund sites are the volatile aromatic constituents of petroleum products (BTEX): toluene at 28% of NPL sites; benzene, 26%; ethylbenzene, 13%; and xylene, 13%. In addition, both Federal and state regulations now mandate a scheduled installation of monitoring systems for underground storage tanks, and above ground tank regulations are being developed; most of these tanks contain hydrocarbon products. Therefore, it is clear that monitoring for hydrocarbons represents one of the largest environmental needs in industry today.

Currently Available Methods

There are several sensors currently in use or under development which are designed to detect volatile hydrocarbons. These include:

1. Metal oxide sensors,[3,4] intended for detection of volatile liquid hydrocarbons, also respond to other oxidizable species such as methane and carbon monoxide. In addition, they are subject to interferences from water vapor. They are not reported to operate in the liquid phase, either water or hydrocarbon.
2. Adsistors[3,4] are based on changes in electrical resistance of a composite material as it sorbs hydrocarbons from the surrounding vapor phase. While the sensor is effective at low concentrations, at higher concentrations it can experience irreversible adsorption such that it will not recover sensitivity after the concentration is reduced. The sensor is not reported to operate in liquid water or hydrocarbon.
3. A developmental side coated fiber optic sensor[5] responds to changes in the index of refraction of the optical fiber cladding when exposed to hydrocarbon vapors. Optical effects cause it to respond very differently under water, although adjustments by calibration changes are reported. No data are reported for hydrocarbon liquids.
4. Commercial liquid hydrocarbon sensors use a conductive polymeric strip which swells and increases resistance with liquid contact. They are not designed for detection of vapor.

Therefore, at present, there appear to be no fieldable (on site) volatile hydrocarbon sensors that can operate in soil vapor, in groundwater, and in contact with liquid phase organics.

Walt[6] at Tufts University developed a technology using fluorescent reagents for detecting volatile hydrocarbons, with an optical fiber serving simply as a light pipe. Ariano Technologies, Inc. licensed this technology from Tufts, and developed a sensor which is now in field testing. The sensor can detect volatile hydrocarbons in soil vapor, in water, and when in contact with organic liquid product. It therefore appears to show promise as a versatile sensor for on site use both at remediation sites and for storage tank monitoring. The basic technology behind the sensor as well as performance data are presented in this chapter.

TECHNICAL APPROACH

General Characteristics of Fiber Optic Chemical Sensors

Fiber optic chemical sensors utilize a transparent thin fiber to transmit a light signal from a source at the near (proximal) end, to a set of chemical reagents bonded to the fiber tip at the far (distal) end. The chemical reagents react in some way with the analyte to cause a change in the light signal. That changed signal is transmitted back up the fiber to a detector, which usually converts the signal to an electrical output. The electrical signal, often after further processing, can be read by an analog or digital monitor, sound an alarm, or produce a desired control response. These so called "intrinsic" sensors carry their own chemical reagents to produce the required signal. "Extrinsic" fiber optic sensors primarily use the optical fiber as a light pipe to bring spectral characteristics (of the analyte present at the distal end) back up to the detecting instrument.

The proximal end of the fiber is usually connected to an electro-optical instrument which provides the source of the activating light signal, and also contains components to separate and convert the light signal returning from the sensor. In on site field instruments, the distal end of the fiber is fixed at the sensing point, remote from the instrument. If desired, that location can be 100 meters or more from the instrument, depending on the acceptable degree of signal attenuation per unit fiber length.

Optical sensing instruments of this kind employ elements of advanced technologies that are now well established in the communications industries, such as in telephone signal transmission. A consequence of this is the availability of equipment components with high reliability and low cost, and it has been a major factor in accelerating development of fiber optic chemical sensors.

Solvent Polarity Effects and Their Use in Fluorescence Based Sensors

In intrinsic fluorescent sensors, the input light signal excites a fluorescent response from chemical reagents placed at the distal end of the fiber. A major advantage is that fluorescence is emitted at wavelengths higher than the input signal. Because of this effect, the signal can be filtered from interferences which may be caused by reflection and return of the input signal.

When a fluorescent material is placed in chemical environments with different polarities, significant changes in the fluorescence spectrum can occur.[7] Portions of the spectrum are shifted, and/or relative intensities at different points on the spectrum change. The magnitude and type of change depends on whether the chemical environment surrounding the fluorescent species is made more or less polar.

This polarity effect of the chemical environment around fluorescent dyes forms the basis for the volatile hydrocarbon sensor technology developed by Walt. In its simplest form, it uses fluorescent dyes in a solid solution fixed to the distal end of an optical fiber. In the absence of the hydrocarbon analyte, the dyes emit a base fluorescent spectrum. When the solution absorbs hydrocarbon, the fluorescence spectrum shifts, and the magnitude of the shift is related to the amount of non polar (hydrocarbon) material present.

The sensor design is illustrated in Figure 7.1. What is shown is the end of an optical fiber coated with the fluorescent reagents. Excitation light from a source of a specified wavelength travels the length of the fiber. It stimulates fluorescence from the reagents, the nature of which is a function of the hydrocarbon concentration surrounding the sensor tip. The emitted fluorescence returns back down the fiber and is read as a quantitative indicating signal.

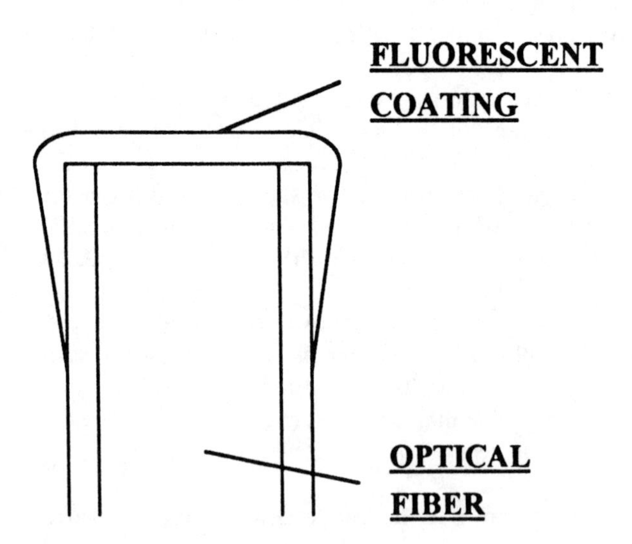

Figure 7.1. Fiber optic chemical sensor (end-coated)

The electro-optical instrumentation needed for the sensor is shown in Figure 7.2. The excitation light source can be either broad spectrum or monochromatic, depending on the availability of sources with adequate power. The source light is typically collimated and filtered to the optimum wavelength, passed through a beam splitter and refocused on the sensor fiber. The returning fluorescent light from the sensor is reflected from the beam splitter to a detector such as a photodiode, which converts the light intensity to an analog signal. That signal is sent to an analog/digital converter, and processed via a microprocessor chip to give a vapor concentration for readout, files, and potential alarm.

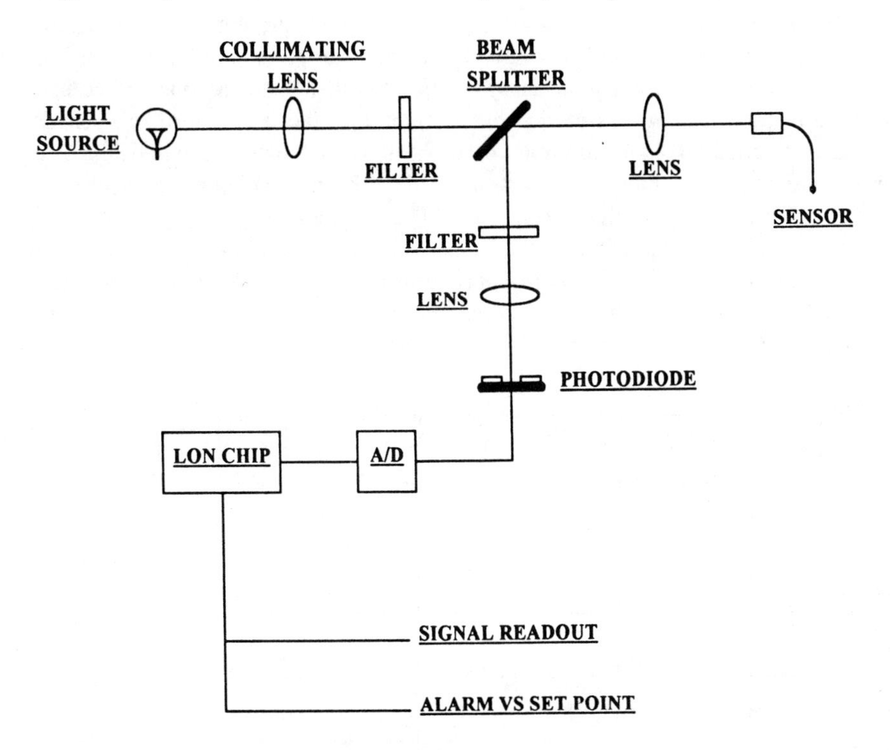

Figure 7.2. Fiber optic Sensor Fluorimeter Block Diagram

This instrument was used in the studies described below, except that the analog signal was read directly without further conversion.

PERFORMANCE OF THE SENSOR

The initial goal in developing a sensor and instrument product from this technology has been to meet the need for detection of:

- vadose zone contamination by leakage from underground or above ground storage tanks;
- vapor or liquid spills or leakage into sumps at fuel marketing and transfer locations;
- contaminants dissolved in or floating on water.

Specific sensor and instrument objectives include: accuracy and reversibility over the entire range from zero to 100% saturation concentration; minimal interferences from temperature and humidity; and long life for remote operation.

Response to Pure-Component Hydrocarbons

Benzene, toluene, and xylenes (BTX) are present at significant concentrations in gasoline. They have toxic characteristics, and are reported to be resistant to natural biological decay relative to other hydrocarbons [8]. Because of these factors, testing was carried out to determine the response of this sensor to the full range of concentrations of each of these volatile aromatics. The results are given in Figures 7.3, 7.4, and 7.5. The data are plotted as percent signal increase over base fluorescent signal (i.e., in the absence of hydrocarbon), as a function of percent of saturation concentration. Measurements were made in the vapor phase. The sensor response to each of these aromatics is similar: about a 25% increase in the base fluorescent signal for a concentration of about 50% of saturation.

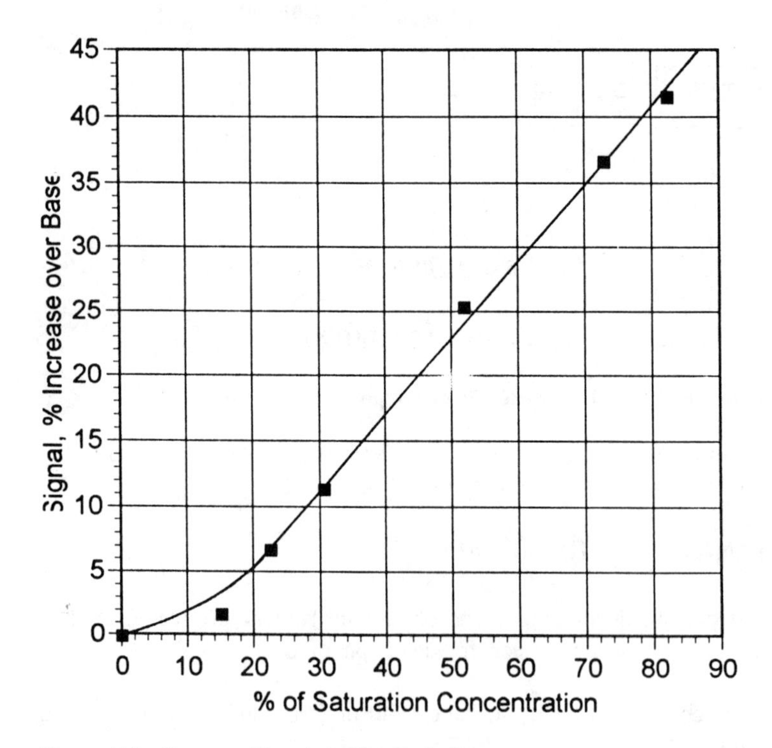

Figure 7.3. Benzene Signal vs. Concentration.

Isopentane (2-methylbutane) is one of the most volatile liquid-phase constituents of gasoline, and as a paraffinic compound, chemically different from the aromatics. Sensor response for isopentane is shown in Figure 7.6. The relative signal for the same saturation level is about an order of magnitude lower than for aromatics, probably due to a weaker solvent effect in this portion of the fluorescent spectrum. It may be possible to distinguish aromatic from paraffinic hydrocarbons using two different excitation or fluorescent wavelengths. This might be used also to discern new contamination, characterized by the presence of highly volatile paraffinic components of gasoline, from older contamination dominated by the more stable aromatics.

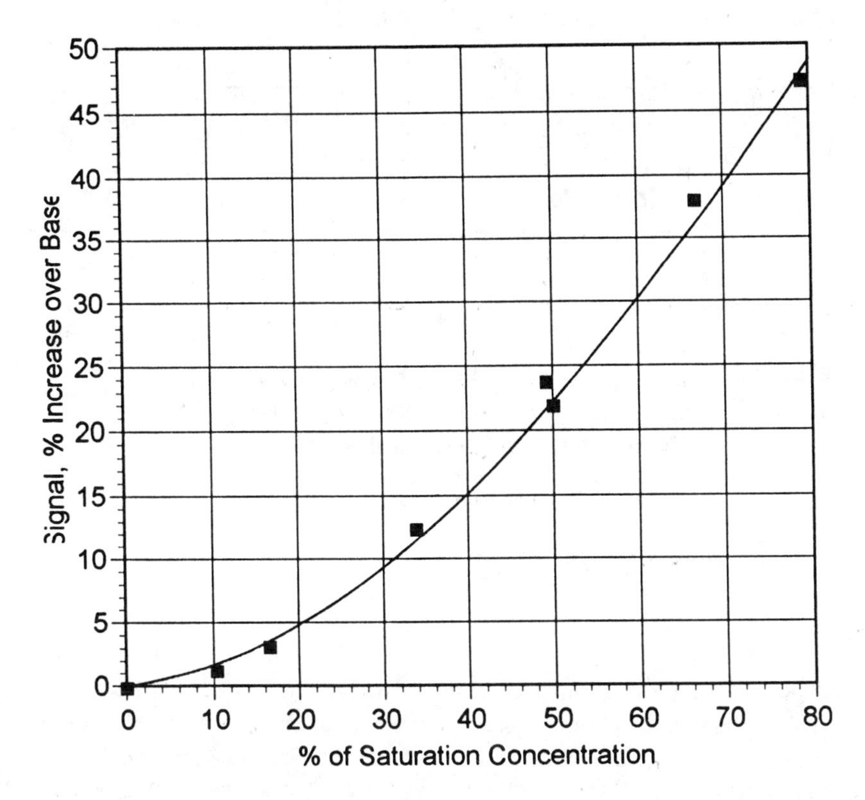

Figure 7.4. Toluene Signal vs. Concentration.

Response to Hydrocarbon Fuels

Similar vapor phase tests were run using common petroleum fuels: gasoline (regular unleaded); kerosene (as a surrogate for jet fuel); and diesel fuel. The results are shown in Figure 7.7.

The magnitude of the signals for all fuels is less than those for pure aromatics, on the order of about one quarter to one third for gasoline and kerosene. This may reflect the fact that both fuels are only partially aromatic in character. The signal level for diesel is still less, but readable even at fairly low levels. It is of interest to note that the effect of fuel volatility is not major: the response for diesel fuel is significantly greater than that calculated from gasoline by volatility ratio alone.

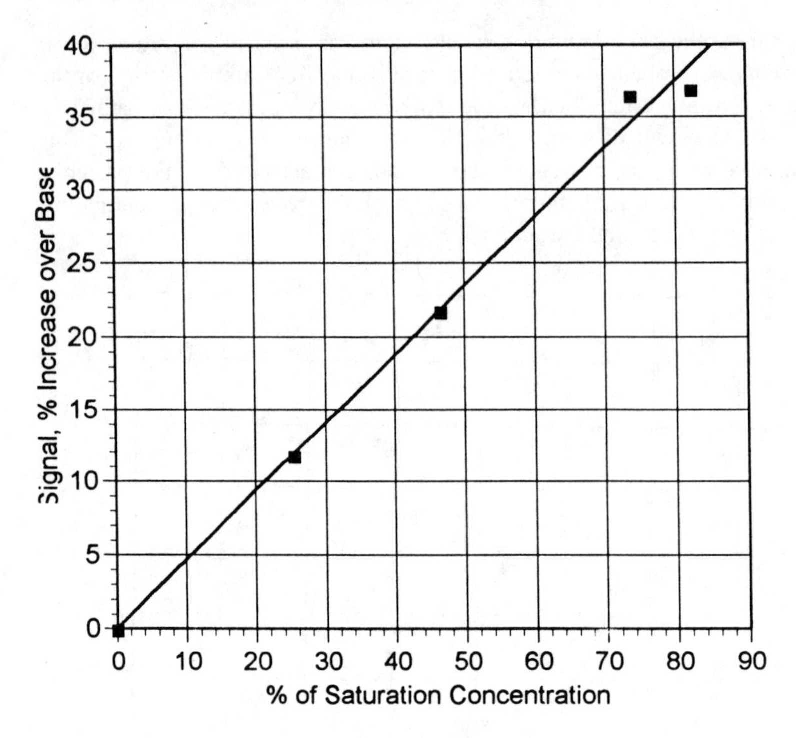

Figure 7.5. P-Xylene Signal vs. Concentration.

Response to Environmental Factors

Temperature

When used as a long term in-dwelling monitor, the sensor will be placed down well either in the vapor space above the groundwater level, below groundwater level (probably close to the surface), or floating at the surface to determine if floating product is present. Where the sensor is in contact with groundwater, temperature changes during a daily cycle should be small. Depending on the local climate, temperature changes of 10°C or more could be expected through an annual cycle. Greater fluctuation in temperature could occur in the vapor space, where changes in atmospheric pressure can bring about displacement of the well vapor volume due to incoming or outgoing flow.

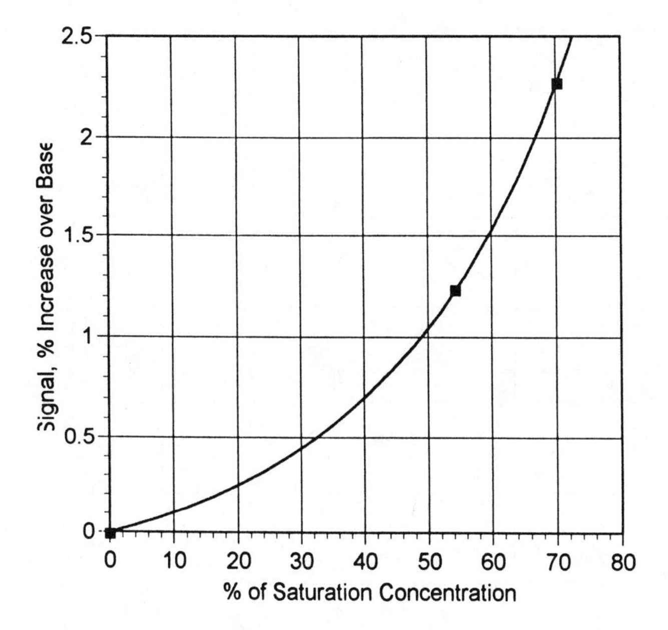

Figure 7.6. Isopentane Signal vs. Concentration.

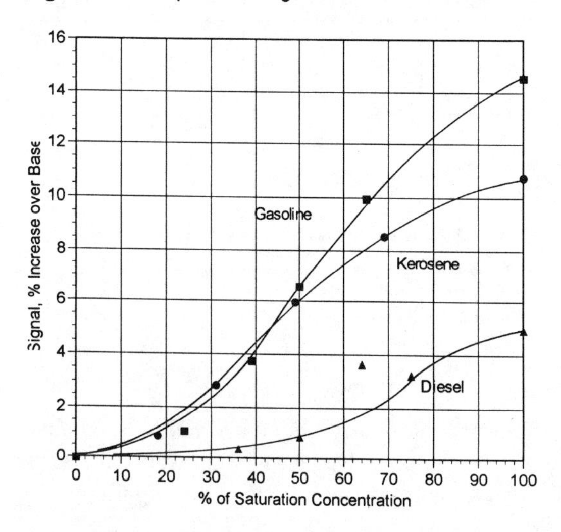

Figure 7.7. Petroleum Fuels Signal vs. Concentration.

Figure 7.8 shows the change in baseline (zero concentration) signal as a function of temperature at zero humidity. These data show that a temperature increase of 10°C causes a signal decrease of about 3.5%. At low hydrocarbon concentrations, or for heavier fuels, this would be a substantial offset, and would require an adjustment. Because of this, a temperature adjustment to the calibration curve is being made.

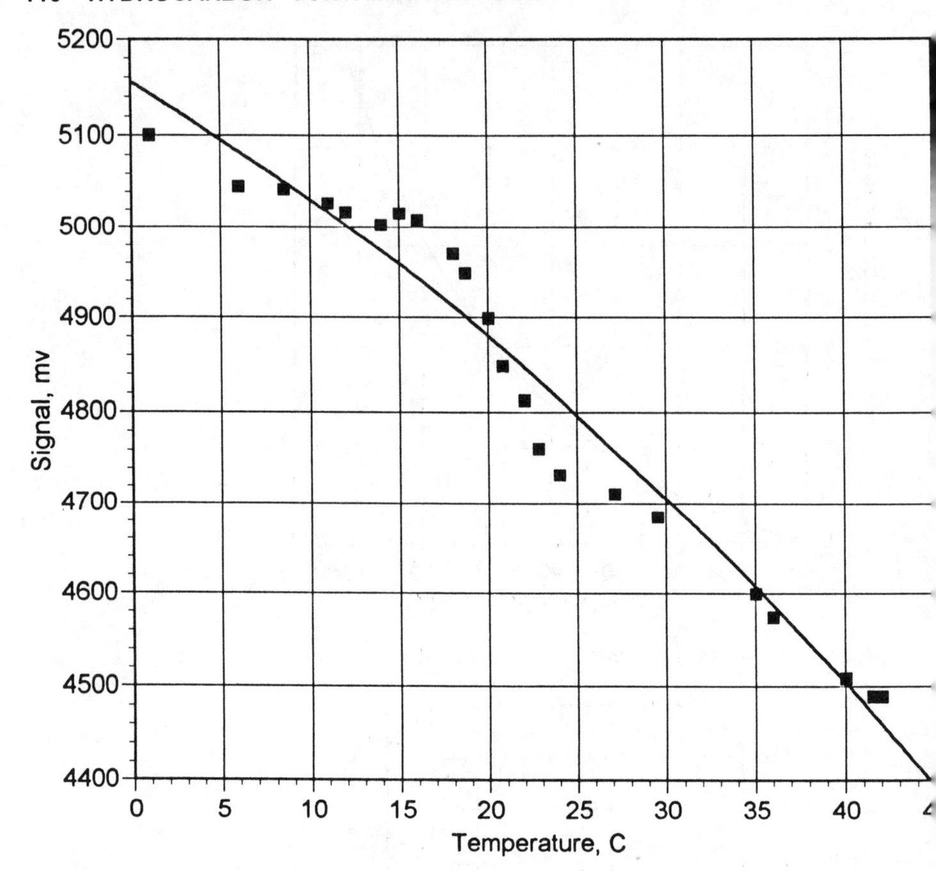

Figure 7.8. Temperature Effect on Signal at Zero Humidity.

Stability and Longevity

Humidity

In most monitoring circumstances, the relative humidity below a depth of twelve inches is essentially 100%.[9] Air volume displacement in wells caused by changes in atmospheric pressure would alter this temporarily, but high humidity may be restored reasonably quickly.

The effect of humidity on the sensor baseline signal is shown in Figure 7.9. Decreasing relative humidity from 100% to 90% causes an increase in baseline signal of about 1%. This is sensitive enough to require an adjustment when the sensor is used in the vapor phase. When in contact with groundwater, humidity changes would not be an issue.

The importance of a temperature adjustment is emphasized by these responses to humidity, which are chemical polarity effects of absolute water vapor concentration. Temperature adjustments must account for both the zero humidity influence of temperature change and the effect of temperature on water vapor concentration in the air (absolute humidity).

Methane

Methane gas is a product of anaerobic biodegradation of organic matter, and therefore can be present in soils at almost any location. Concentrations of course vary significantly; however, it is expected that levels will rarely exceed 5% by volume.[10] When tested at these levels, the sensor response was small, so the methane concentration was increased to the range of 15-20%. The results, from testing two different sensors, are shown in Figure 7.10.

At 5% methane content by volume, the signal change is about 0.4%, which would represent an interference only at very low concentrations of hydrocarbon fuels. In the concentration range of 0-1% by volume, the methane effect on the sensor signal would be unimportant.

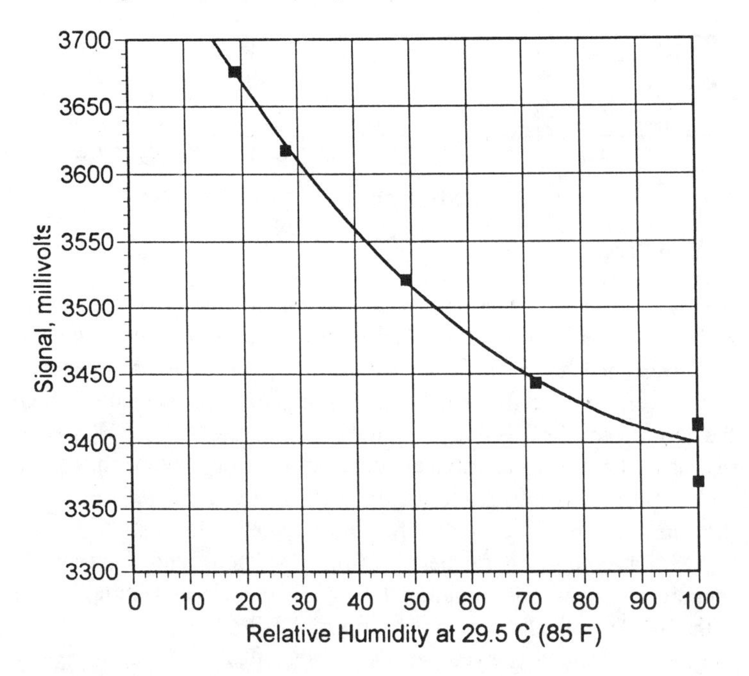

Figure 7.9. Humidity Effect on Sensor Signal.

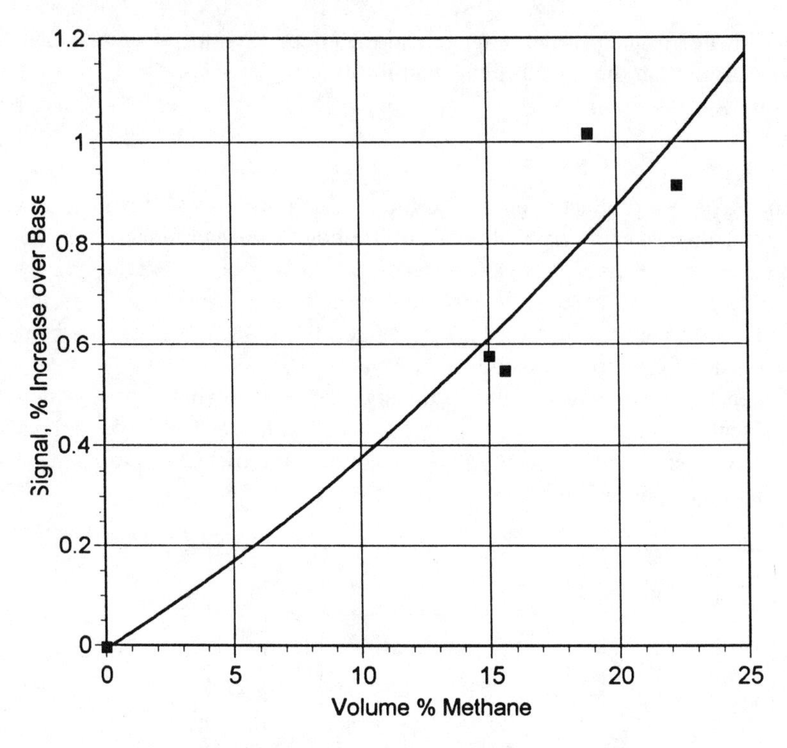

Figure 7.10. Methane Effect on Sensor.

It was reported earlier[11] that a decrease in signal intensity of this sensor was experienced over a time period equivalent to several months of use, and the mechanism was presumed to be photobleaching of the fluorescent reagents. Additional development has been carried out, leading to improvements which have eliminated any detectable decline in signal.

When used as a monitoring instrument, the sensor will be battery-operated, often placed in locations that are remote and/or difficult to access. To preserve battery life, the current design provides for intermittent illumination by the excitation light, with a monitoring frequency of once per hour, and a duty cycle averaging 2 minutes per day (illumination 0.14% of the elapsed time). It is estimated that this cycle will allow a battery life of 1.5-2 years.

A test program is planned to cycle sensors systematically through this and other duty cycles. To date, several sensors have been operated intermittently in irregular cycles, and have provided preliminary data on longevity and stability of the signal:

1. A sensor was operated in the laboratory for a total of 15.1 hours intermittently over 142 days (0.44%), most of the exposure to light taking place in a hydrocarbon vapor atmosphere. There was no measurable decline in signal. Tests are continuing.

2. A second sensor was also run in the laboratory for a total of 12.4 hours over 55 days (0.95%), exposed to vapor, with no decline in signal.
3. A third sensor has been in place for three months to date in a monitoring well in the vadose zone. No hydrocarbon contamination has been found. The sensor has had only spot checks (a total of about 3 minutes' exposure to light), and there has been no decline in signal.
4. A fourth sensor has been placed under the groundwater level in a monitoring well (about ten feet below surface). No decline in signal has been seen after one month, and there is no sign of obstructive biological growth on the sensor.

If the limiting factor on life is sensor illumination time due to photobleaching, the laboratory tests show that greater than one year can be achieved (equivalent exposure of 1.2 years for the first sensor, and 1.0 years for the second). These and other tests are continuing to verify the design goals.

CONCLUSIONS AND ONGOING WORK

The results of these studies have led to the following conclusions:

1. The sensor responds stably and reversibly to concentration levels over the entire range of hydrocarbon vapor concentrations (to saturation levels).
2. Sensitivity is better than 1% of saturated-vapor concentration for benzene, toluene, and xylene (BTX) vapors, equivalent to the order of magnitude of one hundred parts per million, vapor volume concentration, or less. Sensitivity to petroleum fuels is about one half to one third that for BTX, depending on the specific fuel: sensitivity to diesel is less than that to gasoline.
3. Humidity and temperature have small and adjustable effects on the sensor response.
4. The effect of methane on the sensor signal is negligible.
5. The sensor operates under water. Related test data are not presented here, but they show that the same response as vapor is achieved, when expressed as percent of saturation concentration (water solubility in this case). This is equivalent to a sensitivity on the order of 10 ppm by weight for many hydrocarbons in water solution.

Field testing of these sensors is currently underway at locations in the Boston area, to verify performance data and help determine stability under real weathering conditions. Most of these sites are owned by Massport, the Authority which operates Boston's Logan Airport as well as several commercial ship and truck transport terminals. Specific sites include vapor and groundwater wells, at locations were there is potential for contamination from gasoline, jet, and diesel fuel, as well as heating oil. Related sensors were used at Pease Air Force

Base in New Hampshire,[6] and provided data that correlated with samples measured with a photo-ionization detector.

Commercialization of this sensor/instrument system is being pursued by Ariano Technologies, Inc..

REFERENCES

1. Spittler, T. M., *Field Instrumentation Uses and Needs of U.S. EPA,* presented at the Symposium on Field Screening for Environmental Pollutants, Massachusetts Institute of Technology, Cambridge, MA, October 26, 1992.
2. Devitt, Dale A., et al, *Soil Gas Sensing for Detection and Mapping of Volatile Organics*, National Water Well Assn., Dublin, OH, 1987, 3.
3. M. A. Portnoff, R. Grace, A. M. Guzman, and J. Hibner, *Measurement and Analysis of Adsistor and Figaro Gas Sensors Used for Underground Storage Tank Leak Detection*, presented at the American Institute of Chemical Engineers 1991 Summer National Meeting, Pittsburgh, PA, August 18-21, 1991.
4. G. B. Wickramanayake, R. E. Hinchee, J. A. Kittel, N. G. Reichenbach, and B. J. Nielsen, *Evaluation of External Vapor Monitoring Devices for Underground Petroleum Products Storage Tanks*, Hazardous Materials Control, Sept/Oct 1991, P. 32-40.
5. Klainer, S. M., et al, *Proceedings of the Symposium on Field Screening Methods for Hazardous Waste Site Investigations*, October, 1988, Las Vegas, P. 25.
6. Barnard, S. M., Walt, D. R., Environ. Sci. Technol. 1991, 25, 1301-1304.
7. Lakowicz, J. R., *Principles of Fluorescence Spectroscopy*, Plenum Press, New York, 1983, P. 189-208.
8. Devitt, Dale A., et al, op.cit., P. 75.
9. Devitt, Dale A., et al, op.cit., P. 64.
10. Prof. Gary Robbins, University of Connecticut, Storrs, CT; personal communication.
11. de Filippi, R. P., and Cody, T. J., *A Monitoring System for Hydrocarbon Leakage from Petroleum and Petrochemical Products Sites*, Presented at the Third International Symposium on Field Screening Methods for Hazardous Wastes and Toxic Chemicals, Feb. 26, 1993, Las Vegas, Nevada.

CHAPTER 8

Bias Associated With the Use of EPA Method 418.1 For the Determination of Total Petroleum Hydrocarbons in Soil

Scott George, PG, CHMM, Environmental Science & Engineering, Inc., St. Louis, MO

INTRODUCTION

EPA Method 418.1, originally intended solely for use with liquid waste, has been one of the most widely used methods for the determination of total petroleum hydrocarbons (TPH) in soils. At last count, approximately 19 states use or permit the use of Method 418.1 for the determination of "action" or cleanup levels for petroleum contaminated soils.[1] In some cases, Method 418.1 is the sole criteria for verification of site cleanup. Method 418.1 has been "modified" for determining TPH concentrations in soil between states or laboratories with no consistency to the modifications. The EPA had proposed draft Method 9073, which was expanded to include soils, that specified Soxhlet extraction for solid samples and suggested the use of the petroleum product in question as a standard. EPA has withdrawn this method. Draft Method 9073 clearly stated that the method is not applicable for the measurement of gasoline range organics.

Several areas of concern are associated with the use of Method 418.1, as it is commonly used. The concerns can be broken into two principle areas: (1) inherent inaccuracies in the method (i.e., positive and negative biases); and (2) the high degree of interlaboratory variance in standard operating procedures. Although Method 418.1 can still be useful in some site assessments, great care must be taken in the selection of the extraction and cleanup procedures and in the interpretation of the analytical results. All analytical procedures have a degree of variance and problems associated with interpretation of results. Method 418.1, however, has a greater degree of variance among laboratories and more uncertainty in interpretation than most analytical procedures.

This chapter presents some of the problems associated with Method 418.1 and briefly describes the reasons for the use of the newer gas chromatographic (GC) methods for TPH determination in soil. As part of this study, the Method 418.1 standard operating procedures (SOPs) from five laboratories in two states were reviewed. A limited study of analyses of split samples was performed among three laboratories to determine if natural organics or industrial waste products could cause positive biases in Method 418.1. Results obtained from other studies of Method 418.1 are also presented.

PETROLEUM CHEMISTRY

Petroleum products consist of complex mixtures of organic compounds. The individual constituents cover a broad range of boiling points, carbon numbers, chemical families, and structural isomers. The typical petroleum fractions, carbon ranges, and distillation temperatures are presented in Table 8.1 and Figure 8.1.[2,3] The hydrocarbon groups present in petroleum products include: alkanes, alkenes, alkynes, aromatics, polynuclear aromatics, and complex hydrocarbon compounds containing oxygen, nitrogen, and sulfur. Petroleum products also contain trace amounts of elements such as bromine, cadmium, nickel, and vanadium. The hydrocarbon groups present in petroleum products are presented in Figure 8.2.

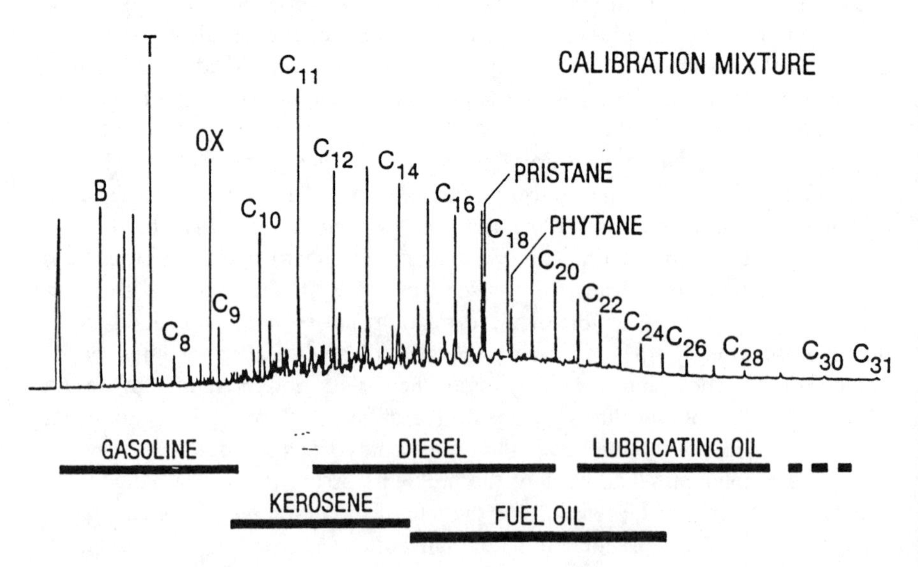

Figure 8.1. Approximate carbon number ranges for individual hydrocarbon products[3].

8293511OMISC

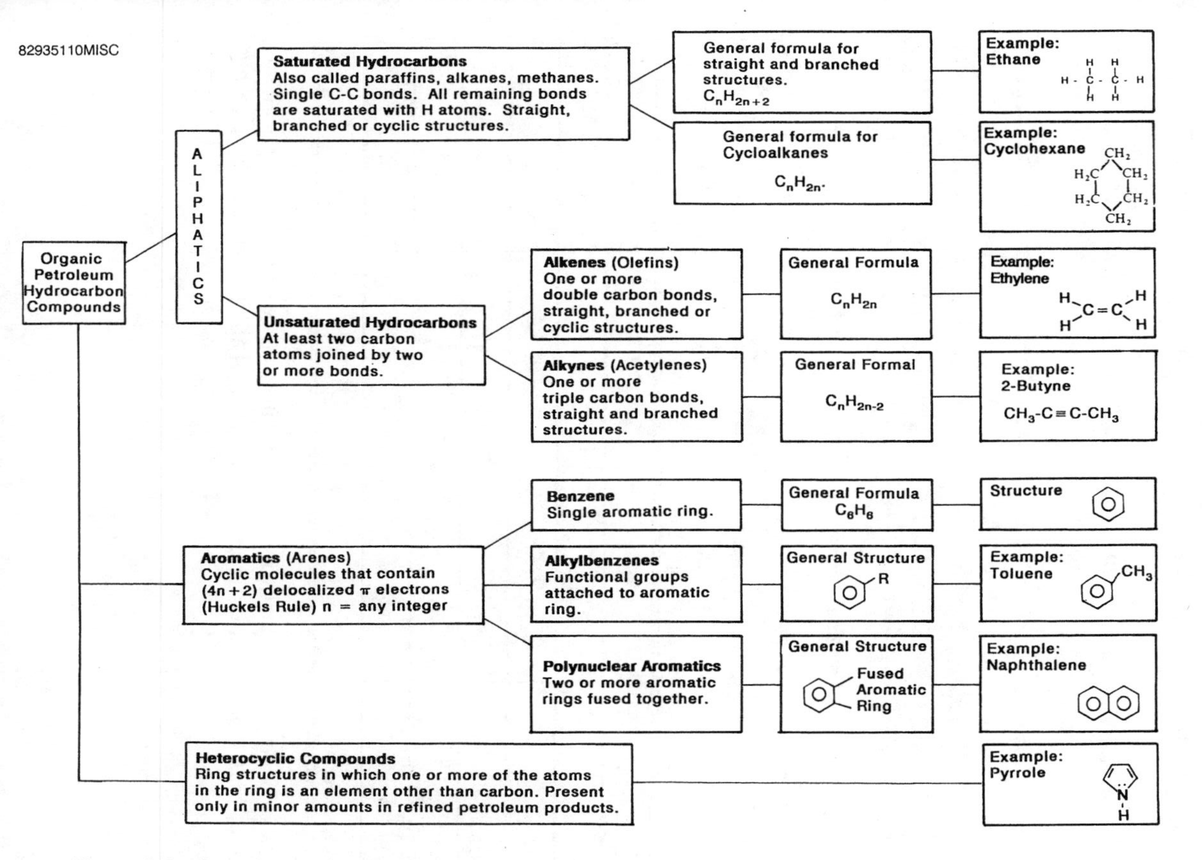

Figure 8.2. Organic petroleum hydrocarbon compounds.

Table 8.1. Petroleum Distillation Products[2]

Fraction	Distillation Temperature, °C	Carbon Number
Gas	Below 20	C-1 to C-4
Petroleum Ether	20 to 60	C-5 to C-6
Ligroin (light naphtha)	60 to 100	C-6 and C-7
Natural Gasoline	40 to 205	C-5 to C-10 and Cycloalkanes
Kerosene	175 to 325	C-12 to C-18 and aromatics
Gas Oil	Above 275	C-12 and higher
Lubricating Oil	Non-volatile liquids	Probably long chains attached to cyclic compounds
Asphalt or Petroleum Coke	Non-volatile solids	Polycyclic structures

Upon distillation of petroleum crude, specific families of organic compounds will concentrate into each of the fractions. Petroleum "cracking" and other refinery processes are also used to alter the petroleum constituent structures into more useable compounds. General ranges of hydrocarbon groups in petroleum products are shown in Table 8.2[4]

Table 8.2. Hydrocarbon Group Types in Petroleum Products[4]

Product	% Composition		
	Saturates (Alkanes)	Olefins (Alkenes)	Aromatics
Gasolines	36 to 71	5 to 13	22 to 54
Jet fuels	78 to 85	<.1 to 4	16 to 25
#2 fuels	48 to 57	?	33 to 38
Diesel fuel	78	2	20
Kerosene	68.6	?	19.4
Lube oils	68 to 90	?	10 to 32
Residual fuels	?	?	?

Although general ranges for boiling points, carbon numbers, and petroleum hydrocarbon groups in the different petroleum distillates can be given, a high degree of chemical variability exists in refined petroleum products. The sources of this variability include:

- Origin of the crude oil;

- Different distillation and refinery processes;
- Blending of additives and octane boosters;
- Seasonal changes in formulation designed to moderate fuel volatility;
- Blending of products by independent retailers; and
- Structural isomers of the individual petroleum constituents.[5]

In addition, several factors will affect the composition of petroleum products when released into the environment (volatilization, partitioning between liquid and solid phases, and biodegradation).

Therefore, chemical analysis for the determination of petroleum products released into the environment poses complicated analytical challenges. Each of the hydrocarbon groups mentioned can have different solubility in extraction solvents and different responses to analytical instrumentation. EPA Method 418.1 has been used as a "catch-all" to cover the broad range of possible chemical constituents in the various petroleum products. As will be discussed, no single method can be considered a reliable test for TPH concentrations in soils. If at all possible, the type of petroleum distillate (i.e., gasoline, diesel, cutting oil) that has been released should be known before an appropriate analytical method can be chosen.

DESCRIPTION OF METHOD 418.1 WITH INTERLABORATORY COMPARISON

An evaluation of the biases associated with Method 418.1 begins with a description of the test procedure. Method 418.1 was originally intended only for aqueous samples not soils. It has been widely modified, however, for the determination of TPH in soil. There has been no standard set of modifications used, allowing for significant differences between laboratories in SOPs. The following is a general description of the test procedure with some of the variances discovered among laboratories.

Step 1--Sample Preparation and Extraction

The first step performed by most laboratories in the extraction procedure is homogenization of the sample by grinding or mixing. The determination of the moisture content is performed on a separate aliquot of the sample. Sample sizes range from 20 to 50 grams with smaller aliquots taken if the concentration of petroleum is high. One of the laboratories in this study adds 1.0 milliliter (ml) of 1:1 hydrochloric acid (HCl) to an approximate 40 gram sample reportedly to enhance the Freon-113 solubility of polar hydrocarbons. All of the laboratories add granular anhydrous sodium sulfate (Na_2SO_4) to remove moisture. Generally, no specifications are given on the mass of Na_2SO_4 added other than a sufficient amount to form a sandy texture. One laboratory adds 50 grams of Na_2SO_4 to a 50-gram sample. Another laboratory adds 10 grams of Na_2SO_4 to a 20-gram soil sample.

The common solvent used for extraction is Freon-113 (1,1,2-trichloro-1,2,2-trifluoroethane). As a nonpolar solvent Freon-113 will preferentially extract nonpolar constituents from the soil matrix (i.e., petroleum hydrocarbons). However, it will also extract some polar organic compounds. A variety of polar organic compounds are present naturally in soils and will codissolve with the non-polar petroleum hydrocarbons. Many of the heavy weight petroleum fractions have poor solubility in Freon-113. The extraction of the heavy weight petroleum can be ameliorated if the Soxhlet extraction method is used [at the expense of losing low boiling point (LBP) fractions].

After the initial sample preparation, the extraction procedures vary widely between laboratories and are probably the single greatest factor affecting interlaboratory variability. Four different types of extraction procedures were found to be in use under the generic Method 418.1: chromatography column, tumbling, sonication, and Soxhlet extraction.

Column Method

One of the laboratories placed the mixture of Na_2SO_4 and soil into a 19 mm x 30 mm glass chromatograph column with glass wool and a stop-cock valve at the bottom. One hundred ml of Freon-113 are poured through the column and collected into a beaker. In general, this method appears to be a poor extraction procedure. The Freon-113 does not contact the soil matrix in a uniform manner. "Channeling" of Freon-113 as it passes through the column can prevent sufficient contact time.

Rotary Agitation

One of the laboratories extracted the soil samples by rotation for four hours. A 20-gram sample is mixed with 10 grams of Na_2SO_4 and 100 mL of Freon-113 in a 250-ml glass bottle. The mixture is rotated end-over-end for four hours, followed by decanting the solvent into a 20-ml scintillation vial. Three-tenths gram of silica gel (specified only as 60-200 mesh) is added to the vial prior to the solvent addition. The vial is loaded onto a mechanical shaker and agitated for five minutes. No specification is given for settling time. The sample is filtered into a clean, dry scintillation vial.

Sonication

The sonication methods are based on EPA Method 3550. After sample preparation, the sample is mixed with Freon-113 and disrupted with an ultrasonic probe. The length of sonication is two minutes. Method 3550 specifies a two minute extraction time for high concentration samples and three minutes for low concentration samples. A study performed by Orion Laboratories found this to be an ineffective extraction method for some petroleum products.[5] The EPA has also found this to be ineffective, leading to the requirement of Soxhlet extraction in the draft Method 9073 (withdrawn).

Soxhlet

The Soxhlet extraction method is based on EPA Method 9071. The prepared sample is placed into an extraction thimble. A glass wool plug is placed on top of the sample. A Soxhlet extractor allows heated Freon-113 to reflux through the sample in a partially closed system repeatedly at approximately 20 times an hour for a minimum of four hours. One laboratory specified that if the Freon-113 filtrate from the thimble was not colorless after four hours, the extraction should continue until the Freon-113 appeared colorless.

Step 2--Sample Cleanup

Since polar organic compounds, such as grease, vegetable oils, fats, waxes, and polyfunctional compounds, are co-dissolved with the petroleum hydrocarbons in Freon-113, a silica gel cleanup step is required to remove the interferences. If the cleanup step is not performed, the results are reported as total recoverable oil and grease (EPA Method 413.1). The silica gel consists of precipitated silicic acid in the form of lustrous granules. The chemical formula is H_2SiO_3.

The silica gel specified in Method 418.1 is 60-200 mesh (Davidson Grade 950 or equivalent). Davidson Grade 950 has been out of production for approximately 10 years. Davidson Grade 923, with a surface area of 500 m^2/gm, is a common replacement.

Many factors will affect the efficiency of the silica gel in removing the interferences:

- Grade of silica used--One of the laboratories used Davidson Grade 62 with a surface area of 343 m^2/gm. Using silica gel with less surface area could cause the silica gel to be less efficient in removing the polar compounds.
- Quantity of silica gel--the laboratories added between 1.5 grams for a 20-gram sample to 3 grams for a 50-gram sample. It is possible that the absorption capacity of the silica gel could be exceeded. The original 418.1 method suggested that the absorbance capacity of the silica gel "could" be tested by adding additional gel and redetermining the infrared (IR) absorbance. The draft Method 9073 (withdrawn) specified that the silica gel absorbance **must** be tested. **None** of the laboratories connected with this study determined if the absorbance capacity of the silica gel had been exceeded. One of the laboratories does not perform the silica gel cleanup, but reports the results as TPH, not oil and grease.
- Deactivation--The test procedure calls for the silica to contain 1 to 2 percent water as defined by a residue test at 130°C. Most laboratory

SOPs contain no information on the preparation of the silica gel. If the silica gel is not deactivated, it could remove small quantities of petroleum hydrocarbons as well as the interferences. If the silica is deactivated with too much water, it may not remove any of the interferences.

- Settling time--Most of the laboratories did not specify the length of time allowed for the silica gel to absorb interferences and settle. One laboratory specified a two hour minimum waiting period. Most laboratories run the sample analysis five minutes after addition of the silica gel, which may not be a sufficient time period for the silica gel to act.

Step 3--Quantification

After the silica gel has been added, the Freon-113 absorbance of TPH in Freon-113 is measured on an IR spectrophotometer at a wave length of approximately 2,950 cm^{-1}. Several of the laboratories specify 2,930 cm^{-1}. Several of the laboratories set the IR at 2,930 cm^{-1} (or 2,950 cm^{-1}) and read the percent transmission. The other laboratories scan a general region around 2,930 cm^{-1}, find the maximum peak in the standard, and use this response in calculating the calibration curve and sample results. If the IR is set at one specific wavelength, it may not be reading the maximum absorbance peak, but one of the peak shoulders. The use of one setting could lead to high or low results depending on the sample curve in the region of that specific wavelength.

Step 4--Standards

For comparison, a mixture of 15.0 mL n-hexadecane (normal chain alkane), 15.0 mL isooctane (branched alkane), and 10.0 mL chlorobenzene (aromatic) is used. Draft Method 9073 (withdrawn) specifies that a sample of the product in question be used, if possible, as the standard (i.e., diesel, fuel oil, etc.). If a sample of the petroleum product is not available, the above mixture is used. All of the laboratories contacted in this study used the standard mixture, not the petroleum product in question.

POSITIVE AND NEGATIVE BIASES

Extraction Methods

The type of soil in which the petroleum hydrocarbons are contained will have an effect on the extraction process and the percent recovery of the petroleum. This problem is, of course, not unique to Method 418.1. Any type of extraction will tend to be more effective in a sandy soil compared to a high clay content soil due to the difficulty in disbursing the clay sized particles.

Sonication and column extraction methods are commonly used with Method 418.1 and tend to be inefficient with tight soils.

A limited study by Orion Laboratories performed with soil affected by heavy weight petroleum products obtained the results shown on Table 8.3 when comparing sonication versus Soxhlet extraction.[6]

Table 8.3. Comparison of Sonication and Soxhlet Extractions[6]

Soil Description	TPH mg/kg by Method 418.1	
	Sonication	Soxhlet
Sand/Petrol Odor	<10.0	595.0
Clay	<10.0	342.2
Silt/Sheen/Petrol Odor	<10.0	132.5
Sand/Gravel	<10.0	211.7
Wet/Petrol Odor	<10.0	81.7
Gray Sand	<10.0	<10.0
Moist Sand	<10.0	<10.0
Clay/Sand	<10.0	84.6
Fine Sand	<10.0	837.7
Silty Clay	<10.0	42.4
Clay	<10.0	234.8

Clearly, the Soxhlet method obtains a more thorough extraction. The problem is that most (if not all) of the LBP hydrocarbons are removed in the extraction process, making this an inappropriate extraction method for LBP hydrocarbons. The draft Method 9073 (withdrawn) which calls for a Soxhlet extraction for soils states, "This method is not applicable to the measurement of gasoline." The chromatographic column is likely the most inefficient process of the commonly used extraction methods. As stated earlier, "channeling" of the Freon-113 as it passes through the column and failure to disburse the soil particles can prevent proper Freon-113/soil contact.

Distinctly different results will be obtained depending on the extraction method chosen. Negative biases for high boiling point hydrocarbons can occur if an ineffective extraction method (chromatography column) or extraction time (sonication -- 2 minutes) are chosen. Negative biases for LBP hydrocarbons will occur if a thorough extraction method (Soxhlet) or a long extraction time is used.

Biases Due to Standards

The relative response of the IR spectrophotometer is based on the amounts of the different hydrocarbon types present (i.e., aromatics, alkanes, etc.). The reference oil standard is a constant mixture of 37.5 percent n-hexadecane (normal chain alkane), 37.5 percent isooctane (branched alkane), and 25 percent chlorobenzene (aromatic) (Figure 8.3).[7] Therefore, if a disparity exists between the chemical composition of the calibration standard and the sample, positive or negative biases will result. The reference oil standard has the best comparison to a middle distillate petroleum product (i.e., diesel, with approximately 75 percent alkanes and approximately 25 percent aromatics). The more the petroleum product component groups (alkanes, aromatics) vary from the reference oil, the higher the analytical biases.

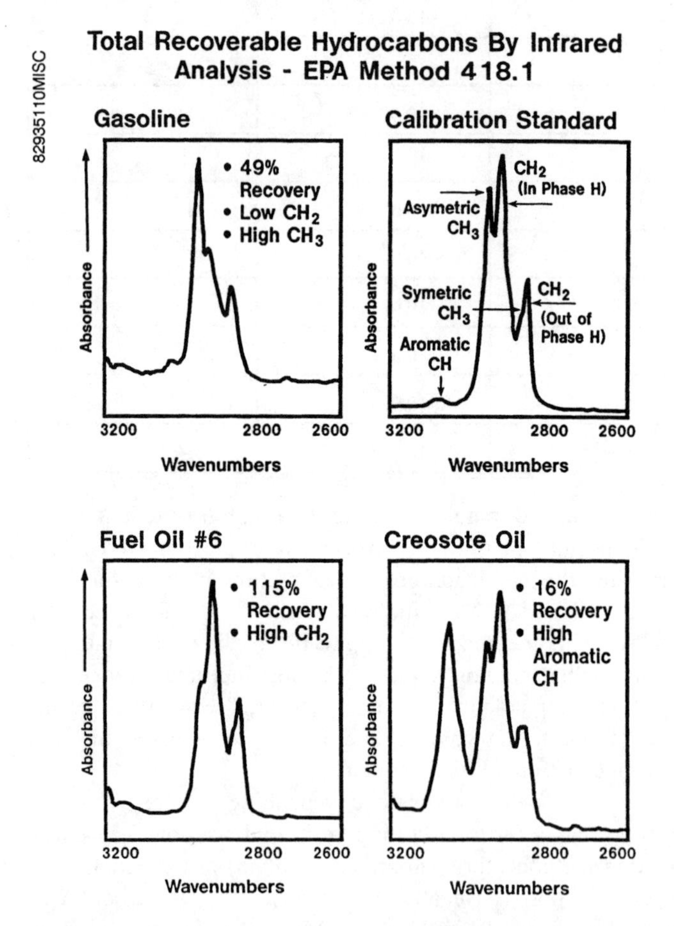

Figure 8.3. IR absorbance patterns of a calibration oil, gasoline, fuel oil #6, and creosote vs. wavenumber (2600 to 3200 cm^{-1}). These samples were prepared in Freon and analyzed according to EPA Method 418.1 using a quantification absorbance at 2930 cm^{-1}.[7]

A limited study conducted by Groundwater Analytical, Inc. demonstrated accuracy errors attributed by the authors to the IR spectral disparity between the product sample and the standard (Table 8.4)[8]. As can be seen, the lowest percent relative error is for diesel fuel.

Positive and Negative Biases Due to the Silica Gel Cleanup

As stated above, silica gel effectiveness will depend on the type and quantity of silica gel used, preparation procedures, and the time allowed for the gel to absorb interferences. In addition, both nonpolar (normal alkanes) and relatively polar compounds are present in petroleum (aromatics and aromatics with functional groups attached). Therefore, it is possible that negative biases could be introduced by the removal of relatively polar hydrocarbons by the silica gel. The degree of bias will depend (in addition to the silica gel factors listed above) on the percentage of nonpolar to relatively polar compounds present in the petroleum product. The author is unaware of any studies of negative biases due to silica gel removal in Freon-113 extracts of soils. Groundwater Analytical, Inc. performed a study of the effects of silica gel suppression on Freon-113 extracts of petroleum saturated aqueous solutions (Table 8.5).[8] The silica gel negative biases would be expected to be higher in aqueous solutions due to the preferential solution of the polar hydrocarbons in water. The results of the Groundwater Analytical, Inc. study indicate significant negative biases. The bias appears to be greatest in high molecular weight (long chain and aromatic hydrocarbon) products.

The author is unaware of studies showing the effectiveness of the silica gel in removing nonpetroleum interferences. Several studies, however, have reported the ineffectiveness of the silica gel.

Biases Due to the Presence of Industrial or Natural Materials

IR spectroscopy quantifies the vibration (stretching and bending) that occurs when a molecule absorbs electromagnetic energy in the IR region of the electromagnetic spectrum.[9] The IR absorption spectrum between 5,000 and 1,250 cm^{-1} is attributed to vibrational stretching and bending of various functional groups.

The IR absorption wave length depends on the bond type and the strength of the bond (i.e., single carbon bonds absorb at 1,200 cm^{-1} and triple carbon bonds absorb at approximately 2,200 cm^{-1}). Different functional groups and bond types have different IR absorption wave lengths and intensities. For example: aromatic Ar-H stretching exhibits an absorption at approximately 3,300 cm^{-1}, and carboxylic acids absorb IR radiation at 2,500 to 3,000 cm^{-1} (O-H stretching).[10] The range of approximately 2,900 to 3,000 cm^{-1} corresponds to stretching of C-H bonds. Therefore, an IR spectrum over a wide range is unique for a given compound and can be used to finger print unknowns.

Table 8.4. Accuracy evaluation of the reference oil standard and the TPH-IR Method (modified from reference #8).

PETROLEUM PRODUCT	CONCENTRATIONS (mg/L)		RELATIVE % ERROR
	ACTUAL	MEASURED (AFTER SILICA GEL ADDITION)	
PREMIUM UNLEADED GASOLINE	30	15.2	-49%
FUEL OIL NO. 2	30	34.1	+14%
DIESEL FUEL	30	31.6	5.3%
FUEL OIL NO. 4	30	22.0	-27%
TRANSMISSION OIL	30	39.8	+33%
10W-30 MOTOR OIL	30	40.4	+35%
80W-90 GEAR OIL	30	39.7	+32%

1. Each solution was prepared by adding 30 mg of petroleum product to 100 mL of Freon-113. Concentration of each Freon-113 solution was measured prior to the addition of silica gel and after the addition of silica gel.

2. Measured concentrations were calculated on the basis of the absorbance of the Reference Oil at 2930 cm^{-1} .

Table 8.5. Effect of silica gel on freon-113 extracts of petroleum saturated aqueous solutions (modified from reference #8).

PETROLEUM PRODUCT	CONCENTRATIONS (mg/L)		RELATIVE % ERROR
	PRIOIR TO SILICA GEL ADDITION	AFTER SILICA GEL ADDITION	
PREMIUM UNLEADED GASOLINE	34.4	12.6	-37%
REGULAR UNLEADED GASOLINE	40.8	27.4	-33%
FUEL OIL NO. 2 (A)	16.9	12.3	27%
FUEL OIL NO. 2 (B)	10.6	10.4	-1.8%
DIESEL FUEL (A)	7.8	5.0	-36%
DIESEL FUEL (B)	6.0	3.9	-35%
FUEL OIL NO. 4	3.1	1.3	-58%
TRANSMISSION OIL	5.1	1.9	-63%
10W-30 MOTOR OIL	30.4	4.3	-86%
80W-90 GEAR OIL	38.8	5.3	-86%

1. Saturated aqueous solutions of each petroleum product were prepared. Each saturated aqueous solution was then extracted with Freon-113. The concentration of each Freon-113 extract was measured prior to the addition of silica gel and after the addition of silica gel.

2. Measured concentrations were calculated on the basis of the absorbance of the Reference Oil at 2930 cm^{-1}.

One of the principle problems of Method 418.1 is that many compounds have IR absorption peaks in the 2,950 cm^{-1} region of the spectrum. Any scan of a book of IR spectra will show innumerable compounds with a positive IR absorption around 2,950 cm^{-1} (Figure 8.4).[11] Many of these compounds (principally carboxylic acids and hydrocarbons) have been found at high concentrations occurring naturally in soil.[12] The IR spectra of humic acids from terrestrial soils and marine sediments is presented in Figure 8.5.[13] The IR region around 2,950 cm^{-1} clearly shows absorbance for humic compounds.

Since only the IR region around 2,950 cm^{-1} is scanned in Method 418.1, a fingerprint of the compound cannot be obtained and identification is not possible. The IR absorbance spectra in the region of 2,950 cm^{-1} of several materials are shown in Figure 8.6. Although the relative intensity may vary, there are no distinctive characteristics that would allow the analyst to make a judgement on the nature of the material.

Polar compounds are theoretically removed with the silica gel cleanup, leaving behind only nonpolar petroleum hydrocarbons. The silica gel cleanup, however, appears to be inefficient. None of the laboratories in this study routinely check if the absorbance capacity of the silica gel has been exceeded. To test the theory that naturally occurring organics and commonly encountered industrial products will cause positive biases by Method 418.1, a group of these materials was collected, mixed thoroughly in a stainless steel bowl, and separate aliquots sent to three laboratories. The samples were marked to indicate normal soil boring samples (i.e., Boring 5 at 12 to 15 feet). The results of the study are presented in Table 8.6.

Table 8.6. Total Petroleum Hydrocarbons (mg/kg) by Method 418.1 of Natural Organic and Industrial Materials.

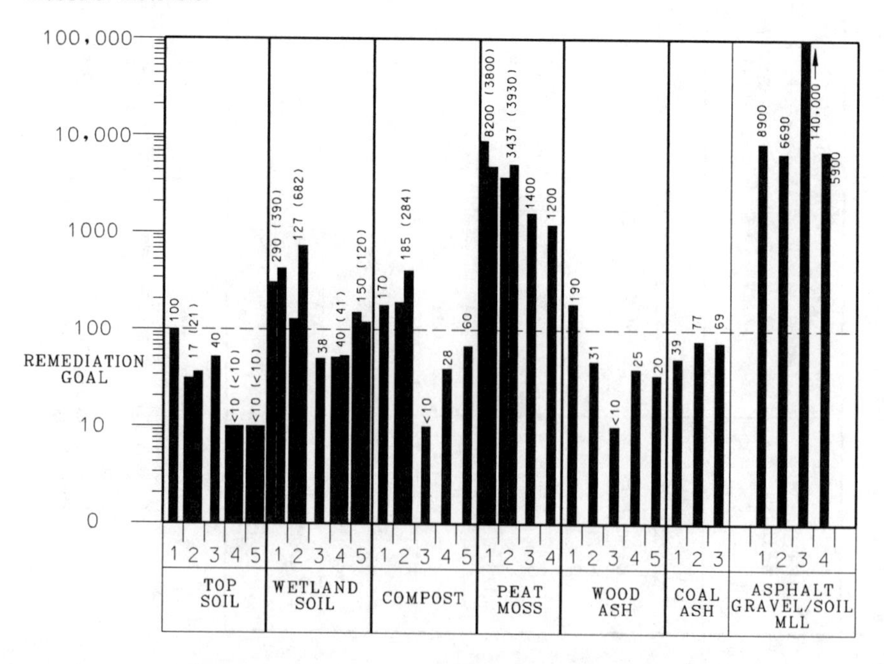

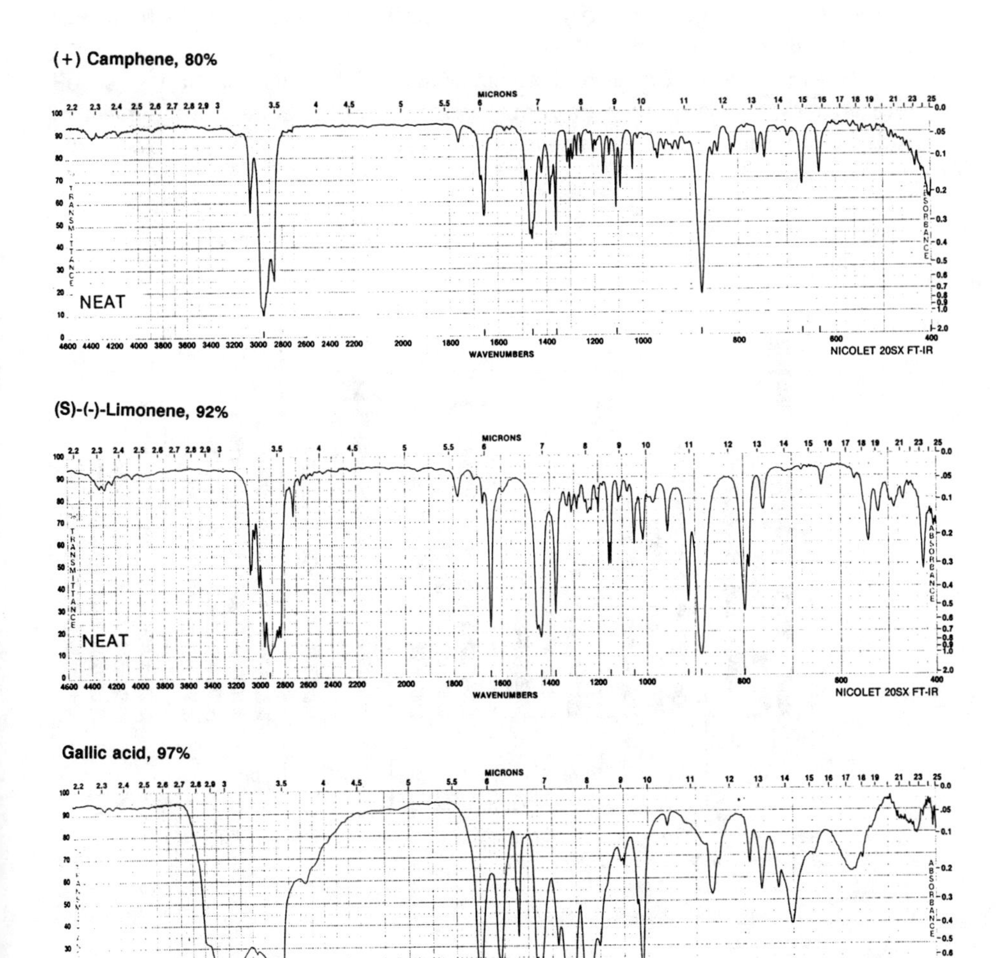

Figure 8.4. IR spectra of naturally occurring organic chemicals.

As can be seen from Table 8.6 and Figure 8.6, it is possible for nonregulated industrial materials and natural organics to be confused with regulated petroleum products.

Other studies have also noted the occurrence of false positives due to natural organics. A study performed by Groundwater Analytical, Inc. showed significant false positives in natural materials (Table 8.7).[8]

Although sequential additions of silica gel did tend to lower the TPH concentrations, some materials still contained high levels of TPH after three additions of silica gel (i.e., dried grass). Clearly, the silica gel is inefficient at removing these interferences.

Block, Clark & Bishop did a comparison of TPH concentrations in soil measured by IR and GC as part of the assessment of the biological treatment of soils. The results of the comparison are shown in Table 8.8.[14] The GC results were consistently lower.

Table 8.7. Effect of silica gel on freon-113 extracts of vegetative materials (modified from reference #8).

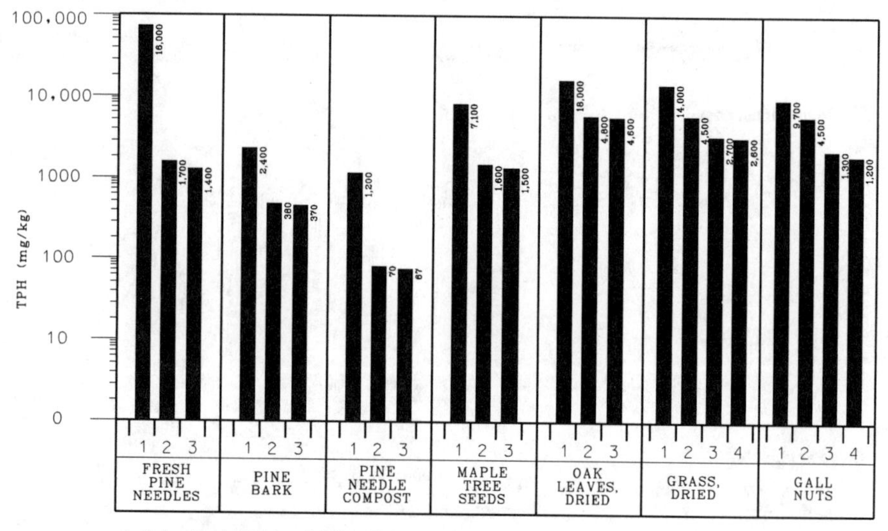

1. Prior to Addition of Silica Gel
2. After First Addition of Silica Gel
3. Second Addition of Silica Gel
4. After Third Addition of Silica Gel

NOTE:

Each vegetative material was extracted with Freon-113. The concentration of each Freon-113 extract was measured prior to the additional of silica gel, and after the addition of silica gel, and then agian after a second addition of silica gel. A third addition of silica gel was performed only for the Dried Grass and Gall Nuts extracts, due to the significant change in concentration caused by the second addition of silica gel. Measured concentrations calculated on the basis of the absorbance of the Reference Oil at 2,930 cm^{-1}.

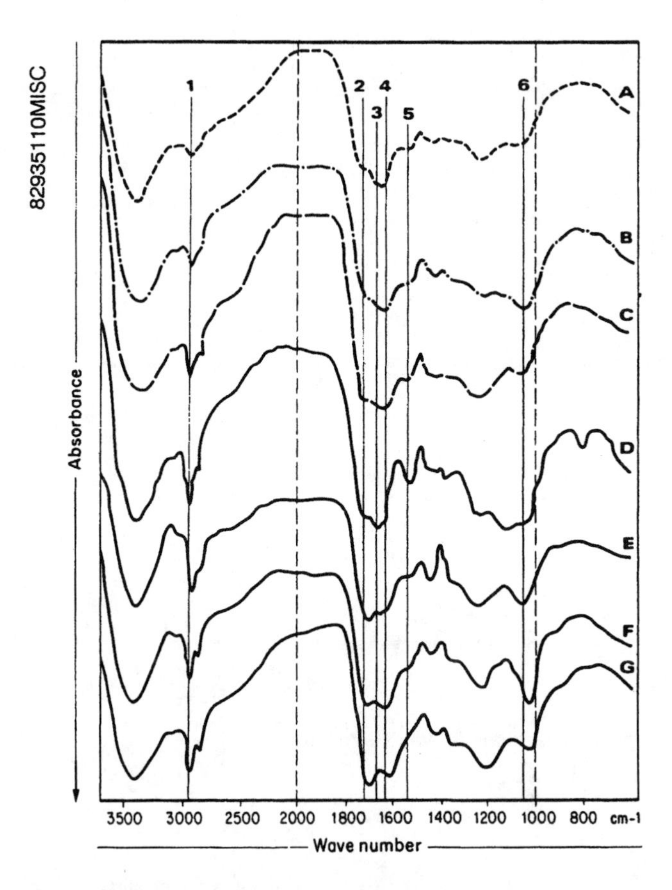

Figure 8.5. Comparison of IR spectra of humic acids from terrestrial soils, and humic acids from recent marine sediments. Identification of humic acids: *Terrestrial soils*: *A* rendzin, *B* brown soil, acid, *C* podzol. *Marine sediments:* *D* and *F* France, Atlantic coast, *E* Eastern Mediterranean, *G* West Africa. *Identification of IR bands:* *1 aliphatic C-H,* *2:* C = O, *3* and *5* amides, *4* aromatic C = C, *6* C-O of polysaccharides.[13]

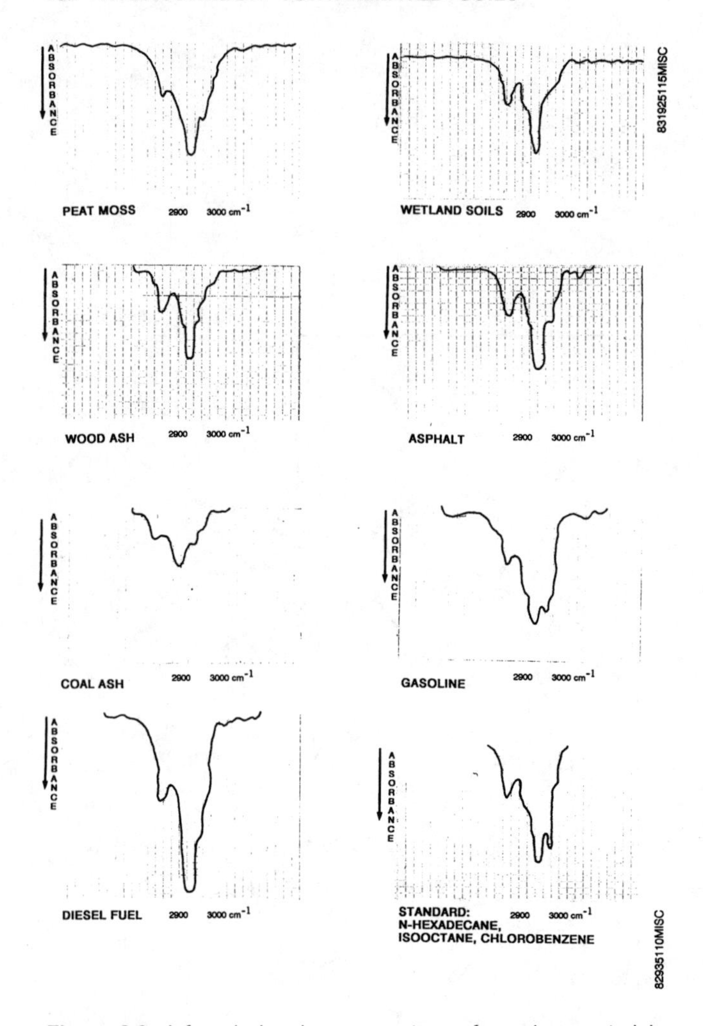

Figure 8.6. Infrared absorbance spectrums for various materials.

Table 8.8. Comparison of TPH analyses IR and GC methods.[14]

Sample	Location	TPH (mg/kg)	
		By IR	By GC
1-AB.1.5	Treatment window	317	69
1-CD.1.5	Treatment window	148	109
1-EF.1.5	Treatment window	136	48
1-GH.1.5	Treatment window	160	65
1-IJ.1.5	Treatment window	167	105
1-K.1.5	Treatment window	172	60
1-L.1.5	Treatment window	110	67
1-M.1.5	Treatment window	153	114
5-A.1.1	Treatment window	250	75
5-B.1.1	Treatment window	144	109
PBGD-4	Park adjacent to site	76	9
PGCD-5	Park adjacent to site	nd	10
PBGD-6	Park adjacent to site	33	10

Block, Clark & Bishop made the following interpretation of the results:

"Many soils contain low level nonpetroleum hydrocarbon interferences. These interferences are presumed to be either naturally occurring humic materials or by-products of the petroleum hydrocarbon biodegradation process. The interferences are not effectively removed by the silica gel cleanup, but they do contain carbon hydrogen bonds. The presence of this interference falsely indicated that a healthy treatment process had stalled at some low to medium petroleum hydrocarbon level."[14]

In another paper by Block, Clark & Bishop, the following quote was found:

"Method 418.1 will measure any Freon-113 extractable, non-silica gel removable compound containing carbon hydrogen groups. This method does not provide any qualitative contaminant information other than the presence of the carbon hydrogen bond."[15]

Nyer and Skladany made the following statement:

"All materials (contaminants or benign materials) that are soluble in the solvent will be extracted. These materials may create positive or negative interferences with the hydrocarbon quantitation."[2]

Another factor to be considered is the possible interference of industrial materials or other contaminants. Many older urban/industrial areas contain significant amounts of fill materials which contain coal ash/cinders, asphalt, ash, decomposing lumber, etc. These materials will also generate high TPH values by Method 418.1 (Table 8.6). It can be stated that asphalt, as a petroleum based product, is accurate in showing positive TPH concentrations. There is a distinct difference, however, in the solubility, mobility, and regulatory classification of solid petroleum based products and liquid refined petroleum distillates.

Soil Matrix

Thomey, Bratberg, and Kalisz conducted a comparison of TPH in soil by 418.1 and GC/FID methods.[16] They found fair agreement in sandy soils between 418.1 and GC/FID methods, but poor correlation with silt and clay soils. In addition, Thomey, Bratberg, and Kalisz theorized that colloidal and clay sized particles could remain in suspension in the Freon-113 extract, absorb infrared light, and cause a positive reading in the absence of petroleum hydrocarbons. The conclusions of the report stated:

"It is apparent that EPA Method 418.1 is not an appropriate technique for measuring TPH concentrations in certain types of soils. These types of soil can be categorized as weathered limestone, clays, and silts."[16]

Potter and Bruya also have reported false positives due to suspended solids (Figure 8.7).[4] Some laboratories determine the IR absorbance at a fixed specific wavelength, therefore the analysts could not distinguish between a petroleum product and suspended clay particles.

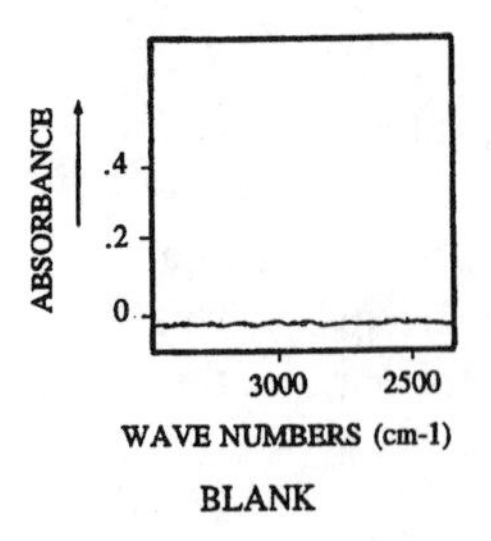

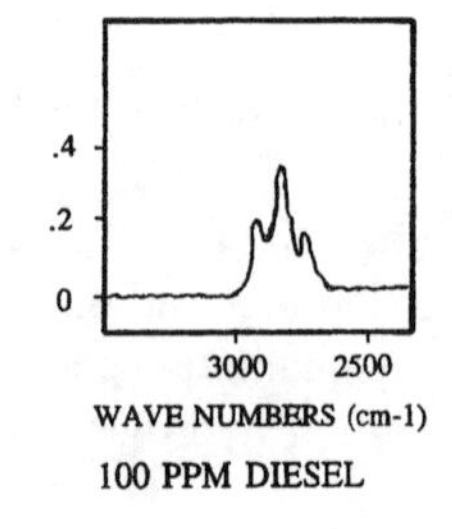

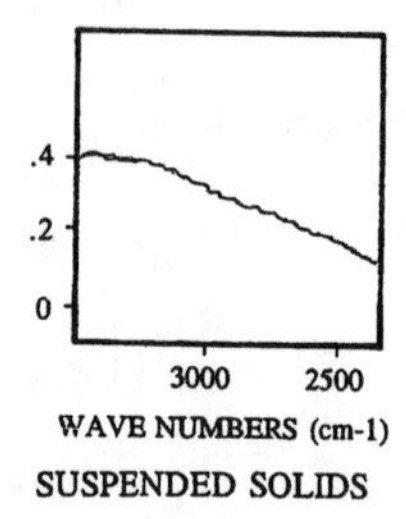

Figure 8.7. IR absorbance due to suspended solids[4].

Alternative Methods

A full discussion of alternative methods to determine TPH concentrations in soil is beyond the scope of this chapter. GC methods are now widely used to determine TPH in soil.[2,3,16-28]

The most commonly used technique is GC with flame ionization (FID) or photoionization detector (PID). Gas chromatography is based on a mixture separation of gas phase compounds (analytes) by the stationary phase (column). Different petroleum products will have different affinities for the stationary phase and elute at different times. After separation in the column, the analytes are either burned by an FID or ionized by ultraviolet light in a PID. Quantification is by direct comparison of the sample with the same petroleum distillate fraction (i.e., gasoline contaminated soil with a gasoline standard).

The GC methods are usually divided into gasoline range (carbon range of C_6-C_{10} and boiling point range of 60°C - 220°C) and diesel range (carbon range of C_{10}-C_{28} and boiling point range 170°C - 430°C).[24]

The gasoline range soil samples are analyzed by purge and trap with water or methanol as the purge fluid. The diesel range organics are extracted with a solvent (usually methylene chloride) followed by GC analysis.

There are several distinct advantages to GC methods. FIDs have similar responses for almost all petroleum hydrocarbons. A correlation can be made between elution time in the GC column and boiling points and carbon numbers of the sample.[26] If the type of petroleum fraction present in an environmental sample is unknown a fingerprint scan can be run to determine distillate type. A comparison is made directly between similar compounds (i.e., diesel to diesel) which helps to minimize the disparity between standards and samples.

Problems do exist with GC methods. As part of the quantification of petroleum distillates, an elution "window" is established for comparison. Due to the highly variable nature of petroleum products, a specific product may contain constituents that fall outside of this window. In turn, other compounds not intended to be quantified can elute in the same window. Heavy distillates (lubricating oils, residual fuels) are not easily separated or quantified by GC methods. In addition, industrial materials and soils with very high levels of organics may also test positive with the GC methods. The GC chromatograms by Iowa's OA-1 (gasoline range) and OA-2 (diesel range) for various petroleum products and organic materials are shown in Figure 8.8.

Although positive results were reported for the nonpetroleum organic materials by the GC/FID method, the "characteristics" of the chromatograms differ significantly from refined petroleum products. A significant departure from normal petroleum product chromatograms could signal the need for additional analytical work. These chromatograms should be compared to the IR spectra in Figure 8.6. The IR spectra offer no opportunity for identification of the material in question.

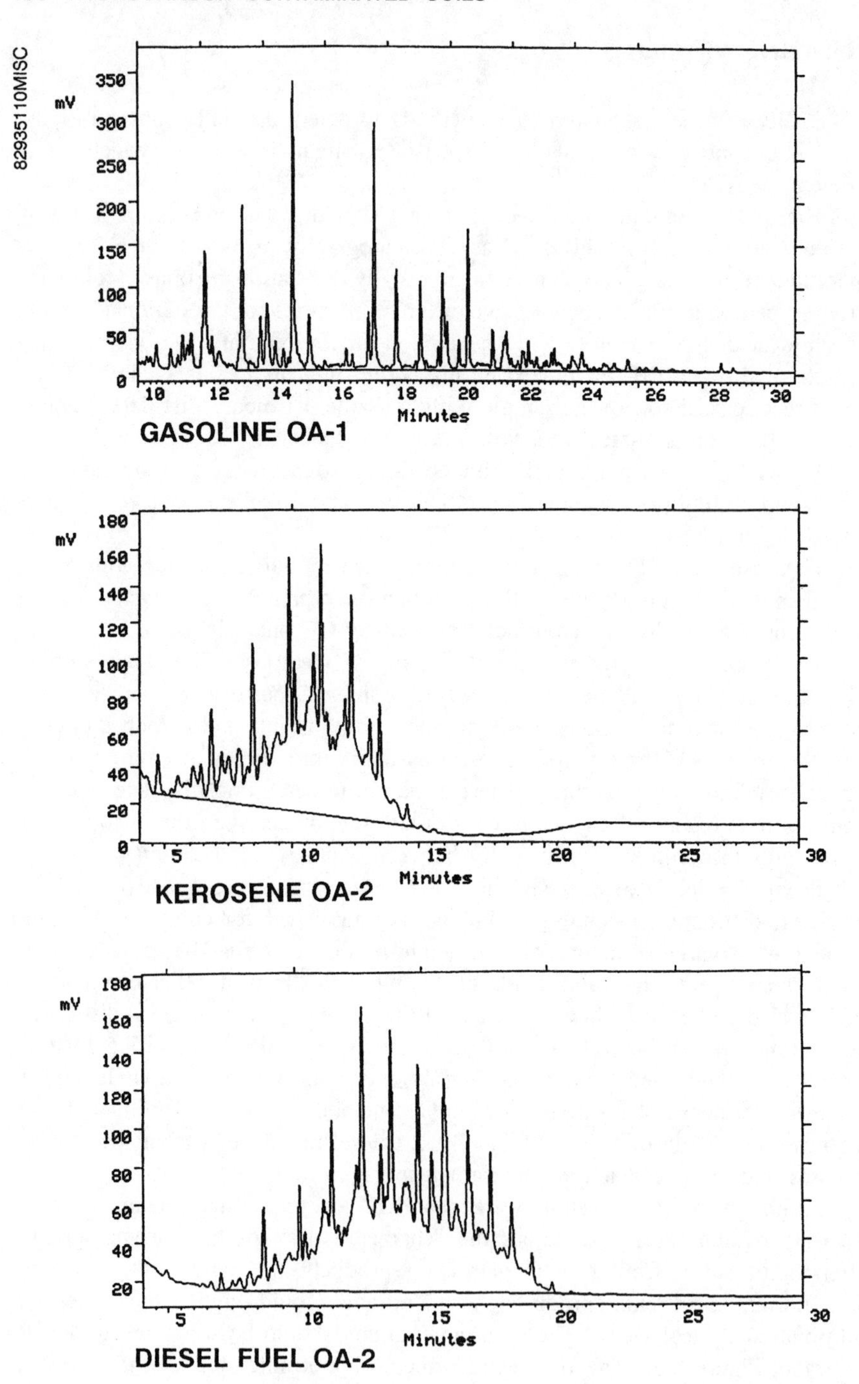

Figure 8.8.1. Gas chromatogram of various petroleum products and organic materials.

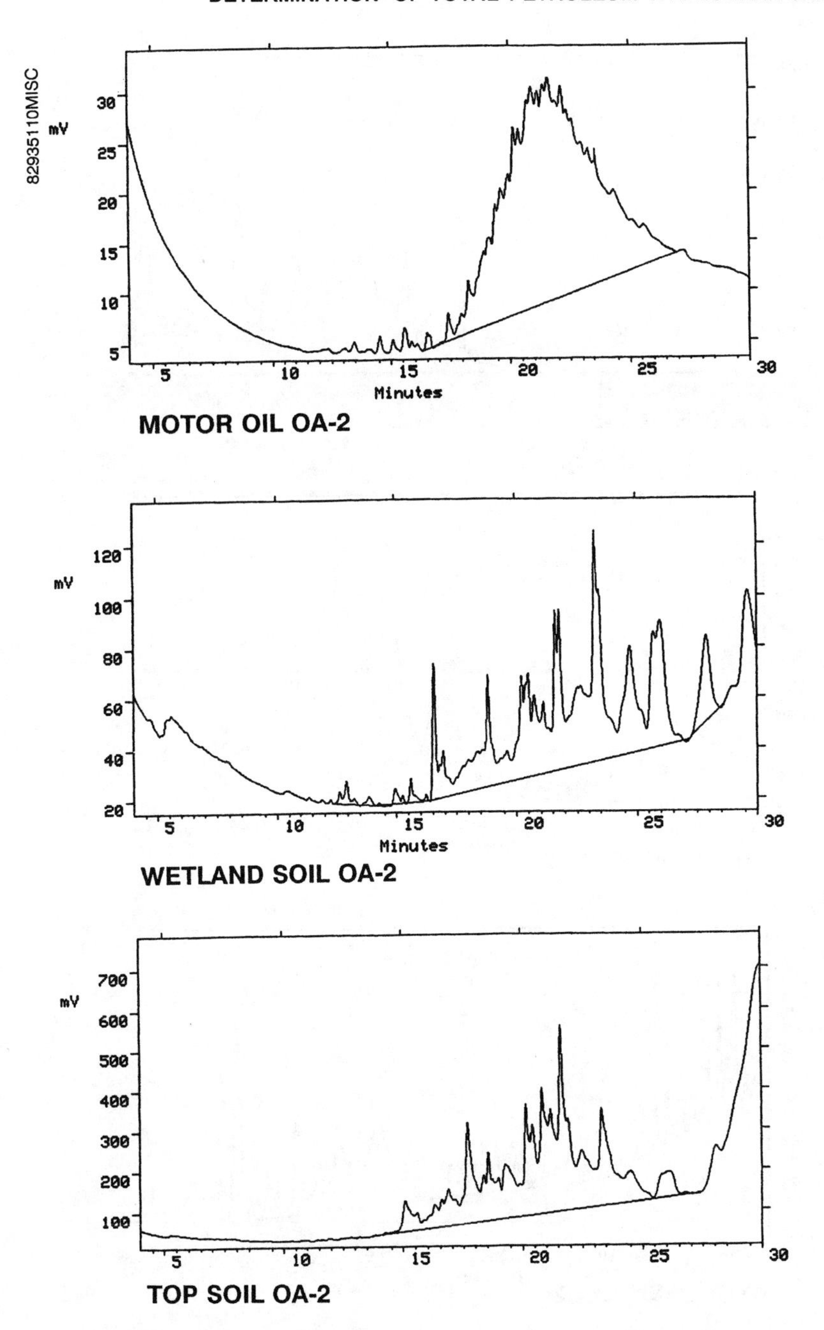

Figure 8.8.2. Gas chromatogram of various petroleum products and organic materials.

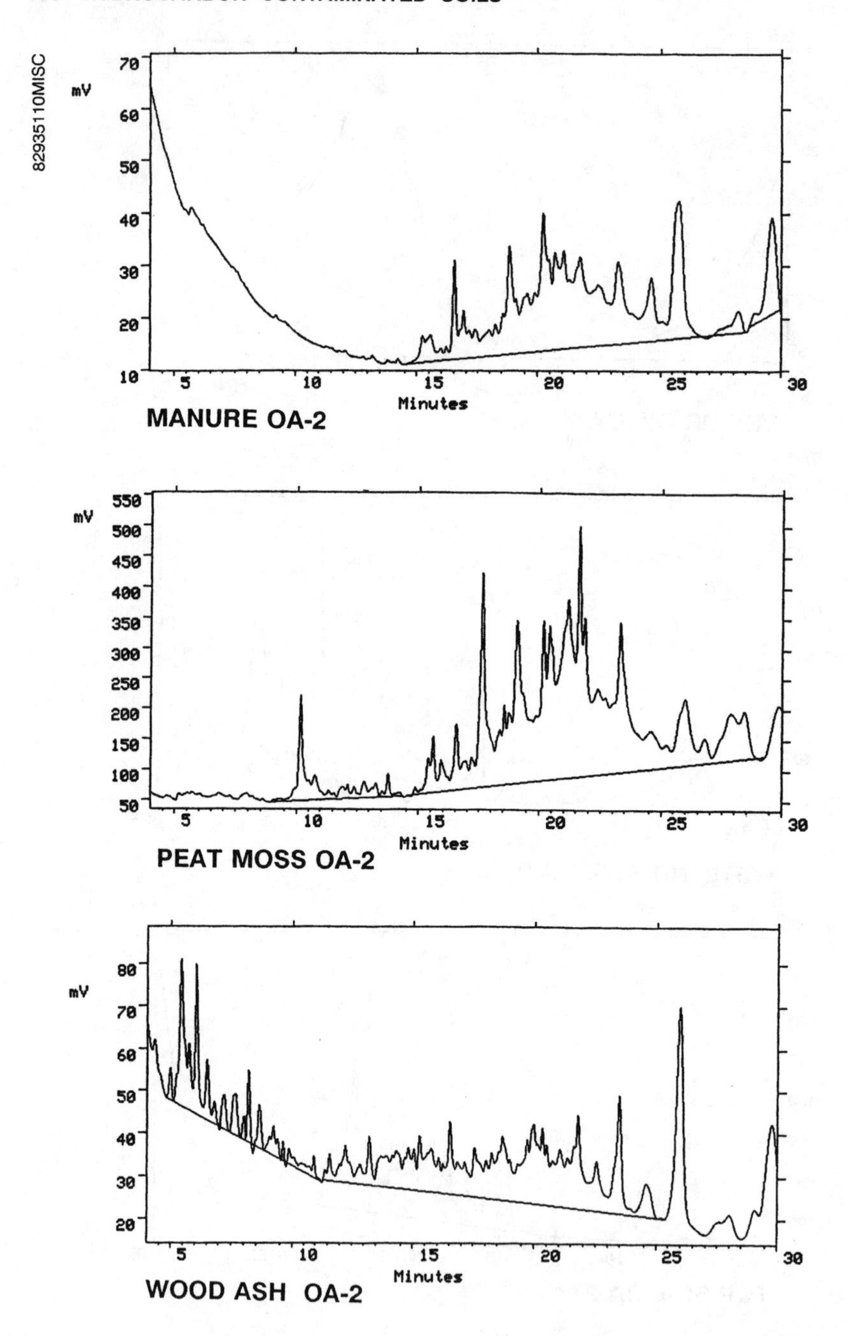

Figure 8.8.3. Gas chromatogram of various petroleum products and organic materials.

CONCLUSIONS

EPA Method 418.1 has been one of the most widely used procedures to determine TPH concentrations in soil. Studies performed by numerous groups have found the procedure to be prone to significant positive and negative biases. The key factors causing the biases are:

- Interlaboratory variations in analytical procedures;
- Negative bias due to volatization of low boiling point compounds;
- Negative bias due to poor extraction of high molecular weight hydrocarbons;
- Positive or negative bias due to disparity in absorption between the sample and the standard;
- Negative bias due to the removal of polar hydrocarbons in the silica gel cleanup;
- Positive bias due to the measurement of naturally occurring organics or nonregulated petroleum based materials;
- Positive bias due to the suspension of clay particles in the Freon-113 extract; and
- Lack of petroleum type determination, preventing an accurate risk assessment.

The following statement appears in the definition section of Method 418.1:

> "As in the case of oil and grease, the parameter of petroleum hydrocarbons is defined by the method. The measurement may be subject to interferences and the results should be evaluated accordingly."[29]

The analysis of petroleum products in soil (as well as other analytes) is a complicated problem. The complex chemistry of petroleum products and the soil matrix make the development of an inexpensive, quick and accurate analytical procedure for TPH in soil almost impossible. Method 418.1 may be used in select site investigations, but the limitations and biases must be understood. Method 418.1 should not be used to assess soils affected by LBP petroleum products. Due to the high analytical variance, the procedure should not be used for remediation verification. The GC/FID procedures offer significant improvements in both quantification and the identification of interfering compounds. At this time, the GC methods appear to offer the best hope for standard TPH tests in soil and groundwater. The problems of heavy weight petroleum product quantification and the selection of suitable standards remain.

In addition to the problems which can be solved by the use of the more specific GC methods, a case can also be made that a solvent extraction method to determine TPH in soil has little relationship to the potential of the petroleum products to leach to groundwater, one of the principle exposure routes for petroleum releases. A more appropriate method may be a modified total characteristic leaching procedure (TCLP) or distilled water extraction method to determine leachability of the petroleum constituents.

ACKNOWLEDGEMENTS

The material in this chapter is a revision of material copyrighted by the National Groundwater Association, reprinted with their permission. The author wishes to thank Dr. Zwicker and Linda Stites of Environmental Science & Engineering, Inc. (ESE) for their assistance during the preparation and review of the manuscript; and also wishes to thank Jessica and Ellen George for their assistance in the collection of the samples.

REFERENCES

1. Oliver, T., and Kostecki, P., Ph.D., State-by-State Summary of Cleanup Standards, *Soils*, 1992.
2. Nyer, E.K. and Skladany, G.J., Relating the Physical and Chemical Properties of Petroleum Hydrocarbons to Soil and Aquifer Remediation, *Groundwater Monitoring Review*, Winter 1989.
3. Senn, R.J. and Johnson, M.S., Interpretation of gas chromatography data as a tool in subsurface hydrocarbon investigations, in *Petroleum Hydrocarbons and Organic Chemicals in Groundwater - Prevention, Detection, and Restoration.* 1985.
4. Potter, Thomas L. and Bruya, J., Analytical Techniques for Determining Petroleum Products in Soils, presented at the 7th Annual Conference on Hydrocarbon-Contaminated Soils, University of Massachusetts at Amherst. 1992.
5. Bergamini, T., Petroleum Product Chemistry and Analytical Tests for Petroleum Hydrocarbons, *Underground Tank Technology Update*, University of Wisconsin - Madison, April 1992.
6. Martin, Michael J., *Sonication Versus Soxhlet Extraction for Soil Analysis*, Environmental Lab., 1992.
7. Douglas, G.S.; McCarthy, K.J.; Dahlen, D.T.; Seavy, J.A.; Steinhauer, W.G.; Prince, R.C., and Elmendorf, D.L.; The use of hydrocarbon analyses for environmental assessment and remediation, in *Journal of Soil Contamination*, Vol. 1, No. 3, 1992.

8. EPA Method 418.1, total recoverable petroleum hydrocarbons by IR, in *Groundwater Technical Analytical Bulletin*, Groundwater Analytical, Inc., Buzzards Bay, Maine, 1992.
9. Wingrove & Caret, *Organic Chemistry*, Harper & Row, 1981.
10. Solomons, T.W., *Organic Chemistry*, John Wiley & Sons, Inc., 1980.
11. Pouchert, C.J., *The Aldrich Library of FT-IR Spectra*, Edition 1.
12. Dragun, James, *The Soil Chemistry of Hazardous Materials*, Hazardous Materials Control Research Institute, Silver Spring, Maryland, 1988.
13. Tissot, B.P., Welte, D.H., Petroleum formation and occurrence, Springer-Verlag, 1984 from Huc, A.Y., *Contribution al'etude de l'humus marin et de ses relations avec les Kerogenes*, thesis, Univ. Nancy, 1973.
14. Block, Clark, and Bishop, *Biological Treatment of Soils Contaminated by Petroleum Hydrocarbons in Petroleum Contaminated Soils*, Volume 3, 1990.
15. Block, Clark, and Bishop, Biological remediation of petroleum hydrocarbons, in *6th National Conference on Hazardous Wastes and Hazardous Materials*, 1989.
16. Thomey, Bratberg, and Kalisz, A comparison of methods for measuring total petroleum hydrocarbons in soil, in *NWWA/API Conference on Petroleum Hydrocarbons and Organic Chemicals in Groundwater*, 1989.
17. American Petroleum Institute - 4449, *Manual of Sampling and Analytical Methods for Petroleum Hydrocarbons in Groundwater and Soil*, 1987.
18. Havlicek, Stephen C., *Characterization of Fuels and Fuel Spills*, Central Coat Analytical Services, Inc., 1988.
19. Parr, J. L., Walters, G., Hoffman, M., Sampling and analysis of soils for gasoline range organics in *West Coast Conference on Hydrocarbon Contaminated Soils and Groundwater*, 1990.
20. Walters, G., Zilis, K., Wessling, E.A., Hoffman, M., Analytical methods for petroleum hydrocarbons, in *1990 Superfund Proceedings, "Superfund 90"*, HMCRI, 1990.
21. Testa, S. M., Hydrocarbon product characterization: applications and techniques, *1990 Fourth National Outdoor Action Conference on Aquifer Restoration, Groundwater Monitoring and Geophysical Methods*, 1991.
22. Kostecki, P.T. and Calabrese, E.J., *Petroleum Contaminated Soils*, Lewis Publishers, Volume 2, 1989.
23. Kostecki, P.T. and Calabrese, E.J., *Petroleum Contaminated Soils*, Lewis Publishers, Volume 3, 1990.
24. Wisconsin Department of Natural Resources, *Leaking Underground Storage Tank Analytical Guidance*, April 1992.
25. Iowa Public Health & Environmental Laboratory-University Hygienic Laboratory-Methods OA-1 and OA-2.
26. ASTM: D 2887-84 - Boiling Range Distribution of Petroleum Fractions by Gas Chromatography.
27. ASTM: D 3328-90 - Comparison of Waterborne Petroleum Oils by Gas Chromatography.

28. Potter, Thomas L. 1989. Analysis of Petroleum Contaminated Soil and Water: An Overview, in Petroleum Contaminated Soils, Volume 2, Lewis Publishers, Inc.
29. Environmental Protection Agency, *Petroleum Hydrocarbons, Total Recoverable, Method 418.1 (Spectrophotometric, Infrared)*.

CHAPTER 9

A Comparison Between an Immunoassay Based Detection Method and Gas Chromatography for PAH Measurement

Bharat B. Kikani, Celeste Twamley, James O. Crawford, George C. Hobbib and James H. Rittenburg, Quantix Systems, Cinnaminson, New Jersey

INTRODUCTION

Fuels such as kerosene, diesel fuel, heating oil and jet fuel are obtained as the middle distillate from fractional distillation of crude oil.[1] This fraction often contains potentially toxic compounds such as polynuclear aromatic hydrocarbons (PAH).[2] Due to low volatility of this class of compounds, a discharge of this class of fuels results in persistent PAH contamination in soil and water.[3] The large number of leaking underground storage tanks and subsequent remediation provide the need for rapid and accurate determination of contamination.[4]

The current U.S. EPA methods used for analysis of petroleum products were designed for compliance monitoring in only certain regulatory programs.[5] These methods were not developed specifically for the analysis of petroleum products nor have they been systematically evaluated for this purpose.[3] The least specific analytical approach to the problem usually involves some form of "total petroleum hydrocarbon" measurement. While the infrared spectroscopy based method 418.1 is commonly used, difficulties in calibration and establishing a background level introduce a substantial uncertainty in the measurement. The 8000 series gas chromatography (GC) methods are widely used for detection and measurement of petroleum hydrocarbons. These methods tend to be time consuming and expensive. A complete separation of all the compounds in highly complex mixtures such as diesel fuel, kerosene and other related products is currently beyond the limits of a single gas chromatography column.[6]

Immunoassays offer a cost effective alternative for rapid, on-site analysis.[7-9] They rely on highly specific, animal derived antibody proteins and can quantify a wide variety of target materials in a broad range of matrices. Unlike GC, immunoassays do not require sophisticated instrumentation and operator training. The high specificity of the antibodies combined with the high sensitivity of the immunoassay significantly reduces sample preparation. The advantages of immunoassay for environmental applications are now being realized and have led to the growth in the number of commercial products in a short period of time. The U.S. EPA is adapting to a performance based method system for evaluation of immunoassay methods.[10] Some of the immunoassay methods have received draft approval status while a number of immunoassay methods are at various stages of U.S. EPA review.

This chapter describes the development of an immunoassay for detection and quantitation of PAH in soil. Comparison of the immunoassay to U.S. EPA SW-846 methods 8015 and 8270 is discussed.

MATERIALS AND METHODS

Preparation of conjugates

Immunogens, screening and enzyme conjugates were prepared by using PAH derivatives coupled to either keyhole limpet hemocyanin (KLH), (Pierce, Rockford, Illinois) bovine serum albumin (BSA), chicken albumin (Sigma Chemical Company, St. Louis, Missouri) or alkaline phosphatase (Boehringer Manheim, Indianapolis, Indiana). All conjugates were dialyzed against either phosphate buffered saline (PBS) or tris buffered saline (Tris) to remove unreacted hapten. Conjugation of hapten to protein and removal of unreacted hapten was confirmed by size exclusion HPLC. The protein concentration was measured using the BCA assay (Pierce) and the conjugates were subsequently diluted with appropriate storage buffer prior to use.

Antibody production

The immunogens were diluted with an equal amount of Freund's complete adjuvant and used to immunize rabbits. The animals were bled monthly at approximately ten days following each injection. Antisera obtained from each animal was screened using a sixteen component PAH mixture in an indirect ELISA procedure on 96 well plates (Nunc) coated with various chicken albumin hapten conjugates. Antisera from various animals giving similar antibody characteristics were pooled and purified by protein-A affinity chromatography. The purified IgG fraction was used in a direct competitive flow-through enzyme immunoassay (EIA) format. The antibody and hapten-alkaline phosphatase conjugate were selected based upon the sensitivity to a PAH mixture as described by U.S. EPA method 610. The mixture contained 0.2 mg/mL of each of the following compounds: Acenaphthene, Acenaphthylene, Anthracene, Benz[a]anthracene, Benzo[a]pyrene, Benzo[b]fluoranthene, Benzo[g,h,i]perylene, Benzo[k]fluoranthene, Chrysene, Dibenz[a,h]anthracene, Fluoranthene, Fluorene, Indeno[1,2,3-cd]pyrene, Naphthalene, Phenanthrene and Pyrene (Accustandard Inc., New Haven, Connecticut).

Immunoassay procedure

The procedure described is a direct competitive immunoassay performed on the microporous surface of a porous plastic detector.[11] An open-ended syringe is used as a coring device to quantitatively collect soil samples in an adapted

API procedure.[12] Soil samples are added into tubes containing an equal volume of isopropanol. The mixture is shaken for one minute to extract the PAH components. After a short settling time a piston filter is used to filter the extract. The extract is then diluted ten fold into the assay diluent for quantitating in the 0.7 to 15ppm range (low range). If necessary a second dilution step can be made to expand the quantitative range up to 140ppm (high range). An alkaline phosphatase hapten enzyme conjugate is added to the sample tube and also to a negative control reference solution. The disposable analyte detector has two discrete reaction zones containing latex particles that have been coated with affinity purified antibody. The liquid reagents are applied to the surface of the detector. In order to perform the immunoassay, five drops of the prepared test sample is applied to the sample zone on the surface of the detector. Five drops of negative control reference are added to the reference zone of the detector. As each solution is absorbed into the detector by capillary action it passes through the surface zone of immobilized antibody. Any PAH present in the sample will compete with the hapten-enzyme conjugate for sites on the immobilized antibodies. Two drops of a rinse solution is added to each well on the detector to remove any unbound hapten conjugate. Two drops of BCIP/NBT alkaline phosphatase color forming substrate is added to each zone which reacts with the antibody bound hapten conjugate to produce a purple color. Finally, two drops of a fixing solution is applied to each zone to stabilize the developed color. Color development in the sample well decreases as the concentration of PAH increases. For quantitative results, the detector can be read using a hand held dual beam reflectometer. This meter compares the color intensity of the sample zone to that of the negative control reference zone. The concentration of PAH is calculated from a preprogrammed standard curve and is displayed by the meter.

RESULTS AND DISCUSSION

Sample Preparation

A study was conducted to determine PAH recoveries obtained using various extraction solvents. This study compared extraction efficiency for isopropanol and methylene chloride/acetone (90:10). Methylene chloride/acetone is a solvent of choice for sample preparation in various GC methods. The immunoassay method favors a polar solvent and therefore it was necessary to demonstrate equivalent extraction efficiency.

The Quantix PAH Workstation and the laboratory GC method modified 8015 (FID) were used to analyze split extracts of soils fortified with the sixteen component PAH mixture. One set of soil (6g) aliquots were fortified with varying concentrations of the PAH mixture. Thirty minutes after fortification, the soil aliquots were extracted with 20 mL methylene chloride/acetone mixture (9:1) with sonication. The experiment was repeated using soil (8.4g) aliquots fortified at the same concentrations with the PAH mixture and were extracted with 8.4mL of isopropanol. The two sets of extracts were analyzed by GC method 8015. Based upon the GC results the percent recoveries were calculated for the various soil samples (Table 9.1). The data shows that PAH recoveries with isopropanol were equivalent or better to those obtained using methylene chloride/acetone.

Table 9.1. Extraction Efficiency of Soils Spiked with PAH using Isopropanol and Methylene Chloride/Acetone (90:10) as Extraction Solvents

	Total PAH Concentration in ppm	
	Results Expressed as Percent Recovery	
Spike level[1] (ppm)	Methylene Chloride/ Acetone[2]	Isopropanol[3]
Clay Soil		
0.0	0.0	0.0
50.0	58.2	72.6
100.0	53.7	73.5
200.0	50.5	74.5
Clay Loam Soil		
0.0	0.0	0.0
50.0	83.3	74.8
100.0	74.2	79.4
200.0	77.0	81.0
Sandy Loam Soil		
0.0	0.0	0.0
50.0	80.5	81.2
100.0	71.9	78.2
200.0	83.5	78.0

1. Soil was spiked with varying levels of PAH mixture containing equal amounts of the following 16 components: acenaphthene, acenaphthylene, anthracene, benzo(a)anthracene, benzo(a)pyrene, benzo(b)fluoranthene, benzo(g,h,i)perylene, benzo(k)fluoranthene, chrysene, dibenzo(a,h)anthracene, fluoranthene, fluorene, indeno(1,2,3-cd)pyrene, naphthalene, phenanthrene and pyrene.
2. Soil was extracted with methylene chloride/acetone mixture (9:1) 30 minutes after fortification. The soil-solvent mixture was sonicated. The extract was analyzed by GC method 8015.
3. Soil was extracted with an equal amount (w/v) of isopropanol 30 minutes after fortification. The extract was analyzed by GC method 8015.

Assay performance

Sensitivity and reproducibility

Standard dose response curves were obtained using the sixteen component PAH mix diluted in isopropanol (Figure 9.1). A minimum detection limit of

0.7ppm was determined to be the level of analyte which could be differentiated from a negative sample with 95% confidence (two standard deviations from the mean). The linear quantitative range is defined as the level of analyte required to give between 20 and 80% inhibition in the assay. Quantitative ranges of 0.7 to 15.0ppm and 7.0 to 140ppm were determined for the low and high ranges respectively. Analysis of replicate samples gave relative standard deviations (% cv) of approximately 30%. This is similar to the precision obtained by conventional GC/MS SW-846 method 8270 analysis.

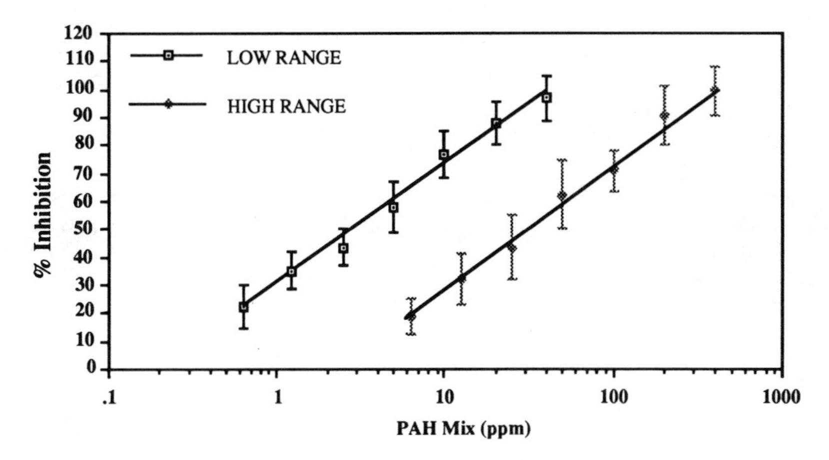

Figure 9.1. Dose response curves for the Quantix PAH assay illustrating quantitation over the range of 0.7ppm to 140ppm.

Specificity and Crossreactivity

Reactivity profiles were obtained for individual components of the PAH standard (Table 9.2). Acenaphthylene was found to be the most reactive with a minimum detection limit (MDL) of 0.2ppm. A six component BTEX standard containing equal amounts of benzene, toluene, ethylbenzene and o-, m- and p-xylene was tested and gave an MDL of 31.2ppm. MDLs of 0.6 and 1.9ppm were obtained for 1-methyl naphthalene and 2-methylnaphthalene respectively. A mixture containing equal amounts of all isomers of dimethylnaphthalenes gave an MDL of 3.1ppm. Gasoline, jet fuel and heating fuel oils #2 and #6 gave MDLs ranging from 15.5ppm to 100ppm total PAH. For diesel, MDLs ranged from 7.8ppm to 38.0ppm while MDLs for kerosene ranged from 62.5ppm to 250ppm. Different levels of PAH were found in samples of the fuels tested by immunoassay and were confirmed by GC method 8270. The immunoassay was particularly sensitive to a sample of creosote and gave an MDL of 1.0ppm. Low reactivities were obtained for certain PAH compounds such as benzo(a)pyrene, chrysene and anthracene due to their poor solubility in an aqueous medium. Toluene, benzene, polychlorinated biphenyls and pentachlorophenol were also not detected in the immunoassay. No reactivity was found for samples of motor oil, waste oil and roofing tar at the concentrations tested in the immunoassay.

Table 9.2. Reactivity profile for various compounds, fuel types and oils.

Analyte	Minimum detection limit[1] (ppm)
PAH mixture	0.7
Phenanthrene	0.3
Naphthalene	1.2
Fluorene	1.6
1-Methylfluorene	2.0
Acenaphthylene	0.2
Acenaphthene	0.6
Pyrene	0.4
BTEX	31.2
o-Xylene	41.4
m-Xylene	103.3
Benzene	>1000
Toluene	>500
1-Methylnaphthalene	0.6
2-Methylnaphthalene	1.9
1,2,3,4-Tetrahydronaphthalene	3.9
Dimethylnaphthalenes	3.1
Biphenyl	31.2
Aroclor 1016	>3.5
Aroclor 1268	>3.5
Gasoline (Exxon 93)	38.3
Gasoline (Exxon 87)	66.2
Gasoline (SU2000)	78.9
Diesel (Shell)	7.8
Diesel (Exxon)	12.5
Diesel (Texaco)	23.0
Diesel (Top Gas)	38.0
Diesel (Getty)	25.0
Fuel Oil #2 (Crystal)	30.3
Fuel Oil #2 (Obergfel)	50.0
Fuel Oil #2	37.0
Fuel Oil #6	62.8
Kerosene (Exxon)	62.5
Kerosene (Texaco-1)	80.0
Kerosene (Texaco-2)	19.0
Kerosene (Shell)	100.0
Kerosene (Westmont)	250.0
JP-4	15.5
JP-5	100.0
Creosote	1.0

[1] Minimum Detection Limit is defined as the concentration of analyte required to produce 20% inhibition in the immunoassay. Anthracene, Benzo(a)pyrene, Chrysene and Pentachlorophenol, were not detected up to their individual limits of solubility in the buffer medium. Samples of motor oil, waste oil and roofing tar were not detected in the immunoassay.

Matrix effects

The frequency of false positive results was determined by spiking sandy loam soil extract at half the detection limit (0.33ppm) with the sixteen component PAH standard and testing 35 replicate samples. An additional 35 replicate results of the unspiked soil extract were also obtained. No false positive results were found for the unspiked matrix while 13 (37%) false positive results were recorded for the PAH spike. The positive bias incorporated into this assay reduces the chance of false negatives.

The frequency of false negative results was determined by spiking soil extract at twice the detection limit and testing 35 replicate samples. Only one (2.8%) false negative result was obtained.

Three different soil sample matrices (clay, clay loam and sandy loam) were spiked in the low and high range at 3.5 and 35ppm respectively with the sixteen component PAH standard and ten replicates of each were tested for matrix effects (Table 9.3). An additional ten replicate results for the respective unspiked soil extracts were also obtained. PAH spikes in isopropanol were also analyzed. Unspiked soil extracts for each sample were negative in the immunoassay. Results for the low range spike averaged between 3.8 and 4.9ppm and between 45.4 and 53.3ppm for the high range spike. Similar results for each matrix in both ranges indicate the absence of matrix interferences.

Table 9.3. Recovery of PAH spikes in various soil types.

	PAH Recovery from Matrix		
Matrix	Isopropanol spike (ppm)	Soil Exact (ppm)	Percent Recovery
Clay Soil			
0	<0.7	<0.7	NA
3.5	4.4	4.9	111.4
35.0	45.4	51.6	113.7
Clay Loam Soil			
0	<0.7	<0.7	NA
3.5	4.4	3.8	86.4
35.0	45.4	53.3	117.4
Sandy Loam Soil			
0	<0.7	<0.7	NA
3.5	4.4	3.8	86.4
35.0	45.4	51.9	114.3

Each result shown above is a mean of ten replicates.
[1] Adjusted %=(PAH recovery from matrix/PAH Recovery from Isopropanol) x 100
[2] Not applicable.

Comparison of immunoassay to U.S. EPA SW-846 Methods 8015 and 8270

Addition recovery experiments for PAH fortification of soil

The soil aliquots were fortified with the PAH mixture at four different concentrations and extracted with an equal amount (w/v) of isopropanol. The extract was split and one aliquot was analyzed by immunoassay and the other by GC method 8015 (FID). An excellent correlation (R^2=0.98) was obtained between the two methods (Figure 9.2).

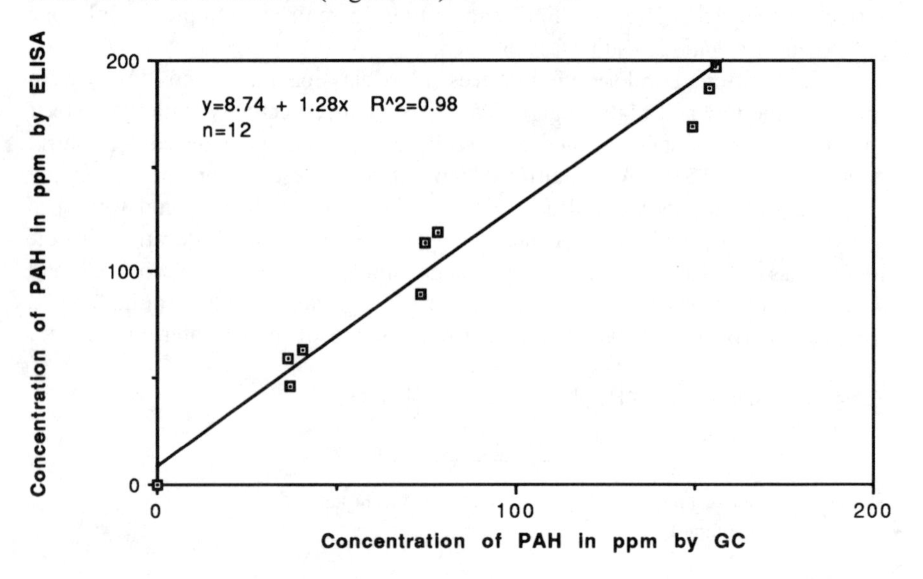

Figure 9.2. Comparison of immunoassay and GC-FID (modified 8015) analysis of isopropanol extracts from PAH spiked soils.

Analysis of various fuel samples by Quantix PAH Workstation and GC method 8270

Samples of fuels such as diesel, kerosene, fuel oil #2 (heating oil) and jet fuel were analyzed using the two methods. The results of this study are summarized in Table 9.4.

The concentration of PAH by immunoassay is the sum of the crossreactivities of individual compounds detected by the antibody. The GC/MS method 8270 data gives the concentration of PAHs corresponding to the sixteen component PAH standard and the other PAHs identified in the sample based upon retention time and the mass spectrum. The results indicate that the PAH concentration varies widely within samples of the same fuel and among various fuels. The percent PAH in the fuel samples as determined by GC method 8270 ranged from 0.4% to 1.7%.

Soil Addition-Recovery Experiments with Kerosene

The Quantix PAH immunoassay and the standard laboratory GC/MS method 8270 were used to analyze split isopropanol extracts of soil samples spiked with kerosene. Excellent agreement was observed between the two methods. Comparison of the total PAH values as measured by both methods for ten kerosene spiked soil samples across the analytical range demonstrated a high degree of correlation with an $R^2 = 0.91$ (Figure 9.3).

Table 9.4. Analysis of various fuel samples by immunoassay and GC method 8270

	Total PAH in ppm and as percent of fuel		
Fuel type	GC Method 8270 (ppm)	Immunoassay (ppm)	[IA]/[GC][1]
JET FUEL			
Sample 1	6510 (0.7%)	28786 (2.9%)	4.42
Sample 2	3752 (0.4%)	8441 (0.8%)	2.25
DIESEL FUEL			
Sample 1	17197 (1.7%)	64421 (6.4%)	3.75
Sample 2	8235 (0.8%)	10643 (1.1%)	1.29
KEROSENE			
Sample 1	4736 (0.5%)	4800 (0.5%)	1.01
Sample 2	11329 (1.1%)	29268 (2.9%)	2.58
FUEL OIL #2			
Sample 1	13039 (1.3%)	32000 (3.2%)	2.45

[1] Ratio of PAH concentration determined by immunoassay to concentration determined by GC method 8270.

Soil Addition-Recovery Experiments with Heating Oil

The Quantix PAH immunoassay and the standard laboratory GC/MS method 8270 were used to analyze split isopropanol extracts of soil samples spiked with fuel oil. Comparison of the total PAH values as measured by both methods for ten fuel oil spiked soil samples across the analytical range demonstrated a correlation of $R^2 = 0.72$ (Figure 9.4).

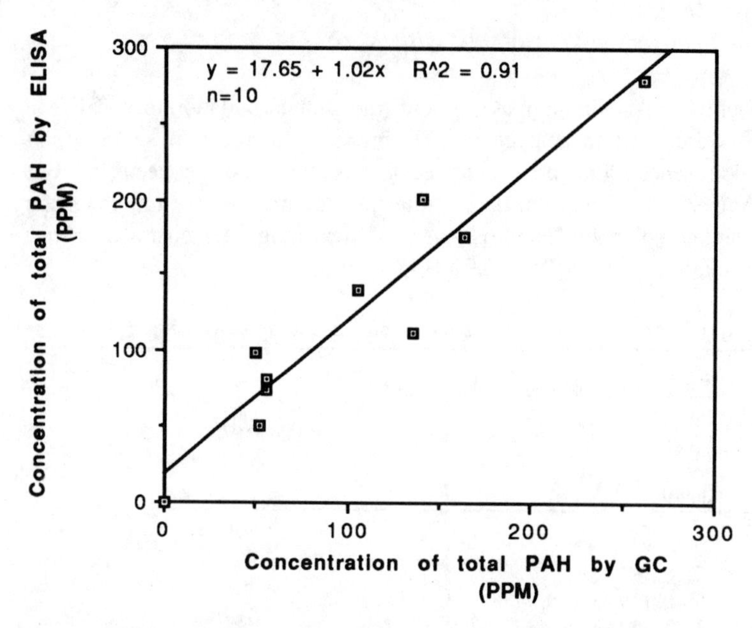

Figure 9.3. Comparison of total PAH analysis using the Quantix immunoassay and EPA method 8270 on isopropanol extracts of kerosene spiked soil.

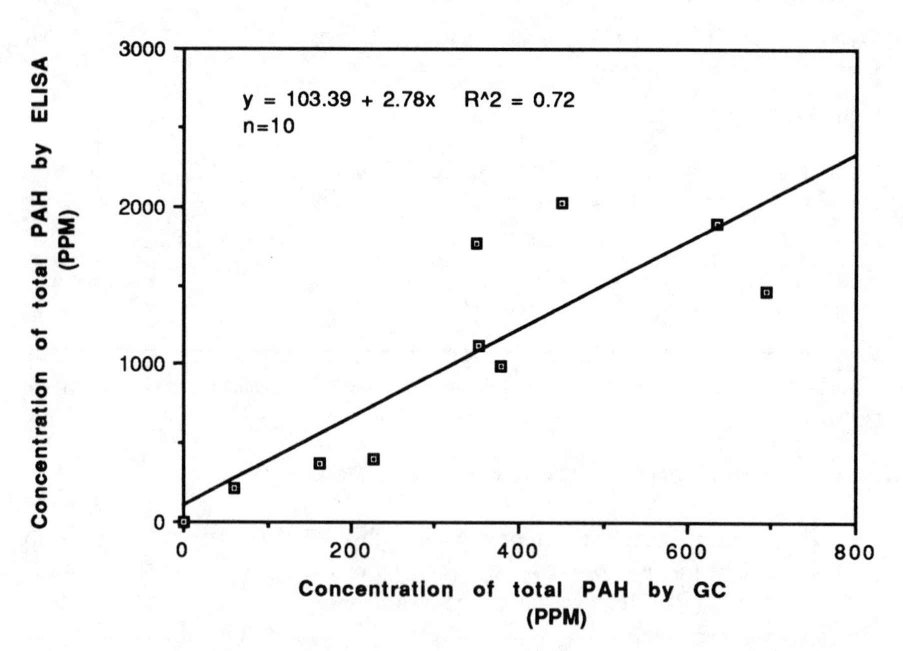

Figure 9.4. Comparison of total PAH analysis using the Quantix immunoassay and EPA method 8270 on isopropanol extracts of fuel oil spiked soil.

Correlation of the immunoassay with GC method 8270 was very good considering the complex nature of the fuels. The concentration of PAH found in the samples of fuels tested is a small percentage of the fuel in all the samples tested. It is often not possible to associate a specific chemical to every peak in the total ion chromatographs. This is particularly evident with fuel oil. The total ion chromatographs for fuel oil indicate the presence of a number of peaks which were not attributable to a specific compound and therefore were not taken into calculation for total PAH concentration. This leads to an underestimation of the concentration of total PAH by GC method 8270. It is likely that some of these compounds may be crossreactive in the immunoassay and may contribute in part to the positive bias for this method.

CONCLUSION

This chapter describes an immunoassay for the quantitation of PAH contamination in soil. The immunoassay enables the user to obtain rapid, on-site quantitation of PAH in a cost effective manner. The entire assay can be used to analyze up to five samples in thirty minutes. The immunoassay system has a detection limit of 0.7ppm for the sixteen component PAH standard. Sensitivities for individual components are even lower. The reproducibility obtained using immunoassay is comparable to that obtained using the U.S. EPA methods 8015 and 8270 over the linear range of the assay. The broad reactivity of the immunoassay is particularly useful as a screening tool and the positive bias reduces the possibility of obtaining false negative results. Additional validation studies with field samples are underway in our laboratory and will be reported in the near future.

REFERENCES

1. Potter, T.L. and Bruya, J.; "Analytical Techniques for Determining Petroleum Products in Soils," *Seventh Annual Conference on Hydrocarbon Contaminated Soils,* Amherst, Massachusetts (1992).
2. Johnson, B.L.; "Public Health Effects of Hazardous Waste in the Environment," *Hazardous Waste: Detection, Control, Treatment,* R. Abbou, Ed., Elsevier Science Publishers, Amsterdam, 1017-1035, (1988).
3. Potter, T.L.; "Analysis of Petroleum Contaminated Soil and Water: An Overview," *Petroleum Contaminated Soils,* E.J. Calabrese and P.T. Kostecki, Ed., Lewis Publishers, Chelsea, Michigan, Vol. 2, 97-110, (1990).
4. Federal Register, Vol. 52(74), 12664 (1987).
5. "Test Methods for Evaluating Solid Waste; Physical/Chemical Methods", SW-846, Third Edition, Office of Solid Waste and Emergency Response, U.S. EPA, Washington, DC, (1986).
6. Duquet, D., Dewaele, C., and Verzele, M.; "Coupling Micro-LC and Capillary GC as a Powerful Tool for the Analysis of Complex Mixtures," *J. High Res. Chromatog. and Chromatog. Commun.,* 11, 252-256, (1988).

7. Stocker, D.R., Miller, S.M., Rittenburg, J.H., Twamley, C., Lal, B.S., and Grothaus, G.D.; "Analysis of Gasoline in Soil and Water using a Rapid On-site Immunoassay System, " E.J. Calabrese and P.T. Kostecki, Ed., Lewis Publishers, in press.
8. Rittenburg, J.H., Fitzpatrick, D.A., Stocker, D.R., and Grothaus, G.D.; "Development of simple and rapid immunoassay systems for analysis of pesticides," *Brighton Crop Protection Conf. Proc.,* Lavenham Press Limited, Lavenham, U.K., Publ., 281, (1991).
9. Rittenburg, J.H., Grothaus, G.D., Fitzpatrick, D.A., and Lankow, R.K.; "Rapid on-site immunoassay systems," *Immunoassays for Trace Chemical Analysis,* Vanderlaan, M., Stanker, L.H., and Watkins, B.E., Ed., ACS Symposium Series No. 451, American Chemical Society, Washington, DC, 28, (1991).
10. U.S. EPA draft communication dated March 1, 1993.
11. Rittenburg, J.H., Stocker, D.R., and McCaffrey, C. R.; "Application of an immunoassay field test kit for measuring BTEX in Gasoline contaminated samples," *Federal Environmental Restoration Conference Proceedings*, 343-348, (1993).
12. Sampling and Analytical Methods for Petroleum Hydrocarbons in Groundwater and Soil, American Petroleum Institute, Washington, DC, 1987.

ACKNOWLEDGMENTS

The authors are grateful to Dr. Viorica Lopez-Avila and Mr. Richard Young of Midwest Research Institute-California Operations for their work with gas chromatography portion of this chapter and their helpful advice in designing the validation study.

CHAPTER 10

The Development of an Analytical Manual for Determining Petroleum Products in the Environment

M.W. Miller and H.T. Hoffman, Jr. New Jersey Department of Environmental Protection and Energy, Trenton, New Jersey

INTRODUCTION

The field of Environmental Analysis began during the 1960s and early 1970s when major oil spills occurred around the world. Analytical methods were needed to determine the type and source of the oil.[1-3] The early 1980s was the time for the development of analytical methods to identify and quantify hazardous compounds in the environment. Soil and aqueous matrices were evaluated.[4-7] These hazardous compound methods were and still are used by chemists to evaluate petroleum contaminated sites. The methods are not specific for petroleum products.

In 1987, the New Jersey Department of Environmental Protection and Energy (NJDEPE), Office of Quality Assurance (OQA) formed a department-wide committee to evaluate analytical methods for determining petroleum products in the environment. The committee found that the department administers seven programs concerned with petroleum products. The programs are Underground Storage Tanks, Industrial Site Recovery Act, N.J. Pollution Discharge Elimination Systems, Resource Conservation and Recovery Act, Superfund, New Jersey Spill Fund, and Sludge Quality Assurance Regulations. The committee found that there was no clear policy to determine which methods were appropriate or required for a given program. In addition, many of the methods did not contain adequate quality control procedures. In the absence of regulatory analytical procedures the committee and OQA has worked to establish a department methods manual. D.M. Stankin, et al. discussed the background studies for the Manual at the 1988 Environmental Protection Agency Solid Waste Conference.[8,9] At the Fourth and Fifth Conferences on Petroleum Contaminated Soils M. W. Miller et al. discussed the organization and content of the Manual.[10,11] The authors emphasized the importance of standard method format, calibration for petroleum compounds, quality control and data deliverables. The papers described specific methods contained in the Manual.

In this chapter the authors will discuss the draft Manual that is ready for peer review by the laboratory community.

OVERVIEW

Methods contained in the draft Analytical Chemistry Manual for Petroleum Products in the Environment are adoptions of existing analytical methods which have been modified to satisfy the need for petroleum product analyses in seven mandated programs managed by the NJDEPE.[12] These methods have been published by the American Society for Testing and Materials, American Public Health Association and the USEPA.[2-7] Authors conducting research for the American Petroleum Institute (API) have presented similar methods.[13-15] The methods presented in this Manual follow the format of the USEPA 600 Series Waste Water Methods.[5] Table 10.1 is an index of the 14 laboratory methods. The table lists the reference method, the techniques, and the EPA data quality objective (DQO). The DQOs are identified as the Analytical Level. Qualitative, semi-quantitative, and quantitative methods for aqueous and solid matrices are included. In most cases separate methods are written for aqueous and solid matrices.

Table 10.1. Petroleum Product Analytical Methods

NJDEPE-OQA#	*REF	ANAL. LEVEL	TITLE	INSTRUMENT DETECTOR	SEPARATION
QAM-001	413.1 SW9070	II	Total Recoverable Oil and Grease from Water	Gravimetric	Extraction
QAM-002	413.2	II	Total Recoverable Oil and Grease from Water	Infrared Spectroscopy	Extraction
QAM-003	SW9071	II	Total Recoverable Oil and Grease from Sludge	Gravimetric	Extraction
QAM-004	418.1	II	Total Recoverable Petroleum Hydrocarbons in Water	Infrared Spectroscopy	Extraction
QAM-005	ERT-IR	II	Total Recoverable Petroleum Hydrocarbons in Soil	Infrared Spectroscopy	Extraction
QAM-008	CAL-602	III	Total Volatile Petroleum Products in Water by GC	GC-PID-FID	Purge & Trap
QAM-009	CAL-luft1 SW5030 API-GRO	III	Total Volatile Petroleum Products in Soil, Sediment and Waste by GC	GC-PID-FID	Extraction
QAM-011	EPA624	III, IV	Determination of Volatile Petroleum Products in Water by GC/MS	GC/MS	Purge & Trap
QAM-012	SW8240	III IV	Determination of Volatile Petroleum Products in Soil by GC/MS	GC/MS	Extraction Purge & Trap
QAM-014	EPA625 SW8270	III	Determination of Polynuclear Aromatic Hydrocarbons in Water, Soil, Sediment and Waste by GC/MS	Gc/MS	Extraction
QAM-15	EPA610	III	Determination of PAH in Petroleum Contaminated Water, Soil and Sediment by HPCL	HPLC/UV- Fluoroscence	Extraction

NJDEPE-OQA#	*REF	ANAL. LEVEL	TITLE	INSTRUMENT DETECTOR	SEPARATION
QAM-018	ASTM3328 SW8310 API-DRO	III	Identification and Quantitation of Total Petroleum Products in Water, Soil and Sediment	GC-PID-FID	Extraction
QAM-019	SW8015	III	Analysis of Oxygen Containing Petroleum Products in Water, by GC	GC-FID	Direct or Distillation
QAM-020	SW3010	II III	Static Headspace Analysis for Volatile Petroleum Products in Water and Soil	GC-PID-FID	Heat

*Ref.#

EPA6--USEPA,	(5)
SW----USEPA	(7)
41-.-USEPA	(4)
CAL California	(12)
ERT USEPA	(7)
API Amer. Petroleum Inst.	(16, 17)

Table 10.2 presents the analytical method outline. All methods are written in this format. Each method is designed to be a complete standard operating procedure. The reporting requirements section was not part of the original methods adapted for use in the Manual. The data deliverable package from a sampling event is critical to the user. There are many laboratories performing the analysis of petroleum contaminated samples. Data packages can vary from one sheet of numbers to a box full of data. For data to be comparable between laboratories the reporting requirements must be similar .

The data needs for site survey, site monitoring or site closure are different. If a case will end up in litigation the data deliverable must be complete. The amount of quality assurance and quality control performed for an analysis must be independent of the extent of the data deliverable.

Method quality control is the key to obtaining quality data. The elements of quality control are tabulated in Table 10.3. The Initial Demonstration of Laboratory Capability is the determination of the precision and accuracy that the laboratory is capable of achieving with the method. This demonstration should be performed each time the method is modified or the analyst is changed. For aqueous methods a QC check sample is spiked into reagent water. In soil methods a QC sample is spiked into reagent silica. The multiple check samples are carried through the entire method.

Table 10.2. General analytical method outline.

INTRODUCTION

Method Scope and Application
- Scope
- Objectives
- Type of Matrix
- Advantages of Method
- Limitations of Method

Method Summary
- Interferences
- Safety

ANALYTICAL METHOD

Reagents
Apparatus
Calibration
Method Quality Control
Sampling, Preservation and Storage
Procedure
Calculations

METHOD PERFORMANCE

Reporting Requirements
References

Table 10.3. Elements of Quality Control

1. Initial Demonstration of Laboratory Capability
2. Daily Instrument Quality Control Check Standard (or 1 per 20 samples)
3. Daily Method Blank
4. Trip and Field Blanks for Aqueous Matrix
5. Determination of Method Detection Limit
6. Weekly Analysis of a Low Level Standard to Confirm MDL (2xMDL)
7. Matrix Spike and Matrix Spike Duplicate
8. Determination of Surrogate Recovery
9. Blanks Spike and Blank Spike Duplicate
10. Maintain Control Charts for Surrogate Recovery, QC Sample Recovery and Spike.

The blanks are Item 3 and 4, Table 10.3. The method blank checks the cleanliness of the laboratory. Contamination of the sample with laboratory solvents is very common. The field and trip blanks check the exposure of the sample bottles and equipment to contaminants. A site cleanup could be falsely triggered by contamination of the sample.

The quality control limits are specified, in each method. The laboratory must experimentally determine the QC limits for every method the laboratory uses. The limits are determined when the laboratory demonstrates the initial ability to generate acceptable accuracy and precision with the method. A laboratory should not be engaged unless the QC requirements of the method can be met.

METHODOLOGY

The Manual contains 14 methods classified by petroleum type. The methods are listed in Table 10.1. There are three oil and grease methods, two total petroleum hydrocarbons methods, five volatile petroleum methods, three semi volatile petroleum methods and one oxygen containing petroleum products method. In most cases a separate method is written for aqueous and soil samples.

Oil and grease analysis is required of most facilities with waste water discharge permits. The methods are included in the Manual because the EPA Methods (413 series) do not contain quality control procedures or data reporting requirements.

The total petroleum hydrocarbon methods were discussed by the authors in a previous paper.[11] These are widely used screening methods because they are inexpensive. They are being replaced by colormetric and immunoassay field methods.[16,17] The drive to replace the methods is accelerating because Federal Clean Air rules require that Freon must be replaced by January 1995.

The five volatile petroleum methods include a headspace GC method, two GC/MS purge and trap methods and two GC/purge and trap methods. The headspace method was discussed in a previous presentation.[11] Headspace methods are becoming widely used. Instrument manufactures have produced several automated units. V.D. Roe et al. have shown that with appropriate calibration the headspace results are equivalent to purge and trap results.[18] Soil and aqueous GC/MS purge and trap methods presented in the manual are used at petroleum and hazardous compound contaminated sites.

Positive identification of specific compounds is required at these sites. The methods are similar to the SW-846 solid waste methods except they include calibration for petroleum products.[6] The manual contains soil and aqueous photoionization (PID) flame ionization (FID), and gas chromatography purge and trap methods for volatile petroleum products. The methods can determine total light fuel hydrocarbons: gasoline (C4-C12), jet fuel (C10-C16) and kerosene (C10-C18). The methods also detect the light components of diesel fuel. The total petroleum hydrocarbons concentration is found by integrating the total FID chromatographic area. Individual quantitative values are obtained from the PID for benzene, toluene, ethylbenzene, and xylene (BTEX), methyl tert-butyl ether (MTBE) and tert butyl alcohol. The soil method was discussed in detail at the Fifth Hydrocarbon Contaminated Soils Conference.[11]

The aqueous method is adapted with modifications from the California Leaking Underground Fuel Tanks Manual and USEPA Method 602.[5,12] Figure 1, is a flow diagram for the method. The key to the method is the calibration of the GC with a petroleum standard that covers the range of volatile petroleum products that can be purged from water. The method suggests the use of the suspected spilled petroleum product for calibration. The normal calibration material is a hydrocarbon blend containing alkanes (C4-C18), alkane isomers and substituted benzenes. The GC is also calibrated for BTEX and MTBE. The FID chromatographic pattern indicates the type of petroleum product that is the source of contamination.

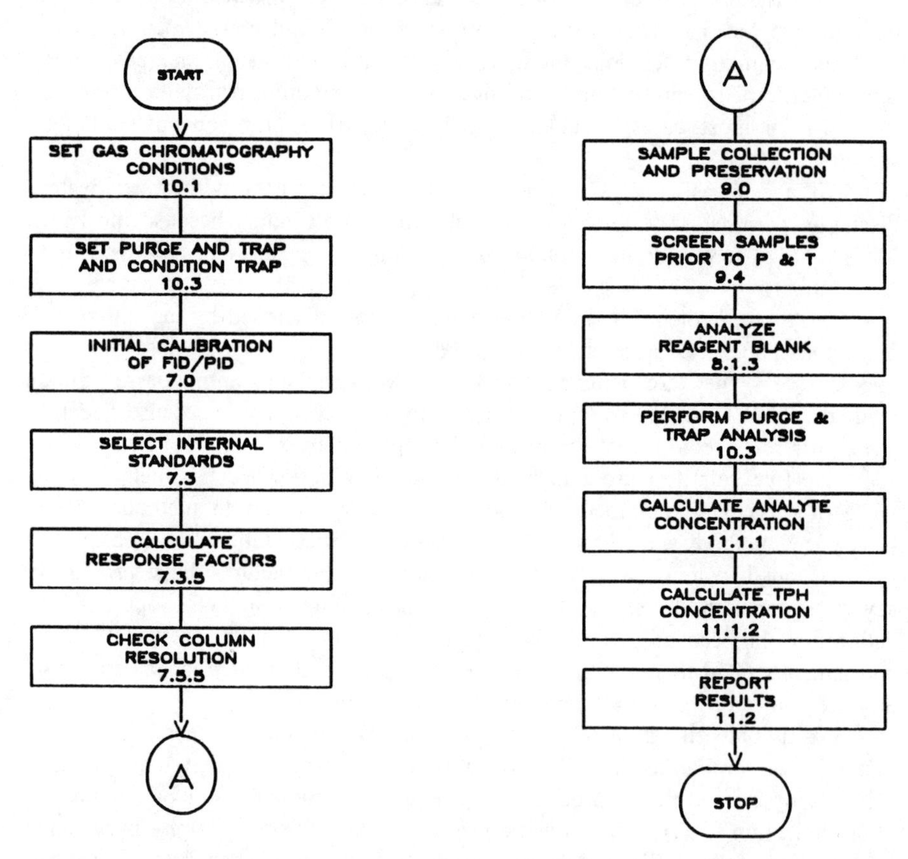

Figure 10.1. Total volatile petroleum products in water by GC analysis OQA-QAM-008.

The American Petroleum Institute (API) has sponsored the development of a GC purge and trap method for gasoline contaminated soil.[14] The gasoline range organics (GRO) method has been subject to an interlaboratory evaluation.[19] The volatile petroleum GC methods in this manual are similar to the API method except they cover volatile petroleum products in addition to gasoline. The methods must quantitate all detected hydrocarbons because the NJDEPE evaluates sites based upon total petroleum hydrocarbons (TPH).

Three semivolatile petroleum methods are presented in the manual. Each method can be used for contaminated water or soils. The high pressure liquid chromatography (HPLC) method is adapted from the USEPA Solid Waste SW-846 Method 8310.[6] The method is a cost effective way of monitoring polynuclear aromatic hydrocarbons in petroleum contaminated water and soil during site cleanup. R. Beach et al. have used a similar method in a mobile laboratory to evaluate a large site.[20]

The most frequently asked question at facilities with underground storage tanks is: What is the level of petroleum contamination of soil and groundwater? Across the United States many efforts are being made to replace the infrared-freon extraction, total petroleum hydrocarbons method with GC methods. The manual contains a photoionization-flame ionization-GC method for semivolatile petroleum products based upon the American Society for Testing and Materials (ASTM) oil identification method, D3328-82 and USEPA Solid Waste SW-846 Method 8100.[2,6] The authors presented the method at the 5th Hydrocarbon Contaminated Soils Conference.[11] The method is designed to determine total semivolatile petroleum contamination (TPH), to obtain a chromatographic pattern for product identification and to quantitative individual aromatic compounds. The method can be used for floating product, petroleum dissolved in water and petroleum contaminated soils. Sealed extractions are used to reduce vapor loss and retain the volatile petroleum products. Aqueous samples are extracted in the sample bottle using vortex mixing with a magnetic stirrer. Soil samples are mixed with anhydrous sodium sulfate and methylene chloride, placed in a sealed flask and shaken on wrist action shaker. Figure 10.2 is a revised flow diagram for the determination of semivolatile petroleum products.

Since the author's presentation in September 1990, ASTM has proposed a revision to method D-3328 to include sediments. G.S. Douglas presented experimental data at the 6th Hydrocarbon Contaminated Soils Conference that is being used in the ASTM revision.[21] API has completed an interlaboratory study of a GC-FID method for diesel fuel contaminated soil, the diesel range method (DRO).[19] The calibration of the method is limited to the carbon range for diesel fuel (C12-C28).

The NJDEPE and ASTM GC methods are broad range methods that include gasoline through heavy fuel oil (C7-C36). The methods detect any compound extractable with methylene chloride. The total area of the chromatogram minus the solvent method blank and leaf hydrocarbons is equal to the total petroleum hydrocarbon concentration. The TPH concentration is used for site evaluations. The use of combined PID and FID produces an aromatic pattern and a total petroleum products pattern that improves the possibility of identifying the contamination source.

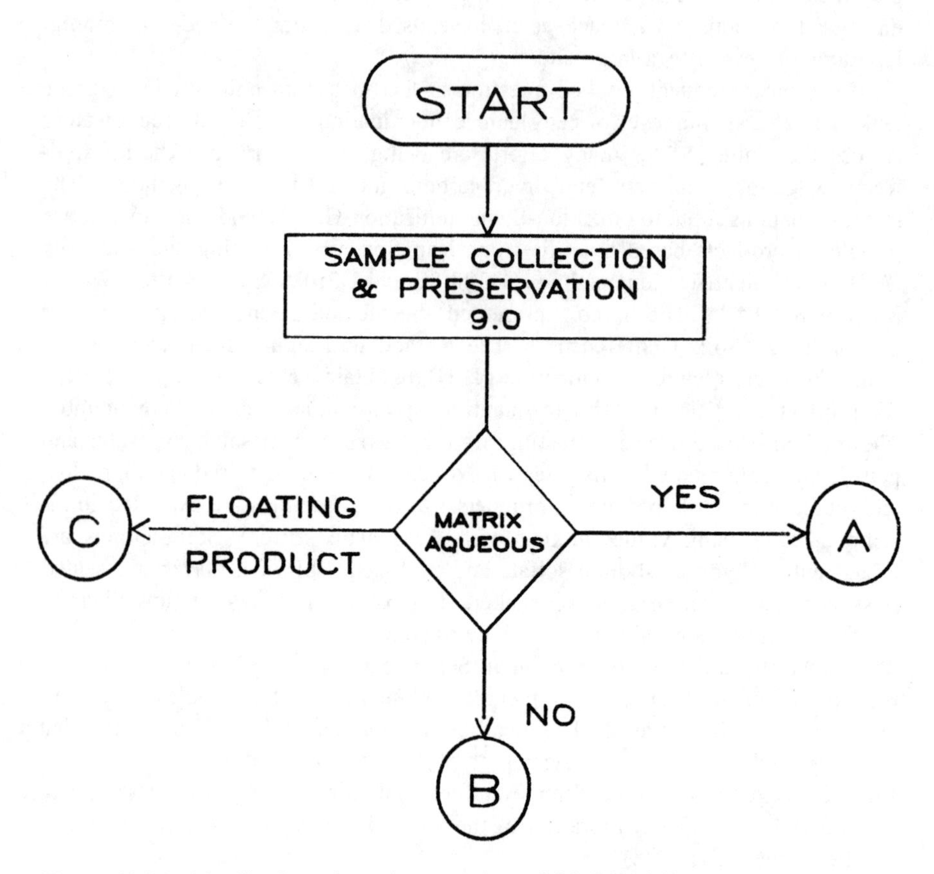

Figure 10.2.1. Identification of petroleum product. OQA-QAM-018.

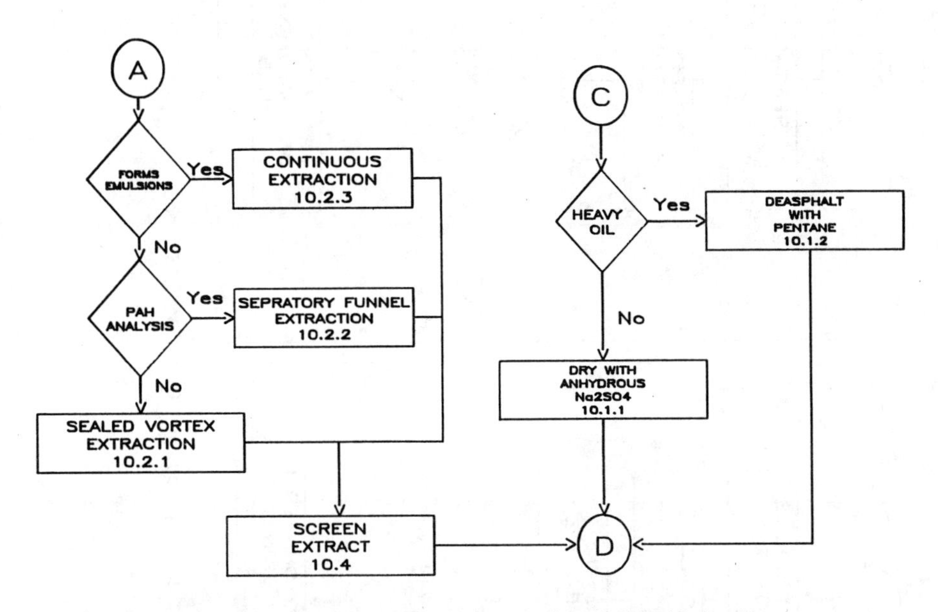

Figure 10.2.2. Identification of petroleum products. OQA-QAM-018 (cont.)

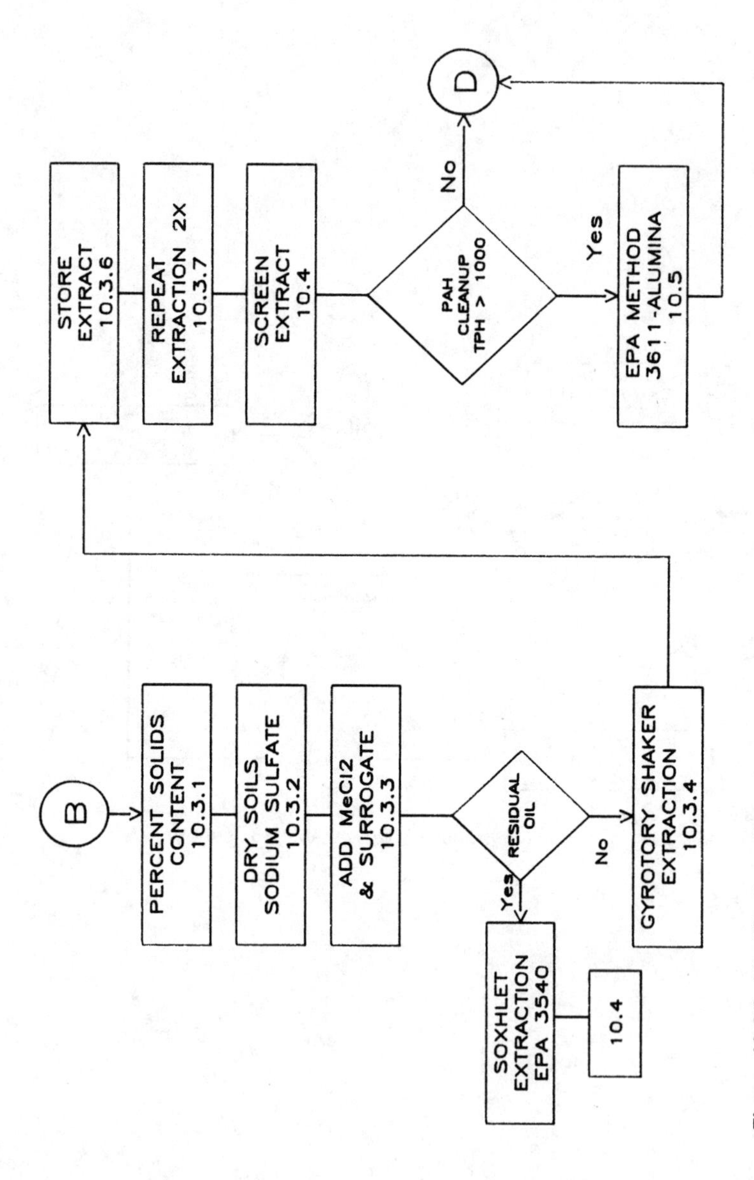

Figure 10.2.3 Identification of petroleum products. OQA-QAM-018 (cont.)

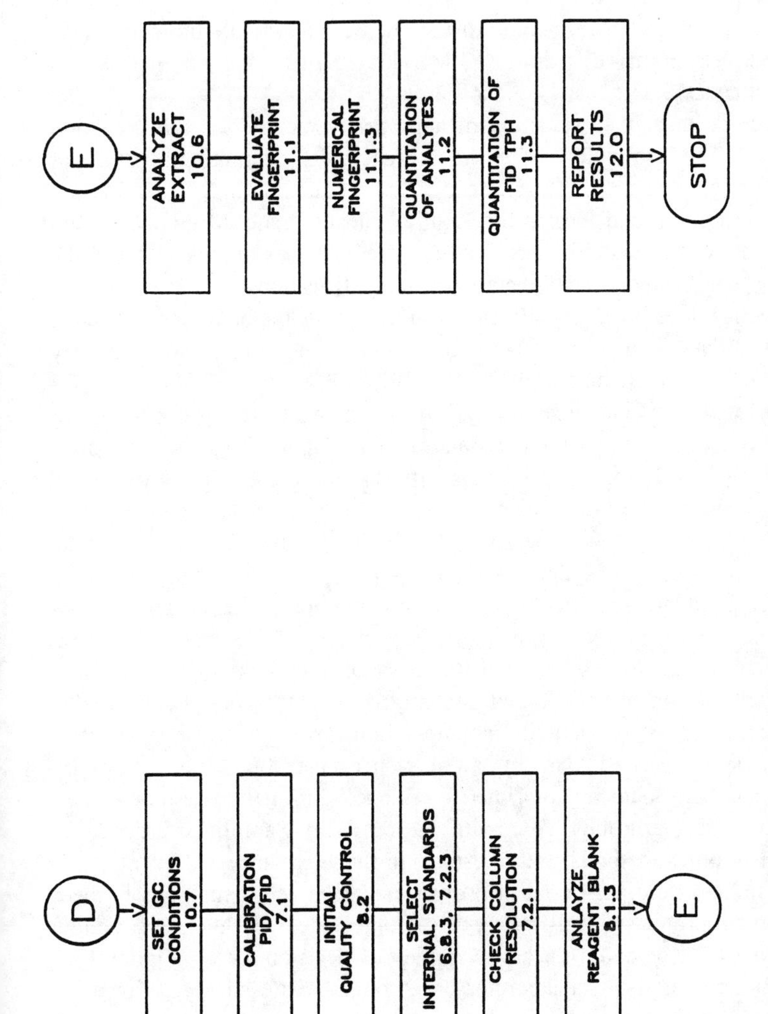

Figure 10.2.4. Identification of petroleum products OQA-QAM-018 (cont.)

The semivolatile petroleum analysis by GC/MS has two key applications; determination of polynuclear aromatic hydrocarbons (PAHs) in petroleum contaminated matrices and determination of the party responsible for the contamination by matching biomarker compounds. The determination of PAHs is important because they are consider hazardous compounds under National Pollution Discharge Elimination and Superfund regulations. These compounds drive the site cleanup conditions. The use of biomarkers to determine the source of contamination has increased in importance in recent years. Several authors have published papers using single monitoring GC/MS to evaluate biomarkers.[21-23] W.A. Saner has prepared a draft GC/MS source identification method for ASTM committee D19.31.[24]

A users guide to help in selection of appropriate methods is a key section of the manual. The evaluation of a site for chemical contamination can be divided into five general areas: Site Survey, Site Contamination Confirmation, Remedial Investigation and Feasibility Study, Cleanup and Monitoring, and Closure. The analytical methods used for the different areas mainly differ in the degree of quantitation and need for compound identification.

The EPA has developed guidelines for determining the analytical methods and the chemical data needed to evaluate contaminated Superfund sites. The key to the system is the establishment of Data Quality Objectives (DQOs). DQOs are statements of the level of uncertainty a decision maker is willing to accept in results derived from environmental data.[25] To support the DQO approach Analytical Levels are defined. The levels differ in the amount of QA/QC and the degree of specific compounds identification. The EPA system contains five levels. The first three levels can be applied directly to petroleum contaminated sites. The fourth levels can be applied directly to petroleum contaminated sites and can be applied to specific petroleum compounds. Level five is for compounds that require the development of a special analytical method. Table 10.1 lists the analytical level of each of the methods presented in the manual.

The current edition of the Manual does not contain the Analytical Level I, field survey methods. These methods include soil gas by organic vapor detector, petroleum by spot tests, PAHs by fluorescence detection, petroleum by immunoassay and petroleum by colorimetry. The soil gas methods are described in the Division of Hazardous Site Mitigation, Field Sampling Procedures Manual.[(26)] The other methods are described in the literature.[(12, 13, 14)]

In order to help field personnel or project managers select methods to meet the DQO of their projects "decision trees" are presented in the Users Guide. Figures 10.3, 10.4, 10.5, and 10.6 are examples of decision trees. Figure 10.3 is the decision tree for using a laboratory method in a site survey. The path taken depends on if the survey is for the total petroleum product concentration or the specific type of petroleum product present.

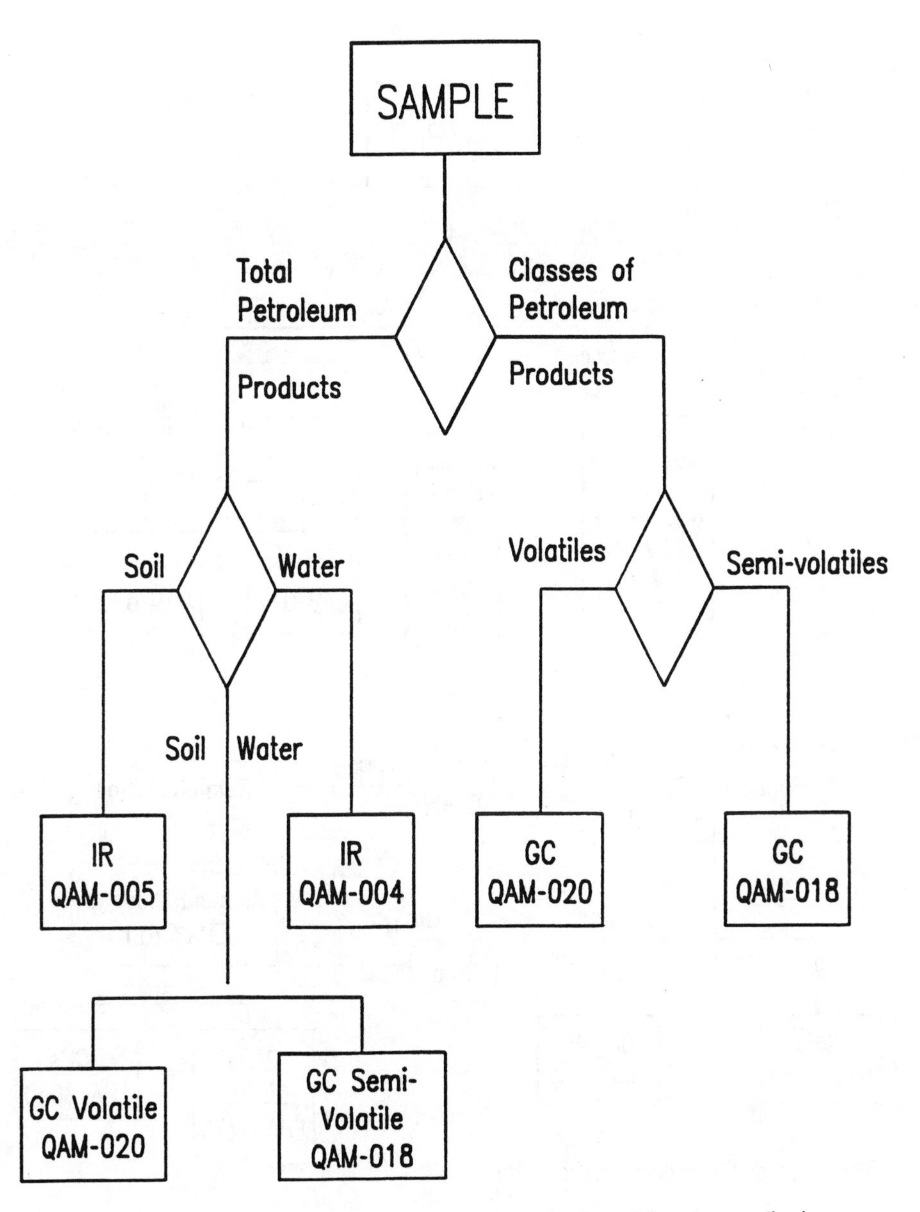

Figure 10.3. Site survey for petroleum product contamination: laboratory methods.

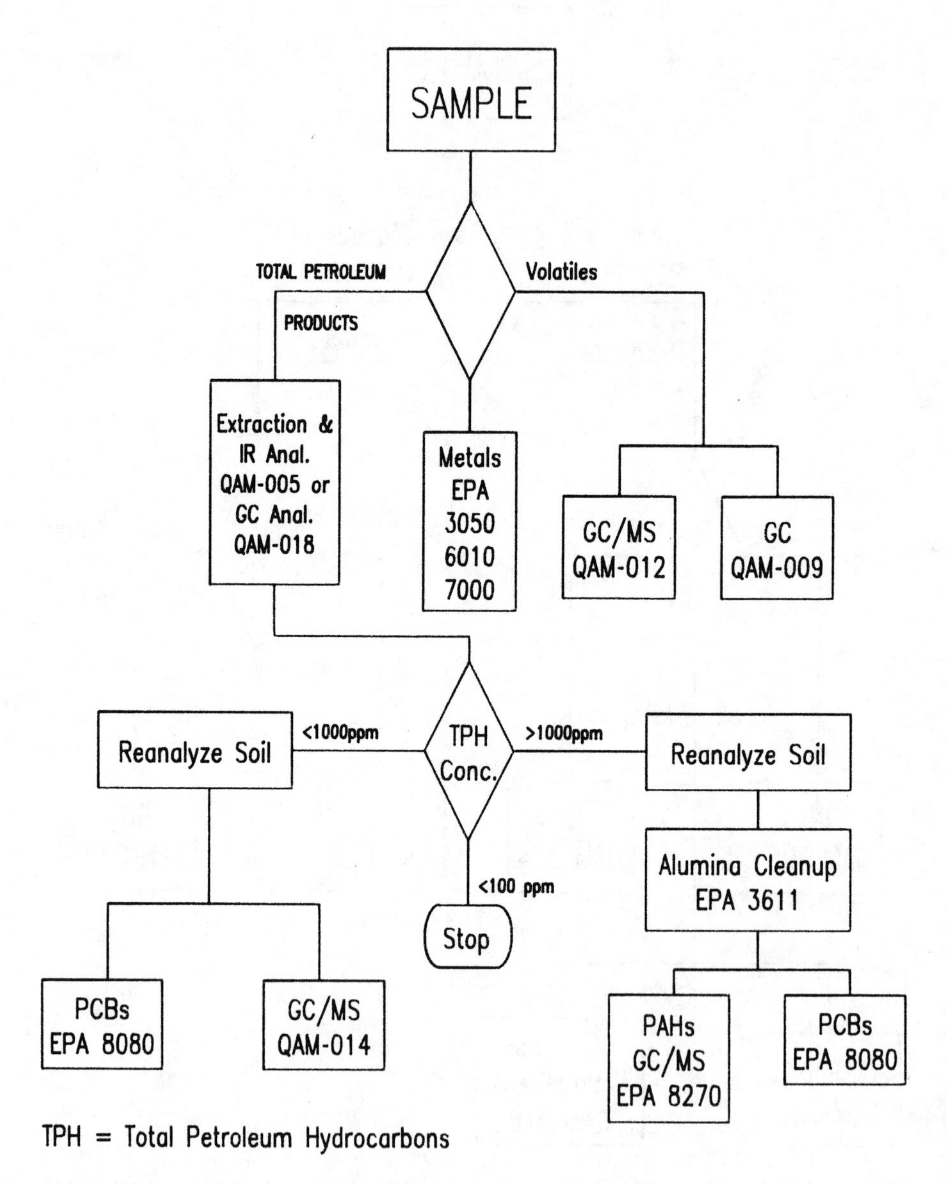

Figure 10.4. Determination of priority pollutants, substituted aromatics and polynuclear aromatics in petroleum contaminated soils.

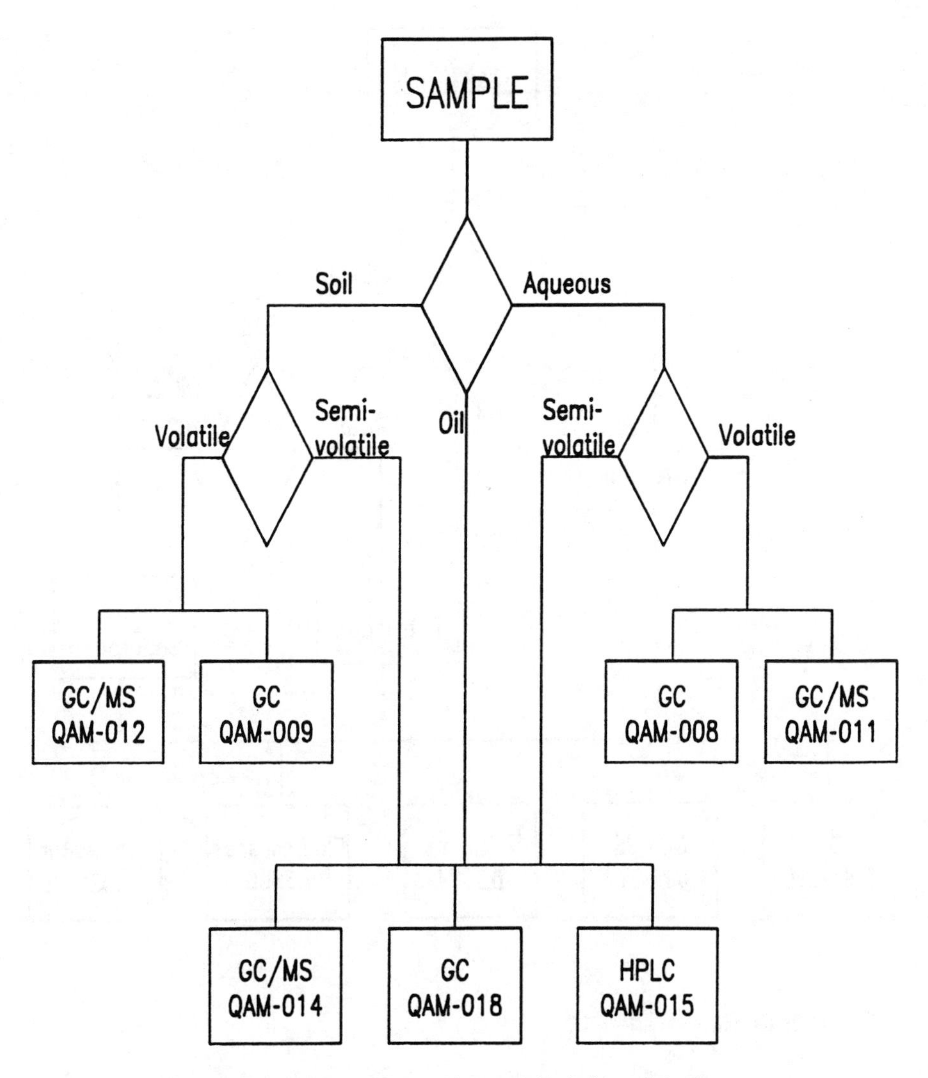

Figure 10.5. Quantitation of petroleum products and priority pollutants.

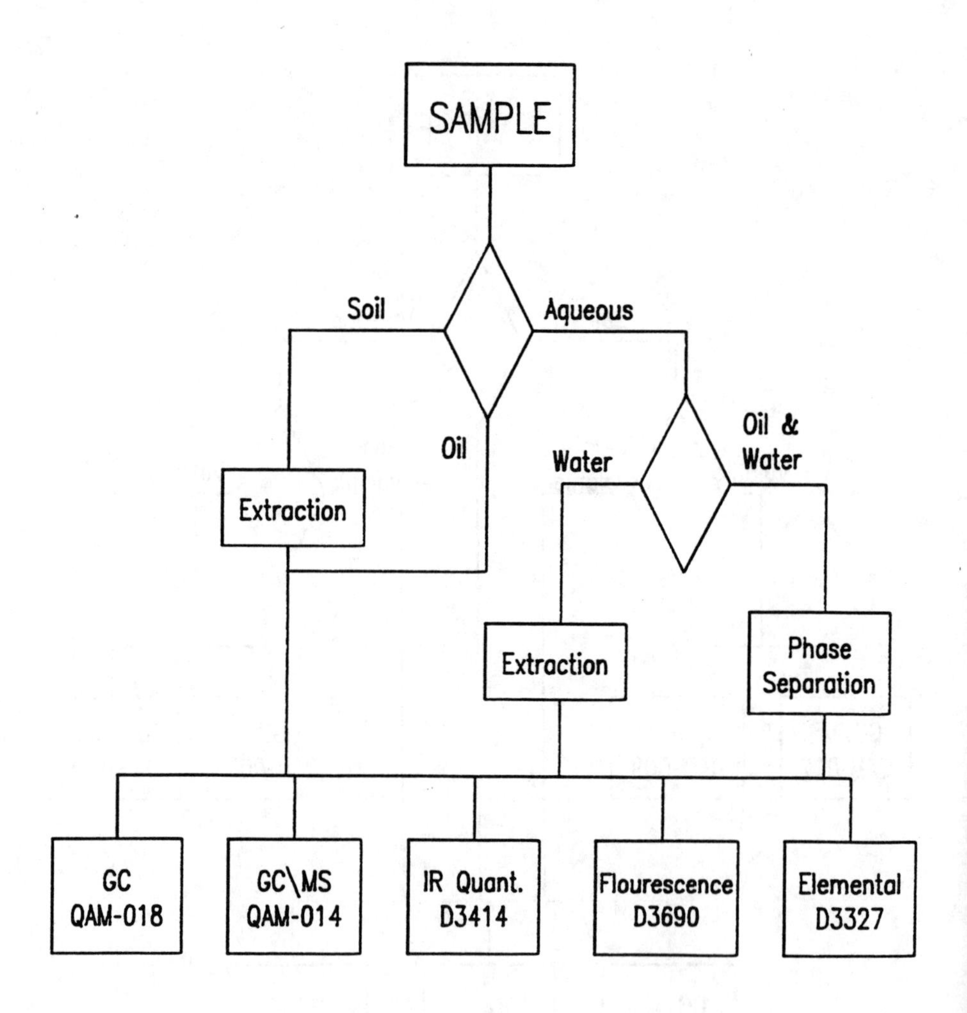

Figure 10.6. Determination of responsible party: pattern recognition.

Figure 10.4 presents the decision tree for determining the concentration of priority pollutants and specific petroleum products in contaminated soil and water. Figure 10.5 is a specific example of using a decision tree to select analytical methods to determine to petroleum product concentration for an underground storage tanks site cleanup. Figure 10.6 is a decision tree used to determine a responsible party.

Useability of the Methods

At this time (September 1993) the methods have not been tested by the Department's laboratory (Bureau of Organic Laboratory Services) due to lack of funding. Ideally the methods which contain changes in procedure should be formally validated. Therefore, these methods are not official petroleum methods of the Department. These are suggested petroleum methods. Appendix A of the Users Guide presents an outline of the procedures necessary to obtain analytical sample data for the petroleum methods so that the methods can be validated. The appendix also contain suggested data reporting forms. Table 10.4 is a summary of the data validation outline.

Table 10.4. Data Requested for Method Validation Study

INSTRUMENTATION

Equipment Description
Operating Conditions

CALIBRATION

Initial Calibration, Summary Table
Continuing Calibration
QC Sample Results

PRECISION and ACCURACY STUDY
METHOD DETECTION LIMITS STUDY

SAMPLE REPORTS

Sample Description; Matrix, Soil Type
Sample Results
Chromatograms
QC Results

The Office of Quality Assurance (OQA) requests that the laboratory community using these methods submit data voluntarily based on the outline. In order for the data from different laboratories to be comparable, the method procedures, calibrations and quality control must be followed closely. The OQA will collect and evaluate the submitted sample data. If the data supports the individual method the method will be added to the *New Jersey Department of Environmental Protection and Energy Directory of Approved Environmental*

Measurement and Laboratory Methods proposed in the revisions to the Laboratory Certification regulations N.J.A.C. 7:18.

CONCLUSION

The analytical objectives of the NJDEPEs that are concerned with the determination of petroleum product contamination are met by the Manual. Problems with current methods are addressed and modifications provided. The methods specify quality control procedures and reporting requirements. This helps the Manual user obtain analytical consistency between laboratories and improves data quality.

ACKNOWLEDGEMENTS

Please note that the interpretations and opinions expressed in this paper are those of the authors and should not be construed as official policy of the New Jersey Department of Environmental Protection. The authors would like to thank the members of the Petroleum Products Analysis Committee and of the Office of Quality Assurance for their contributions to the Manual.

REFERENCES

1. *Standard Methods of Examination of Water and Waste Water.* 17th ed. American Public Health Association, American Water Works Association, Water Pollution Control Federation, Washington DC, 1989.
2. American Society for Testing and Materials, Water (II), Volume 11.02. *Annual Book of ASTM Standards*, Philadelphia, PA, 1992.
3. U.S. Coast Guard Staff, *Oil Spill Identification System,* U.S. Coast Guard R & D Center, GC-D-52-77, 1977.
4. U.S. Environmental Protection Agency, 1979 "Methods for Chemical Analyses of Water and Waste Water," Revised 1983, EPA 600/4-79-020.
5. U.S. Environmental Protection Agency, "Guidelines Establishing Test Procedures for the Analyses of Pollutants Under the Clean Water Act; Final Rule and Interim Final Rule and proposed Rule," Federal Register 40 CFR Part 136, 1988.
6. U.S. Environmental Protection Agency, *Test Methods for Evaluating Solid Waste*, 3rd Edition, Office of Solid Waste Publication SW846, 1986.
7. Remeta, D.P., and Grundfeld, M. "Emergency Response Analytical Methods for Use On Board Mobile Laboratories," Internal Communication, USEPA Hazardous Waste Engineering Research Laboratory Release Control Branch, Edison, NJ, 1987.
8. Stainken, D., Miller, M. "Establishing an Analytical Manual for Petroleum and Gasoline Products for New Jersey's Environmental Program," *Proceedings of Symposium on Waste Testing and Quality Assurance,* Vol. II, USEPA, Office of Solid Waste, Washington, D.C., 1988.

9. Stainken, D., Miller, M., "Establishing an Analytical Manual for Petroleum and Gasoline Products for New Jersey's Environmental Program," *Waste Testing and Quality Assurance,* Vol. 2, American Society for Testing and Materials, STP 1062, Philadelphia, PA, 1990.
10. Miller, M., Stainken, D., "An Analytical Manual for Petroleum and Gasoline Products for New Jersey's Environmental Program," *Petroleum Contaminated Soils,* Vol. 3, p.383, Lewis Publishers, Chelsea, MI, 1990.
11. Miller, M., et al., "An Analytical Manual for Petroleum Products in the Environmental," *Hydrocarbon Contaminated Soils*, Vol. I, p257, Lewis Publishers, Chelsea, MI, 1991.
12. Simmons, B., Ed. *Leaking Underground Fuel Tank Underground Storage Tank Closure.* California Leaking Underground Fuel Tank Task Force, State Water Resources Control Board, Sacramento, CA, 1989.
13. "Evaluation of Proposed Analytical Methods to Determine Total Petroleum hydrocarbons in Soil and Groundwater," prepared by Midwest Research Institute for USEPA Office of Underground Storage Tanks, August 14, 1990.
14. Parr, J.L., G. Walters and M. Hoffman, "A Method for Determining Gasoline Range Organics in Soil and Groundwater," Presentation of the American Petroleum Institute Workshop on Analytical Methods for Petroleum Hydrocarbons, Colorado Springs, CO, February 26, 1992.
15. Parr, J.L., K. Selis and M. McDevitt, method for Determining Diesel Range Organics in Soil and Groundwater," Presentation American Petroleum Institute Workshop on Analytical Methods for Petroleum Hydrocarbons, Colorado Springs, CO, February 26, 1992.
16. Hanby, J.D., "A New Method for the Detection and Measurement of Aromatic Compounds in Water and Soil," Corporate Literature, Handy Analytical Laboratories, Inc., Houston, TX, 1989.
17. Friedman, S.B. "Immunoassay Methods for Environmental Field Screening," *Proceedings 8th Annual Waste Testing and Quality Assurance Symposium,* page 43, July 14-17, 1992.
18. Roe, V. D., Lacy, M.J, Stuart, J.D., 1989, "Manual Headspace Method to Analyze for the Volatile Aromatics of Gasoline in Groundwater and Soil Samples", Anal. Chem., 61, 2584-2985.
19. Jerry L. Parr et al, "Interlaboratory Study of Analytical Methods for Petroleum Hydrocarbons" ASTM Symposium: Analysis of Soil Contaminated with Petroleum Constituents, Atlanta, GA June 24, 1993.
20. Beach R. et al, "A Screening Method for Total Polynuclear Aromatics" Fourteenth Annual USEPA Conference on analysis of Pollutants in the Environmental Norfolk, VA May 1991.
21. Douglas, G.S. et al, "Hydrocarbon Finger Printing Analysis Factor Fiction?" *Proceedings of the Sixth Conference Petroleum Contaminated Soils*, Lewis Publishers, Chelsea, MI, 1992.

22. Sauer, T., Bochens, P., "The Use of Defensible Analytical Chemical Measurements for Oil Spill Natural Resources Damage Assessment," Oil Spill Conference 1991.
23. Butler, E.L., et al "Hopane, a new Chemical Tool for Measuring Oil Biodegradation," *On-site Bioreclamation,* pp 539, Butterworth-Heinemann, Stoneham, MA 1991.
23. Saner, W.A. "Standard Practice for Oil Spill Source Identification by Gas Chromatography and Positive Ion Electron Impact Low Resolution Mass Spectroscopy," Committee D10.31 communication, Draft 3, American Society for Testing and Materials, March 1993.
24. *Data Quality Objectives for Remedial Response Activities*, U.S. Environmental Protection Agency, RPA 540/G-87/003A, 1987.
25. *Field Sampling Procedures Manual,* Bureau of Environmental Measurements and Quality Assurance, Division of Publicly-Funded Site Remediation, NJDEPE, Trenton, NJ, 1992.

CHAPTER 11

A Novel Passive Sorptive Method for Site Screening of VOCs and SVOCs in Soil and Groundwater

Mark Stutman, Environmental Products Group, W. L. Gore & Associates, Inc., Elkton, Maryland

INTRODUCTION

A preliminary site screening is an established means of lowering the overall cost and time required before remediation can commence. Currently available soil-gas methods work best for simple volatile compounds in dry soils. This chapter describes field results from a new site screening service, under development for several years. This service features patented, passive sorbent collection devices, constructed from GORE-TEX microporous polytetrafluoroethylene (similar to Teflon). These devices are inserted directly into the soil or groundwater. All GORE-SORBER Screening Modules contain replicates of specially selected adsorbent materials (i.e. Tenax-TA). No elaborate field tools are required for installation or retrieval. Installation rates, including selection of sample locations, can exceed five per hour. After retrieval, sorbers are thermally extracted, then analyzed via GC/MS, and the results mapped. Case studies from gasoline stations, chemical and asphalt plants are described, and comparisons are made to available soil, groundwater and soil-gas data. These devices have been demonstrated to be effective in detecting both volatile and semivolatile compounds in difficult applications such as clay and saturated soils.

SCREENING FOR ORGANICS IN THE SUBSURFACE

For a thorough review of the art and science of soil-gas sensing for detecting and mapping of volatile compounds, the reader is referred to Devitt et all. Briefly, active, pumped soil-gas samples are snapshots, they require detectable compound concentrations, skilled on-site personnel, and expensive on-site equipment. They are most appropriate for rapid screening of volatile organic compounds (VOCs) in moderately permeable soils. In contrast, passive means rely on diffusion and adsorption. Passive samplers can be installed unobtrusively, allow a dynamic equilibrium to develop between the soil-gases and the sorbent, and integrate the dynamic flux of vapors produced by fluctuations in barometric pressure, rainfall and temperature. Both methods have been demonstrated for the detection of relatively volatile chemicals in drained, permeable soils. However, many locations such as chemical, asphalt and town-gas plants[2] and refineries require the detection of semivolatile organic compounds (SVOCs) such as larger alkanes, substituted aromatics, naphthalenes and polycyclic aromatic hydrocarbons. Conventional active and other passive soil-gas methods are insufficiently sensitive to these substances under most conditions, especially in the saturated zone and in impermeable clays.

Objectives. Some years ago, we experienced the practical limitations of existing active and passive soil-gas techniques in exploring for impacted groundwater in Maryland's wet, weathered-in-place clays and fractured crystalline bedrock. In response, we invented a patented, highly sensitive passive sorbent collection device, which greatly expands the utility of soil-gas techniques for site screening for VOCs and SVOCs in the subsurface. Our goals in developing this technology are to provide:

- extreme sensitivity to VOCs and SVOCs,
- detection anywhere in the soil profile, even below the water table,
- rapid, unobtrusive installation and retrieval, using simple hand tools,
- inert construction materials, allowing thermal extraction and cyrofocusing,
- chemical analysis using chromatographic separation with mass selective detection (GC/MSD),
- replicate sorbers for QA/QC and routine sample archiving,
- clear data presentation using contour maps overlain onto CAD site drawings.

Service Description. All of these features of our GORE-SORBER^{SM} Screening Survey service combine to provide useful information on areal extent and relative abundance of organic chemicals impacting soil and groundwater, under a wide range of conditions. GORE-SORBER Screening Surveys have been successfully demonstrated in impermeable clays, and industrial sites built on filled wetlands. With our sensors, we can detect a wide range of solvents, and petroleum hydrocarbons. Our service includes assistance with survey design, all required Screening Modules, complete analytical service, and maps. Installation and retrieval, using simple hand tools, is performed primarily by environmental consultants and industrial users.

Source areas and plume boundaries are delineated by mapping the compounds or mixtures detected, utilizing computer generated contour plots overlaid onto CAD maps of the site. Our maps can assist hydrogeological engineers in reducing the overall cost of a remedial action. These cost reductions are produced primarily by shifting the role of borings and wells from exploration tools to confirmation tools, subsequently minimizing the number of wells drilled, and subsequent disposal, development and routine sampling costs. Results are illustrated here by three case studies:

- a gasoline/UST source and plume delineation,
- a fracture trace study for placement of TCE recovery wells,
- an asphalt manufacturing plant.

COLLECTOR DESCRIPTION

GORE-SORBER Screening Modules are the passive sorbent collection apparatus which overcomes many of the limitations of existing soil-gas methods. The sorbent containers and insertion/retrieval cords are constructed solely of inert, hydrophobic, microporous GORE-TEX expanded polytetrafluoroethylene (ePTFE, similar to Teflon). Their appearance is that of a white, slippery shoestring. A unique feature of their construction is that the entire sorbent container surface area, as well as the surrounding insertion/retrieval "cord", facilitates vapor transfer. Sorbent containers (sorbers) can be filled with a variety of suitable granular adsorbent materials and resins, including coconut and graphitized carbons, molecular sieves, Tenax-TA, and silica gel.

Screening modules are packaged and shipped to the test site in sealed glass vials. Figure 11.1 shows a schematic of a typical screening module, with two replicate passive sorbent containers within. A typical sorber is 40 mm long, with a 3 mm ID, and holds 40 mg of sorbent. These collectors feature rapid and easy installation and retrieval by field personnel. Simple installation tools, such as slam bars or rotary hammer-drills, can be used to create 1-inch diameter holes for routine deployment of samplers to typical depths of three to four feet. Two technicians can install 60 to 100 modules in a day. In use, a matrix of modules are temporarily inserted into the ground and left for a period lasting several days to two weeks. Sample retrieval simply requires that field personnel remove the cork, grasp the ePTFE cord and pull the module from the ground. Each module is resealed into its vial and shipped on ice back to our laboratory via overnight service.

ANALYTICAL SERVICE

In the field, the individual sorbers remain clean and protected from dirt and soil by the insertion/retrieval cord. In our laboratory, sample preparation simply requires cutting the tip off the bottom of the module, removing the exposed sorbers into sealed desorption tubes. Samples can remain frozen until analysis. Holding time limitations have not yet been determined.

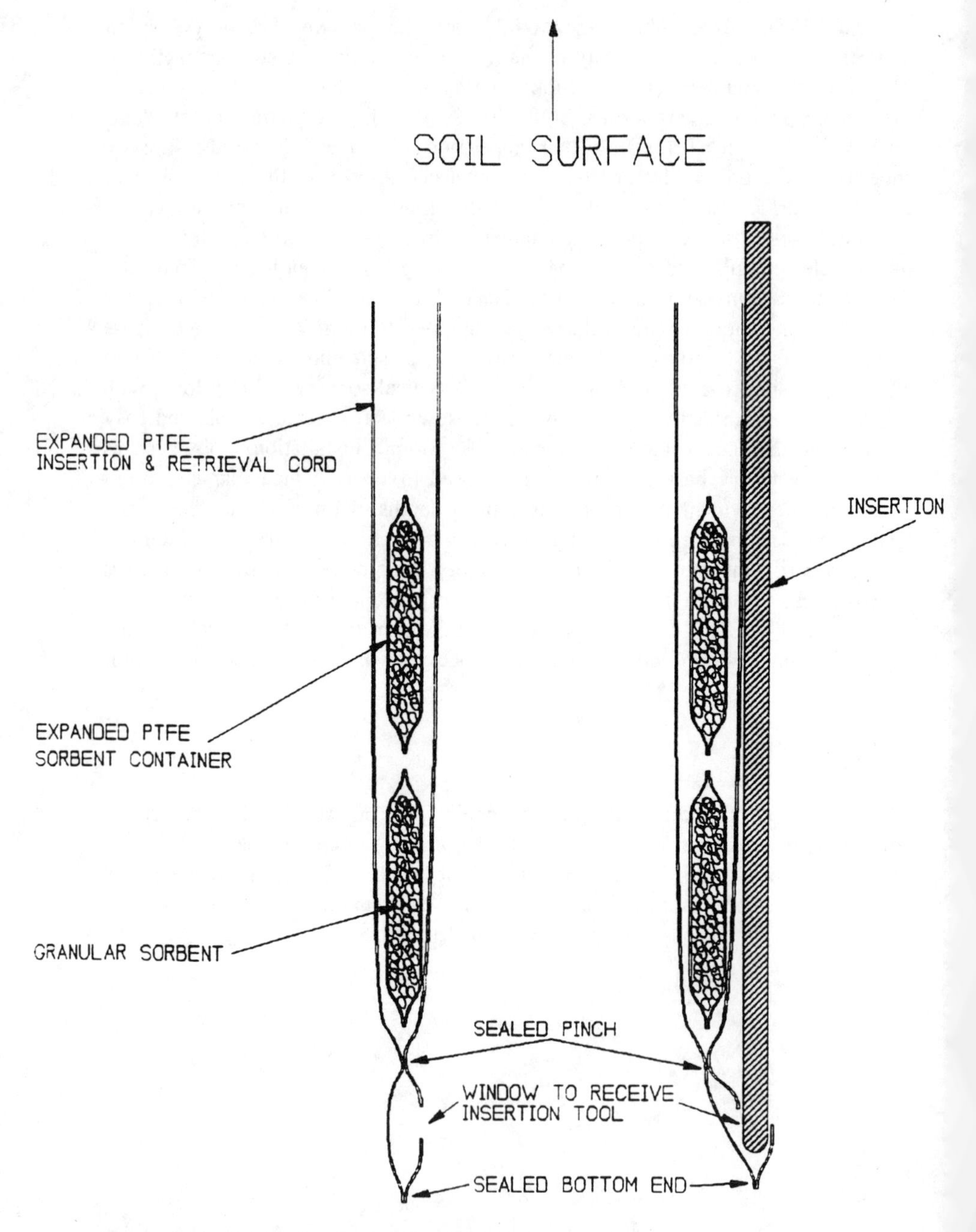

Figure 11.1. Schematic of a GORE-SORBER Screening Module during installation (right) and after installation (left).

Instrumentation consists of a Hewlett-Packard gas chromatograph and mass selective detector. Recently, a Thermal Desorption (TD) unit with cryofocusing has been added to our laboratory as the preferred extraction device for the sorbers. With it we have achieved sensitivity in the low nanogram levels to the most common compounds, and superior separation of VOCs compared to solvent or headspace extraction methods. Standard quality procedures are practiced throughout the laboratory.

Our analytical service is designed to provide a flexible program for the analysis and mapping of individual compounds, or chromatographic fingerprints of common fluids. We can search for proscribed lists of compounds, or provide in depth interpretation of GC/MS data, coupled with IR and other methods as required.

Reports can be provided for individual compounds, common significant ions and hydrocarbon fragments. We can computer match analytical results to customer supplied product samples, or to stored library fingerprints. Finally, we create contour maps of the data collected. The breadth and flexibility of our analyses is due to the combination of chromatographic separation and mass selective detection.

CASE STUDIES AND FIELD RESULTS

Benchtop results. These collectors feature very high diffusive uptake rates into the sorbent bed, on the order of 1000 g of vapor per day. Sorbers exposed to concentrated mixtures of gasoline and chlorinated solvents in water on the bench reach a dynamic equilibrium in less than 48 hours. Current practice calls for two week exposure times, although this is expected to decrease after on-going time-study experiments in the field are completed.

Numerous commercial fluids have been tested in our lab, under dry, wet and saturated soil conditions. Of course, different commercial adsorbents exhibit a wide range of effectiveness in detecting these common fluids under different soil moisture conditions. For the vast majority of fluids tested, our research shows at least one adsorbent material gives good response, at any soil moisture level.

In moist soils, GC/MS fingerprints of commercial gasoline and heating oil range organics, are generally identical to fingerprints recovered from GORE-SORBER Screening Modules exposed to those same products. Experiments with commercially available polynuclear aromatic hydrocarbon contaminated soil reveals a second mass transport mechanism for our sorbers: physical absorption of separate phase products onto the microporous ePTFE cord.

Field Experiences with VOCs. In an earlier paper[3], we described a study correlating soil samples with sorber results for ppm levels of aniline and nitrobenzene in saturated soil. At many UST sites, several distinct plumes have been delineated where the existing groundwater data did not reflect this detail. Fresh and weathered gasolines from USTs have been distinguished at depths of dozens of feet.

The table below summarizes the many VOCS and SVOCs that have been detected with GORE-SORBER Screening Modules. These compounds include most compounds on the EPA Method 8240 and 8270 lists:

- Chlorinated Solvents: PCE, TCE, TCAs, DCEs, DCAs,
- Fluorinated Solvents: chlorofluorocarbons (i.e. Freon) and fluoropolymers (i.e. Fluorinert),
- Petroleum Hydrocarbons: MTBE, BTEX, gasoline, diesel, #2 heating oil, kerosene, jet fuel, #6 heating oil, asphalt, creosote, coal-tar,
- Industrial Chemicals: aromatics, alkanes, ketones, amines, phenols, pthalates, PAHs.

CASE STUDY K: *Delineation of Gasoline from Underground Storage Tanks and Pump.* The site is a vehicle maintenance garage in an urban town in the Piedmont. The building, UST and two dispensing pumps are located at the intersection of two streets.

The site is largely paved or under roof. Pre-construction drawings differed on presence of a second UST on the southern corner of the property. The area surveyed was "L" shaped, and approximately 18,000 sq. ft. A survey of 27 Screening Modules were installed, as shown on the map in Figure 11.2. The map shows a grey-scale contour plot of BTEX detected, in ng. Plumes of BTEX and MTBE (not shown) appear associated with the main gasoline UST and northern pump. A second, much less intense BTEX plume suggests that the hypothesized second tank did exist at one time.

Based on results of survey, five wells were drilled, as shown on the map. During installation, some evidence of hydrocarbons in the soil and a sheen was noticed in MW-2. Soil and groundwater samples were collected. These analytical results are posted on the map, which shows BTEX in the groundwater at MW-2 and MW-3, both located within the larger plume delineated by the GORE-SORBER Screening Survey. No groundwater contamination was evident in the lower (presumably older) delineation. In conclusion, this survey shows MTBE/BTEX plume from UST and dispenser pump, evidence of a second pump and tank.

CASE STUDY E: *Trichloroethylene (TCE) Fracture Trace.* The site is a manufacturing plant in a Mid-Atlantic state, with <200 g/l TCE contamination in groundwater. Degreasing and house cleaning operations had resulted in scattered low levels of chlorinated solvents in soil near the loading docks and outside storage pads at the rear of building. Screening with active soil-gas samples was attempted, but proved impossible due to the very low permeability, weathered-in-place clay. Depth to bedrock and groundwater are both roughly 30 feet. Groundwater flow, is dominated by west-east fractures (not the regional hydraulic gradient), and surfaces at a small spring to the east.

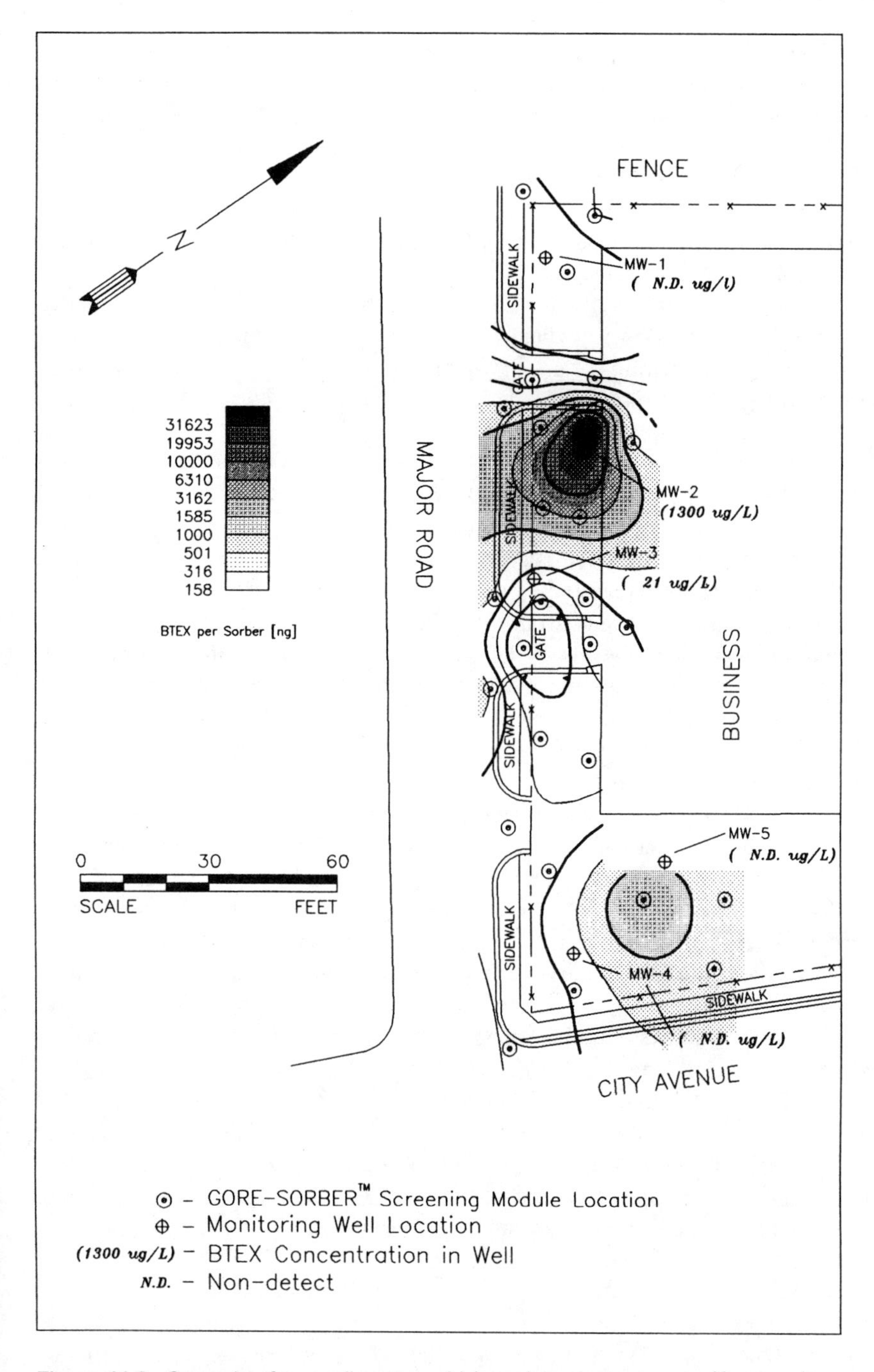

Figure 11.2. Screening for gasoline at a vehicle maintenance garage with an underground storage tank. Contour plot shows results from a GORE-SORBER Screening Survey. BTEX results are posted for monitoring wells drilled subsequent to the survey.

Over a three year period, sixteen wells were bored and the subsurface was explored via seismic and very low frequency techniques. No soil contamination was ever detected outside the suspected source area. Both methods suggested West-East troughs in the bedrock surface, and vertical bedrock fractures. TCE in the up-gradient, on-site wells decreased with time, while those down-gradient rose slowly or remained steady. A passive soil-gas survey done in 1987 showed the probable source area behind the building, but did not reveal the groundwater plume detected by the wells.

Wells placed midway along a 700 foot line connecting the suspected source area with the highest down-gradient monitoring well all contained 140 - 200 g/l of TCE. Elsewhere within the groundwater plume, TCE levels had declined over the five years of monitoring from levels not higher than 40 g/l of TCE, and in some areas was below 1 g/l.

A small Screening Survey, shown in Figure 11.3, was conducted to locate recovery wells in the suspected bedrock fracture. The survey consisted of five North-South "cross-fracture" transects of sensors, located 30 feet apart. A total of 77 modules were installed on four foot centers, to a depth of four feet. Installation equipment consisted of a slide hammer and 3/4" diameter steel rod. The transects varied in length from 40 to 70 feet. Exposure time was 21 days. The contour map shows levels of TCE recovered from each sorber. Recovery wells subsequently bored within the contoured areas yielded much greater water flow than older nearby monitoring wells placed in competent bedrock.

Placement of the recovery wells within the high-yield fracture zone greatly increased the efficiency of the pump and treat program.

CASE STUDY H: *Asphalt Manufacturing Facility.* Site H is an asphalt manufacturing plant, located several thousand meters from a freshwater bay. The plant has been in continuous operation for many years. Forty-four modules were installed over an area of 3.2 hectares (8 acres), to a depth of 1.2 m, utilizing a rotary hammer-drill and 25 mm OD auger bit. Shallow groundwater was noted in most of the drilled holes during module installation. Retrieval occurred after 21 days.

Figure 11.4 shows TICs and mass spectral fingerprints of a sorber, and the headspace of a soil sample also collected from that location. Relatively little contamination elutes from the GC column before 8 minutes or after 16 minutes.

These analyses clearly illustrate the complexity of the SVOC contamination at this site. In this case, maps of specificions were the most appropriate way to map the subsurface asphalt related contamination. Starting at eight minutes, a series of two minute mass spectral fingerprint "slices" were examined for representative ion fragments that could be used for mapping.

Figure 11.5 is a contour map of the distribution of the 169 amu ion, the dominant fragment produced by the mass selective detector during the ionization of hydrocarbon compounds throughout the late (fourteen to sixteen minute) elution range. The maps show that VOCs and SVOCs have similar distributions, with highest impacts around API separator and transfer pipelines, and lowest impacts adjacent to building and eastern tanks. Comparison of sorbers contents and soil samples reveals similar GC/MS fingerprints.

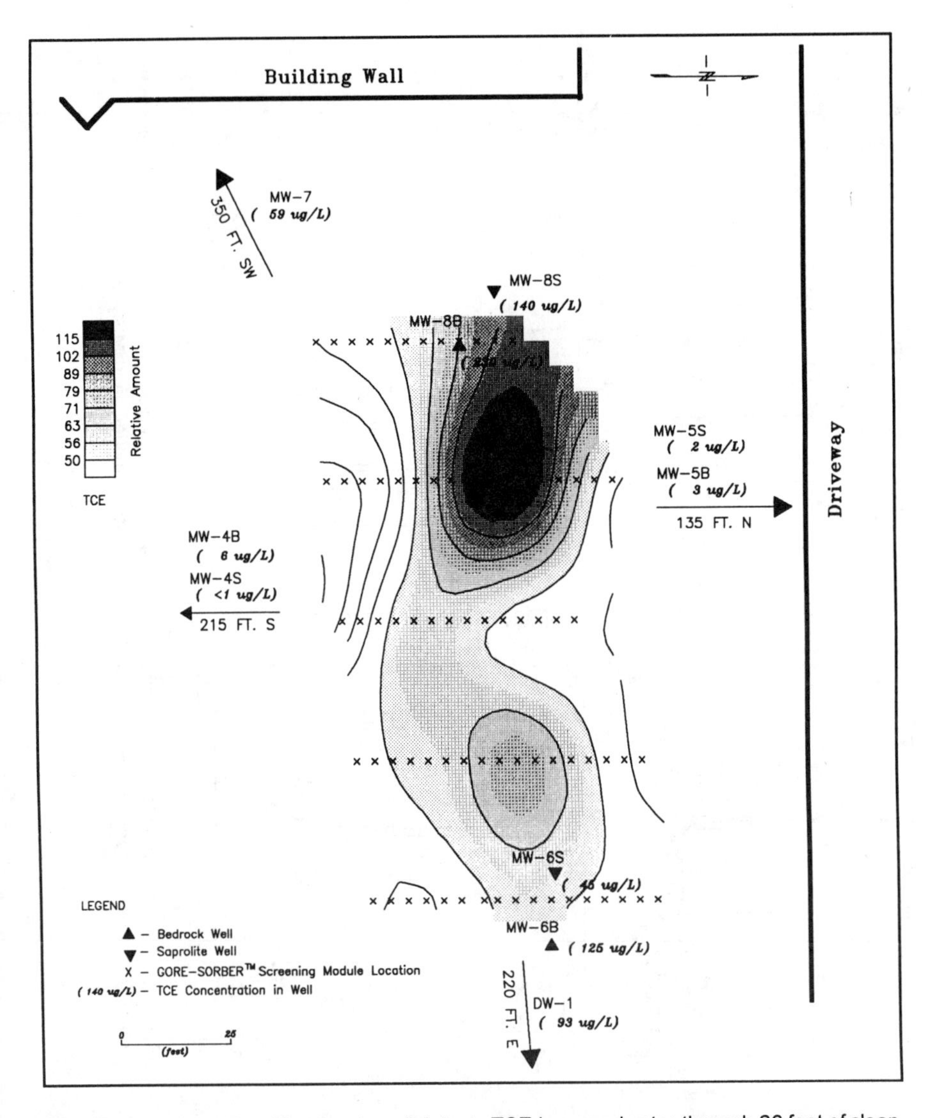

Figure 11.3. West-East "fracture trace" detects TCE in groundwater through 26 feet of clean, weathered-in-place clay. Contour plot shows results from a GORE-SORBER Screening Survey. TCE results are posted for surrounding monitoring wells.

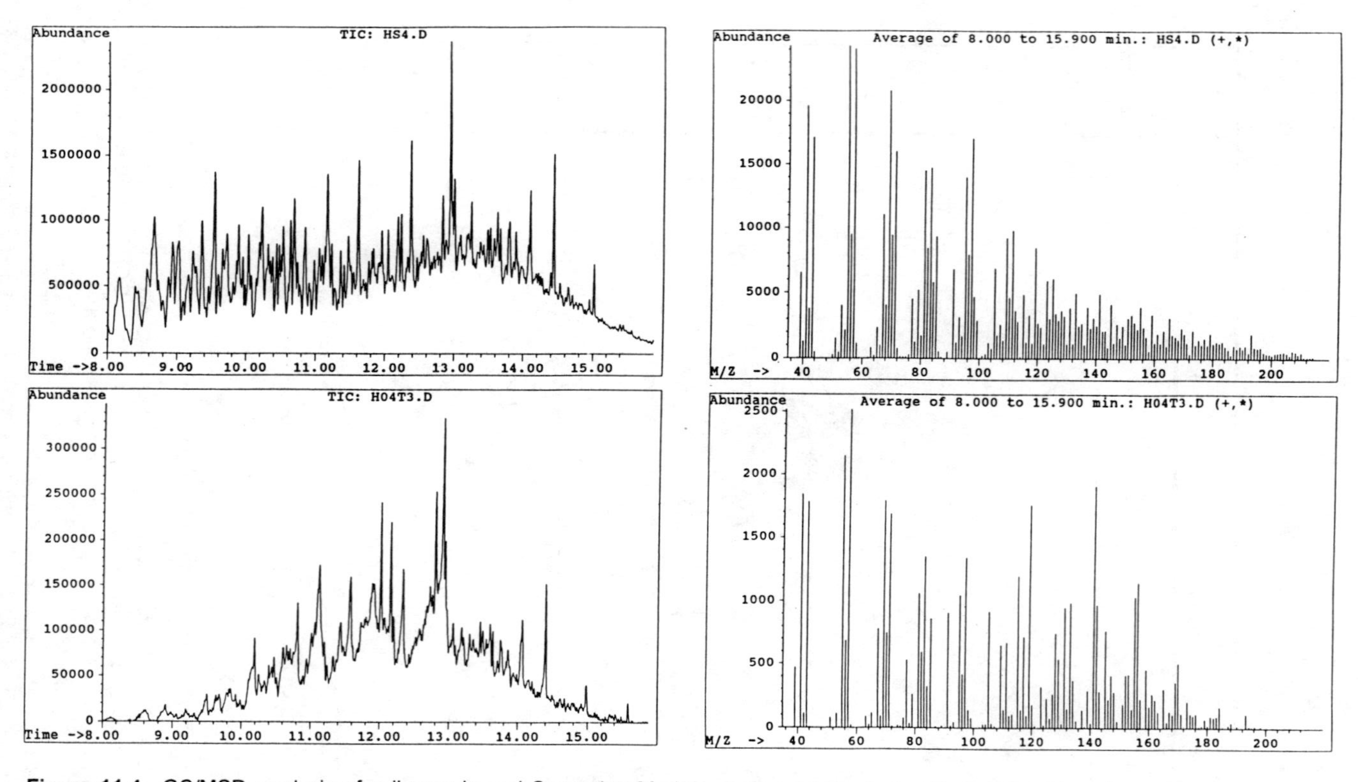

Figure 11.4. GC/MSD analysis of soil sample and Screening Module at an asphalt plant. (Above) Total ion chromatogram (left) and MSD fingerprint (right) of soil sample. (Below) Total ion chromatogram (left) and MSD fingerprint (right) of sorber.

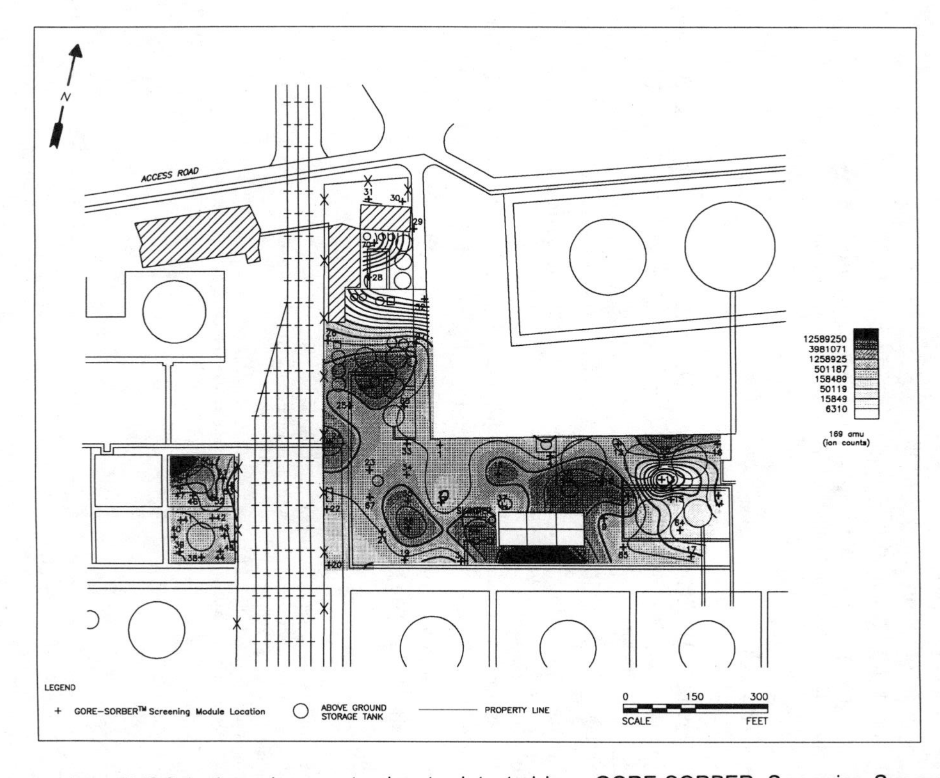

Figure 11.5. Contour map of the SVOC hydrocarbon contaminants detected by a GORE-SORBER Screening Survey, represented by the 169 amu ion, present at an asphalt plant.

CONCLUSIONS

We have described a novel passive sorbent method that can be employed to screen the subsurface for volatile and semivolatile organic compounds. The sensitivity of GORE-SORBER Screening Surveys to TCE, gasoline, and asphalt is documented with several case studies comparing our soil-gas results to subsequent soil borings and groundwater samples. In summary, we have described:

- an improved passive "soil-gas" collector design,
- easy installation and retrieval,
- demonstrated sensitivity to VOCs and SVOCs,
- sensitivity in saturated soils and low permeability clays,
- demonstrated for USTs, surface spills, refineries.

BIBLIOGRAPHY

1. D.A. Devitt, R.B. Evans, W.A. Jury et al., Soil Gas Sensing for Detection and Mapping of Volatile Organics, National Water Well Association, Dublin, OH, 1987.
2. C. Roberson, J.L. Cutler, Jr., Soil Gas Investigations at MGP Sites: An Evaluation of Alternative Compounds, GRI-89/0166, Gas Research Institute, Chicago, IL, 1989.
3. M. B. Stutman, A Novel Passive Sorbent Collection Apparatus for Site Screening of Semivolatile Compounds, Proc. 3rd Int. Conf. on Field Screening Methods for Hazardous Waste & Toxic Chemicals, Las Vegas, NV, Feb 24-26, 1993.

CHAPTER 12

The Use of Immunoassay Technology to Delineate Petroleum Hydrocarbon Contamination

Alex Tracy, Tina Cline-Thomas, William Mills, Woodward-Clyde Federal Services, Rockville, Maryland

INTRODUCTION

Immunoassay technology has evolved into a mature methodology that has been successfully applied to petroleum hydrocarbon contamination. The technique offers speed, sensitivity and selectivity and is rugged enough to be applied in the field. WCFS has used immunoassay field screening to:

- direct field sampling efforts by delineating contaminated areas
- prioritize samples for laboratory analysis
- provide the laboratory with information on the expected range of contaminants

Immunoassay field screening was used to perform two expedited site clearances at an Army base in the Washington D.C. area. The site clearances were triggered by two areas slated to undergo a facilities expansion that would involve construction. The first project involved an area that contained a possible landfill with burn pits and the second project involved "orphaned" underground storage tanks (USTs) that had leaked No. 2 fuel oil and diesel.

The events that led to the first site clearance were as follows: immediately prior to the start of the construction, information became available indicating possible contamination in the area where the construction was to take place. The exact location and extent of contamination were not known. Due to the construction schedule, the site clearance project had to be completed in eight weeks. Normally this type of project would require six months. Using immunoassay, approximately 130 soil samples were screened in the field and approximately 30 of those samples had results verified by laboratory analysis.

The second site clearance again involved an area where new facilities were to be constructed despite possible petroleum contamination from abandoned USTs. The USTs had been removed, and some preliminary work had been performed that verified existence of contamination, but the extent had not been determined. WCFS used immunoassay field screening to perform a rapid contamination assessment by analyzing both soil and water samples. A total of 47 soil and water samples were field screened by immunoassay and nine samples were submitted for laboratory confirmation.

Although some false positives were observed by field screening for petroleum hydrocarbons, no false negatives were observed. The first site clearance showed what appeared to be a higher percentage of false positives but these results may be attributed to the soil sample heterogeneity found at the site and the immunoassay kit's high sensitivity to bi and tri-cyclic polyaromatic hydrocarbons that were found in the burn pit areas. The second site clearance showed a much lower percentage of false positives and neither site clearance had any false negatives. This presentation will discuss time and budgetary savings, QA/QC procedures, and comparability of the field screening with laboratory results.

METHODS-GENERAL

Immunoassay technologies are well established within the medical laboratory industry where they have been used to provide rapid, accurate test results at low target concentrations. In recent years this technology has also started to be used in the environmental analysis field. Immunoassay test kits are available for a wide variety of organic contaminants, including polychlorinated biphenyls (PCB), selected herbicides and pesticides, polyaromatic hydrocarbons (PAH), BTEX (benzene, toluene, ethyl benzene and xylenes) and petroleum hydrocarbons (TPH).

The general protocol for performing immunoassay tests for environmental contaminants is:

- Extract the soil sample with methanol and filter the extract. Water samples are buffered.
- With a pipette, add 30 uL of the clarified methanol extract or one to two mL of the buffered water sample to the immunoassay tube and buffer.
- Incubate the sample at ambient temperature for ten minutes.
- Add enzyme conjugate with dropper bottles.
- Incubate the enzyme conjugate at ambient temperature for five minutes.
- Rinse the immunoassay tube.
- Add substrate and chromogen with dropper bottles and incubate for two and a half minutes.
- Add stop solution (acid) with a dropper bottle and measure absorbance on a spectrophotometer set to 450 nm.

Methanol is the extraction solvent of choice for soils because it is miscible with water (immunoassays require an aqueous environment to react), it does an adequate job of extracting most organic contaminants, and it does not pose a health and safety or handling risk to the analysts. WCFS decided to retain and refrigerate all methanol extracts to ensure that any re-analysis would be performed on the same aliquot of the environmental sample.

Site Clearance No. 1

Site Background

Woodward-Clyde Federal Services (WCFS) was given eight weeks to provide clearance of a site for construction activities. This entailed ensuring that sufficient samples had been analyzed to characterize the site and producing screening data that were accurate. Since the construction contract had already been awarded and the government would face penalties if construction was delayed, the time frame available for the investigation was very short. In addition to the historical information which indicated the presence of a landfill whose size and contents were unknown, there was the possibility that the landfill area contained burn pits where PCB transformers had been burned, presumably with waste oil and solvents. Some preliminary work indicated elevated levels of PCBs, miscellaneous other organics, and metals in the areas where the present playground was located and where the athletic field was to be relocated.

Laboratory analysis takes three to four weeks with normal turnaround times. Faster turnaround times are possible at premium rates but even the fastest analysis requires 24-48 hours before results can be reported. The approach that was developed for this project involved field screening and laboratory analysis with a five day turnaround. Field screening was performed on soil samples for petroleum hydrocarbons using immunoassay technology. The Ensys Petro Risc^{tm} immunoassay which was chosen is designed to provide total petroleum hydrocarbon data and is particularly sensitive to bi and tri-cyclic polyaromatic hydrocarbons. The field screening methods were used to prioritize samples for laboratory analysis, provide information to the laboratory on the approximate concentration range expected to minimize re-analysis, provide extent of contamination information for the areas being investigated and to allow rapid further delineation of concentration distributions near areas found to have high concentration values.

Methods for Site Clearance No. 1

A laboratory facility was set up on base for sample log-in and analysis. All samples were labeled, logged into a sample tracking system set up on a laptop, and screened at this location. All immunoassay data, including balance calibration, extraction weight, and the absorbances of both the samples and the standards were recorded in bound laboratory notebooks.

For the Ensys Petro Risc^{tm} immunoassays, sample absorbances were determined relative to a low concentration standard (0.7 ppm m-xylene) which is equivalent to 100 ppm gasoline and served as the threshold of detection. Two aliquots of each methanol extract were analyzed relative to this standard: the first represented the sample without any dilution and the second was the same extract at a ten fold dilution. Using the results from the sample and its ten fold dilution, approximate concentrations of petroleum constituents were determined with relative ease. While the petroleum kits were calibrated using m-xylene, they were sensitive to a variety of compounds found in petroleum products especially bi- and tri-cyclic aromatics.[1,2] WCFS utilized the Ensys Petro Risc[tm] kits' sensitivity to aromatic hydrocarbons to indicate burn areas where these hydrocarbons remained as products of incomplete combustion. Because the Ensys Petro Risc[tm] kits are sensitive to a variety of compounds, the immunoassay results correlated well with the hot spots as defined by laboratory analysis. Data on the correlation between the two methods are shown in Table 12.1.

Results

Table 12.1. Comparison of laboratory and field values for Ensys Petro Risc[tm] during site clearance no. 1.

Sample Number	Ensys Petro Risc[tm] Value	Sum of PAH Values*
Sample 1-01	ND	ND
Sample 1-02	ND	ND
Sample 1-03	ND	ND
Sample 1-04	ND	ND
Sample 1-05	ND	ND
Sample 1-06	Detect	ND**
Sample 1-07	Detect	>1 ppm
Sample 1-08	ND	ND
Sample 1-09	Detect	ND
Sample 1-10	Detect	ND
Sample 1-11	Detect	ND
Sample 1-12	ND	ND

Table 12.1 (cont.)

Sample Number	Ensys Petro Risc[tm] Value	Sum of PAH Values*
Sample 1-13	ND	ND
Sample 1-14	ND	ND
Sample 1-15	ND	ND
Sample 1-16	ND	ND
Sample 1-17	ND	ND
Sample 1-18	Detect	>1 ppm
Sample 1-19	ND	ND
Sample 1-20	ND	ND
Sample 1-21	ND	ND
Sample 1-22	ND	ND
Sample 1-23	ND	ND
Sample 1-24	Detect	>1 ppm
Sample 1-25	ND	ND
Sample 1-26	ND	ND
Sample 1-27	ND	ND
Sample 1-28	ND	ND
Sample 1-29	ND	ND

*Sum PAH=Sum of all detects for compounds listed in SW-846 Method 8100.

**Dilution at laboratory prevented proper quantitation.

Discussion of Results

While the percentage of immunoassay false positives for this project appeared to be high, it must be noted that very low levels of bi and tri-cyclic PAHs will result in positive test results. Cross-reactivity data from Ensys shows that the Petro Risc^{tm} kits are roughly ten times more sensitive to bi and tri-cyclic PAHs than m-Xylene, which was the compound used to calibrate the kits. For the first site clearance, bi and tri-cyclic PAHs were commonly found as soil contaminants, and sample heterogeneity when investigating the landfill also proved to be a problem.

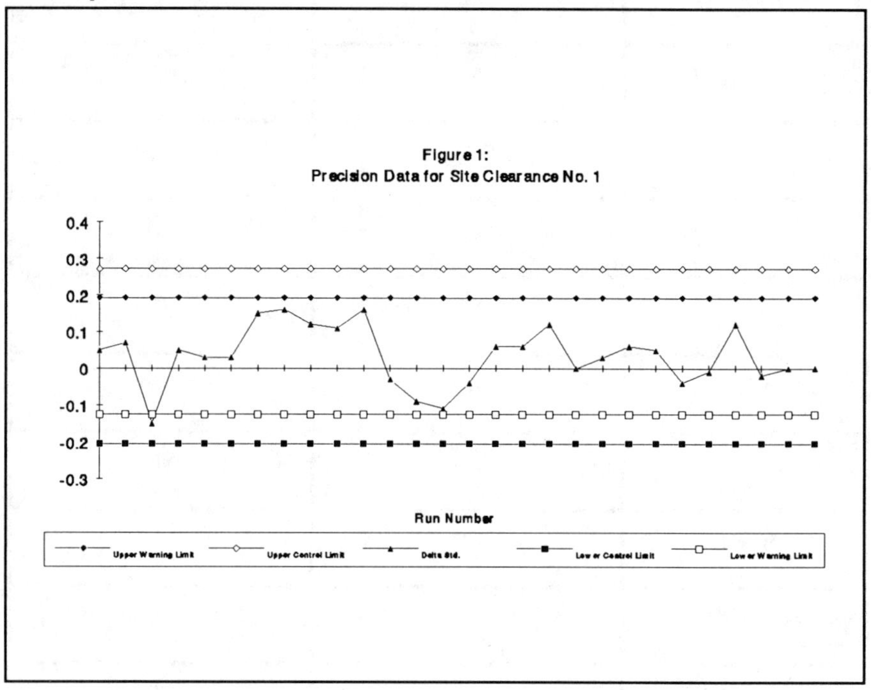

Discussion of Precision Results

The protocol for performing analysis dictated that the difference between duplicate standards (Delta Std, or D Std) could not exceed 0.2 absorbance units (a.u.) or the calibration would be considered invalid and the samples would have to be re-analyzed. Figure 12.1 presents a Shewart plot of Delta Std (D Std.=Std. 1-Std. 2) for petroleum hydrocarbon analysis during Project 1.

At the time of the first site clearance, WCFS felt that the use of dropper bottles rather than a repeat pipettor to add immunoassay reagents was the primary reason for the variability of the method. Ensys can supply the reagents either in dropper bottles or in bulk (for use with a pipettor), but for this site clearance the dropper bottles were used. Based on a review of additional data, the staff concluded that the accuracy and precision associated with the 30 uL addition of the standard or sample extract to the immunoassay tube is more critical because any variability for such a small volume can drastically affect results, whereas volume effects when adding 200 uL (the typical volume of immunoassay reagents such as buffer, conjugate, substrate, etc.) would be less noticeable. Still, the ideal situation would involve the use of a pipette to add the methanol extracts to the immunoassay tube and the use of a repeat pipettor to add the immunoassay reagents.

Site Clearance No. 2

The second project involved two proposed construction sites within the same general area of the base. Construction of a vehicle maintenance building, vehicle storage areas and a mobile equipment shop was proposed for an area where two USTs containing No. 2 fuel oil and diesel had been removed. Nearby, a new Logistics Complex was to be constructed in an area where five USTs containing No. 2 fuel oil and diesel had been removed after leaks were discovered in the system. Both areas had only been partially characterized in previous investigations.

Methods for Site Clearance No. 2

The Ensys' Ensys Petro Risc^{tm} immunoassay was again used to delineate the petroleum contamination at the site, but the test kit was a more sensitive version of the original kit, with a threshold of detection of 10 ppm gasoline rather than 100 ppm. While water samples required a slightly different preparation than soils, the overall protocol for performing both tests was identical. Pipettes were used to add sample, dropper bottles were used to add immunoassay reagents and the concentration range of petroleum hydrocarbons was determined by analysis of a sample followed analysis of its ten fold dilution.

As this second project was smaller in scope, a field laboratory was not set up. Samples were either analyzed off-site, with the results available by the next morning, or were analyzed in a van on-site, to provide information immediately. Neither situation was as ideal as the field laboratory used for the first site clearance. All immunoassay data were recorded in bound laboratory notebooks.

Field Screening For Petroleum Hydrocarbons (TPH)

Although it is more difficult to accurately quantify low concentrations of petroleum products, the immunoassay results still compared favorably with results obtained by fixed laboratory analysis. Headspace analysis using an organic vapor analyzer was also performed on these samples during sampling activities; however, the results from the headspace analysis did not correlate well with the laboratory or immunoassay results. The sporadic results from the headspace analysis are probably a result of a combination of matrix effects, which would induce a negative bias. Additionally, natural organic matter that was decaying was present in the soil and could have been producing methane that resulted in the false positives from the headspace analysis. Table 12.2 presents the comparison of immunoassay and fixed laboratory results.

Results

Table 12.2. Comparison of laboratory and field values for Ensys Petro Risc^{tm} during site clearance no. 2.

Sample Number	Ensys Petro Risc^{tm} Value (ppm)	TPH Result from Laboratory (ppm)*
Sample 2-01	10<Result<100	120
Sample 2-02	10<Result	250
Sample 2-03	>100	3900
Sample 2-04	<10	ND
Sample 2-05	<10	3.3
Sample 2-06	>100	1.40
Sample 2-07	<10	.80
Sample 2-08	<10	1.50
Sample 2-09	<10	1.60

*TPH analysis was performed using modified SW-846 Method 8015.

Discussion of Results

Laboratory quantitation, especially for TPH analysis, can vary greatly but the immunoassay results generally correlated with the laboratory results. Samples 2-01 through 2-03 were correctly identified as having contamination greater than the immunoassay limit of detection, although the actual amount of contamination detected by the immunoassay test for samples 2-01 and 2-02 was different from the laboratory. Interlaboratory method studies will typically show a high degree of variability using identical methods and a well characterized reference material, so it is not surprising to find some variability between the field and laboratory methods. Sample 2-03 was well beyond the analytical range of the test, so quantitation by immunoassay was not possible. Samples 2-04, 2-05, 2-07, 2-08 and 2-09 were under the immunoassay threshold of detection and were correctly identified as such. The false positive for sample 2-06 was probably a result of sample heterogeneity: the contaminant was weathered No. 2 fuel oil and diesel that is hydrophobic and not very mobile, and there had been previous excavation activities at the site. Consequently, it is possible to find some pockets of localized contamination that vary from the site as a whole. In summary, eight of the nine splits had comparable results and although one sample may have been a false positive, that result was probably due to sample heterogeneity.

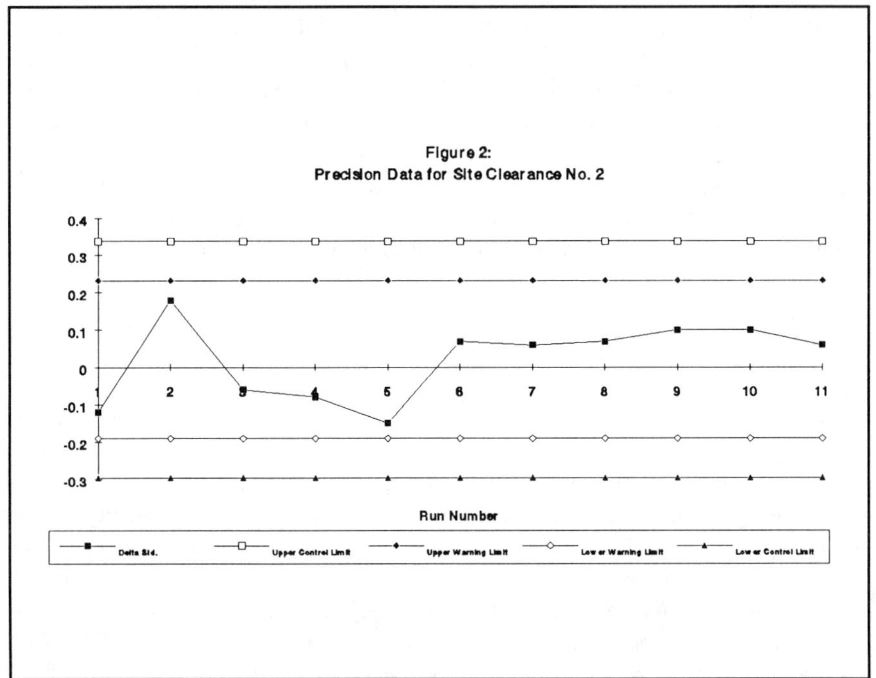

Discussion of Precision Results

The precision data for immunoassay standards during site clearance no. 2 are presented as a Shewart chart in Figure 12.2 The data shows roughly the same variability as the first project, despite adverse site conditions during immunoassay analysis. Roughly half of these analyses were performed in the field at relatively low temperatures (40°F) during high wind.

QA/QC Issues

Field screening can provide either Level I or Level II data[5]. For these projects the field screening data were regarded as Level I data and the laboratory analysis, which was Level III data, was used to make all final decisions regarding site contamination. Specific guidelines for producing Level II data may vary from site to site, and the sampling and analysis program must address the problems of sample heterogeneity, matrix effects, interfering compounds, and sample contamination as a result of improper handling or preparation[3,5].

Although field screening can present additional challenges to the field team, there are many instances where the additional data produced from the lower cost field screening tests can significantly reduce the sampling error in site investigations. Analytical error (bias and variability introduced in the laboratory) typically accounts for only 15% of the total error introduced in the site investigation process. The remaining 85% of the error in site investigations results from an insufficient number of samples or samples that do not accurately represent the contamination at the site[4]. Field screening allows for rapid analysis following sample collection, which reduces problems in sample handling, preservation and transport, and gives the field team the flexibility to employ an iterative sampling strategy to fully characterize the contamination.

IMPLEMENTING FIELD SCREENING INTO PROJECT SCOPING

In keeping with the DQO development process defined by EPA[4], the project should be planned with field screening in mind from the outset, and a chemist familiar with the technology to be employed should be involved during the planning stage. The overall effectiveness of field screening will depend on project specific needs and there are instances where field screening would be an inappropriate methodology. At the time of the first project (April-May 1992), none of the immunoassay techniques had been recognized as methods by EPA. By the second site clearance (January 1993), EPA had granted SW-846 third update numbers of 4010 (pentachlorophenol), 4020 (PCB), and 4030 (Total Petroleum Hydrocarbons) for immunoassay screening techniques. In the draft versions of these methods it states that the actual screening analysis must be carried out by, or under the supervision of, a qualified analyst otherwise; the method has not been followed. This will minimize re-sampling and re-analysis will ensure that results are not used inappropriately.

CONCLUSION

The staff chemist performing immunoassay analysis was able to screen approximately 30 samples per day by immunoassay and despite the different conditions during immunoassay analysis, the precision of the two site clearances was essentially indistinguishable. The use of a repeat pipettor to add immunoassay reagents is preferred rather than dropper bottles: it will speed immunoassay analysis and yield data of better precision and accuracy. For these projects, the correlation between laboratory and field data was good, but the differences in detection limits and problems with sample heterogeneity can make direct comparison difficult

Through the use of immunoassay field screening, WCFS completed the site clearance on time, better characterized the extent and level of contamination, and helped to focus the activities of the field crew for iterative sampling and distribution assessment. In addition to the data provided by the immunoassay and laboratory analysis, remote sensing information such as aerial photography, geophysics and metal detector surveys were used to identify the areas occupied by the former landfill, burn pits and USTs. The information from the remote sensing agreed with the immunoassay and laboratory data.. As shown in these two site clearance projects, immunoassay is a mature screening technology, which, when used properly can be very cost effective tool in the site investigation process.

REFERENCES

1. PETRO RISc™ User's Guide, Ensys Inc, 1992.
2. "Soil Screening for Petroleum Hydrocarbons by Immunoassay," Draft Method 4030, USEPA SW-846 Third Update, July 1992.
3. Kevin J. Nesbitt, "Application and QA/QC Guidance USEPA SW-846 Immunoassay-Based Field Methods 4010, 4020 & 4030;" Ensys Inc, 1992.
4. Francis Pittard, *Principles of Environmental Sampling*: A Short Course Presented Prior to the 8th Annual Waste Testing & Quality Assurance Symposium, July 11-12, 1992.
5. USEPA, *Data Quality Objectives for Remedial Response Activities*, EPA/540/G-87/003, March 1987.

PART III

HUMAN HEALTH AND RISK ASSESSMENT

CHAPTER 13

Effects of Gender on the Bioavailability of Xenobiotics

Mohamed S. Abdel-Rahman and Gloria A. Skowronski, Pharmacology and Toxicology Department, New Jersey Medical School, University of Medicine and Dentistry of New Jersey, New Jersey, and **Rita M. Turkall,** Clinical Laboratory Sciences Department, School of Health Related Professions and Pharmacology and Toxicology Department, New Jersey Medical School, University of Medicine and Dentistry of New Jersey

INTRODUCTION

Gender-related differences in response to toxic substances have been suspected since the early 1900s. In 1985 Calabrese made a comprehensive search of the published literature and found strong evidence for the existence of sex-related responses to drugs as well as to environmentally and occupationally toxic substances. He established that sex-related differences occur in a broad range of species including humans. Furthermore, the number of toxic agents for which gender-related differences have been found to occur is extensive and approaches nearly 200.[1]

Some of the underlying causes of sex-specific responses have been related to differences in a variety of biochemical and physiological factors namely differences in gastrointestinal absorption, plasma protein binding, enzymatic bioactivation and detoxification, tissue distribution, and biliary excretion.[1] Testosterone often plays a key role in sex differences, as is illustrated by the numerous studies in which administering testosterone to female animals had a masculinizing effect and/or in which depriving male animals of testosterone had a feminizing effect.[2-4]

The manner and route by which exposure to chemicals occurs may also be contributing factors. Environmental exposures are more often the result of contact with chemically contaminated soil than with pure chemicals. Soil contamination is a major concern for industry as well as for regulatory agencies and communities living in proximity to contaminated sites. The strength of a chemical-soil interaction can profoundly effect the desorption of a chemical from soil and ultimately the percentage of the chemical in the soil which actually enters the body. Although skin is a major route of exposure to many environmental pollutants adsorbed to soil, ingestion is also a significant route of exposure, particularly in young children 1.5 to 3.5 years of age. Ingestion may occur through inadvertent consumption of soil on the hands or food items, mouthing tendencies, a craving for soil (geophasia) or a combination of these pathways.[5]

All instances and causes of gender differentiation are not yet known. Moreover, it is difficult to predict whether sex differences are likely to be significant in a given situation. Therefore, there is a need for methodologies to accurately quantify the effects of gender on chemical bioavailability and eventually to assess the health risk from exposure. Two approaches were utilized in our laboratory to identify the factors that influence bioavailability so that more informed predictions of potential health risk can be made following exposure to environmental pollutants. The first approach was an *in vivo* method. The ability of each chemical to produce adverse health effects can be related to its concentration and duration in the body which are ultimately determined by absorption, distribution, metabolism and excretion processes. The net result of these processes can be described in mathematical terms by pharmacokinetics. By this method we can obtain the plasma absorption and elimination half-life of a compound as well as the area under the plasma concentration time curve (AUC). Concentration of chemical in excreta and body tissues in addition to the amount, type and appearance of metabolites can also be determined.

The second approach was an *in vitro* method. *In vitro* systems have recently been developed to measure the penetration of radiolabeled chemicals through skin held in diffusion cells. Results from *in vitro* studies have been shown to correlate well with *in vivo* studies.[6,7] *In vitro* studies enable the researcher to measure the rate of chemical movement through skin, the concentration of chemical bound to skin that may subsequently become available systemically and volatilization from the skin surface.

Using the *in vivo* approach we showed that gender effects the dermal bioavailability of phenanthrene. More phenanthrene was absorbed through skin by females than by males as confirmed by a higher peak plasma concentration and AUC in females. The increase in female AUC was consistent with a decrease in skin application site radioactivity.[8]

The influence of gender on the bioavailability of benzene, m-xylene and trichloroethylene (TCE) were also examined and will be discussed here. All three compounds are widely used in industry and commonly found in hazardous waste disposal sites.[9] Benzene is used extensively in industry as a solvent and as a starting material in chemical synthesis.[10,11] Benzene together with toluene and xylene represent the major aromatic compounds of gasoline.[12] Because of its leukemia and cancer causing properties, benzene is often considered to be more hazardous to health than toluene or xylene.[13,14]

Xylene is extensively used as a solvent, a cleaning agent, a degreaser, and a starting material and intermediate in the chemical industry. Xylene is also present in a broad range of consumer products such as aerosols, paints, varnishes, shellacs and rust preventatives.[15] Gerarde reported that xylene may be more acutely toxic than benzene.[16] When inhaled at high concentrations, symptoms included disturbed vision, dizziness, tremors, salivation, cardiac stress, central nervous system (CNS) depression, confusion and coma.[17] Xylene causes dehydration and defatting of the skin which may lead to erythema, blistering or dermatitis.[16]

TCE has been shown to be carcinogenic in mice and is considered a suspected human carcinogen.[18] TCE has also been associated with CNS toxicity and hepatotoxicity.[19] Despite associated health risks, however, it is still used in metal degreasing and in the manufacture of many industrial products such as printing inks, lacquers, and adhesives.[20,21] TCE has also been found as a contaminant in a wide variety of water samples, as well as in mollusks, fish and food products.[22]

MATERIALS AND METHODS

Chemicals

Uniformly labeled ^{14}C-benzene with a specific activity of 60 mCi/mmol and radiochemical purity of ≥98% was purchased from ICN Pharmaceuticals. Both m-(ring-U-^{14}C) xylene and trichloroethylene (1,2-^{14}C) were custom synthesized by E.I. DuPont de Nemours and Co., Inc., New England Nuclear (NEN) Research Products and had a radiochemical purity of ≥98%. The specific activities of m-xylene and TCE were 7.2 and 13 mCi/mmol, respectively. Prior to use, the radioisotopes were diluted, respectively, with nonradioactive HPLC-grade benzene, unlabeled anhydrous (>99% purity) m-xylene, and 99% spectro-photometric grade, unlabeled TCE spectrophotometric to reduce specific activity to a workable range.

Soil

Two soils were examined: (A) an Atsion sandy soil (90% sand, 2% clay, 4.4% organic matter) collected from an aquifer drill site of the Cohansey sand formation near Chatsworth in south central New Jersey[23] and (B) a Keyport formation clay soil (5% sand, 22% clay, 1.6% organic matter) collected from the Woodbury formation near Moorestown in southwestern New Jersey.[24] Mechanical, sieve, organic matter and chemical contamination analyses were performed as discussed previously from our laboratory.[25]

Animals

Male and female Sprague-Dawley rats weighing 225-300g were purchased from Taconic Farms and quarantined for at least one week prior to administration of the chemical. Animals were housed three per cage and were maintained on a 12-hr light/dark cycle at constant temperature (23-25°C) and humidity (50-55%). Ralston Purina rodent chow and tap water were provided ad libitum.

Treatment (*In Vivo* Studies)

The oral administration of chemicals was performed as follows: Either 150 ul of radioisotope (5 uCi) alone, or the same volume of radioactivity added to 0.5 g of soil, was combined with 2.85 ml of aqueous 5% gum acacia and a suspension formed by vortexing. The weight of soil and volume of chemical were selected so that a uniformly contaminated soil could be prepared without an excess of pollutant. Immediately after preparation, chemical alone in gum acacia or chemical soil suspension was administered by gavage to groups of rats which had been fasted overnight.

For the dermal application, a shallow glass cap circumscribing a 13-cm^2 area was tightly fixed with Lang's jet liquid acrylic and powder on the lightly shaved right costoabdominal region of each ether-anesthetized animal one-half hour prior to the administration of radioisotope. Care was taken to prevent any abrasion of the skin during shaving and cap attachment. The glass cap was attached immediately after shaving the animal and remained on the rat for the duration of the study. Three hundred microliters of chemical (40 uCi) alone or after the addition of 750 mg of soil was introduced through a small opening in the cap which was immediately sealed. The weight of soil and volumes of the chemicals were selected so that a uniformly contaminated soil could be prepared without excess fluid.

Absorption and Elimination

Heparinized blood samples were collected by cardiac puncture under light ether anesthesia at selected time points.[26-29] Samples from all studies were processed and radioactivity was measured by liquid scintillation spectrometry as previously discussed.[25]

Tissue Distribution, Excretion and Metabolism

Immediately after the collection of the last blood samples in the oral studies, rats were sacrificed by an overdose of ether and the following tissues were removed and weighed: brain, thymus, thyroid, esophagus, stomach, duodenum, ileum, lung, pancreas, adrenal, testes, skin, subrenal fat, carcass, bone marrow, liver, kidney, spleen, heart and whole blood. Samples of 300 mg or less of tissue and gastric contents were used to determine the distribution of radioactivity as previously reported.[25]

In the excretion studies, groups of six rats each were administered chemical alone or chemical adsorbed to soil as described above. Animals were housed in all-glass metabolism chambers for the collection of expired air, urine, and fecal samples. Expired air was passed through activated charcoal tubes for the collection of the parent compounds, then bubbled through traps filled with ethanolamine: ethylene glycol monomethyl ether (1:2 v/v) for the collection of CO_2.[30] Charcoal was extracted with glacial acetic acid and fecal samples were homogenized in deionized water. Aliquots of the charcoal extracts, ethanolamine: ethylene glycol monomethyl ether mixture, fecal homogenates and urine were then dispensed directly into Aquasol-2 for analysis.[25]

At the conclusion of the dermal excretion studies, rats were sacrificed by an overdose of ether. Then, the surface of the treated skin area was washed with ethyl alcohol to determine the percentage of radioactivity remaining on skin application sites. Glass caps were removed from the rats and specimens collected as in the oral studies. Radioactivity was determined in the alcohol washes, skin application site, and in the untreated skin of the rat (left side). Three areas of fat were examined, namely, fat beneath treated and untreated skin and subrenal fat.

The identity, quantity and time for appearance of metabolites in urine were monitored by high performance liquid chromatography (HPLC).[25,28,31]

Treatment (*In Vitro* Studies)

Silastic capsules (30 mm), commonly used for hormone administration,[32,33] were used to administer testosterone. The capsules were constructed from Dow Chemical Silastic, medical grade tubing, 0.062" i.d. x 0.125" o.d. and were implanted subcutaneously between the shoulders.[32] The experimental groups were identified as follows:

Male

Control: excluded from capsule implantation, castration, and testosterone treatment

Testosterone-deprived: castrated and then implanted with an empty Silastic capsule

Sham: treated as testosterone-deprived group except that testes were not removed

Testosterone-restored: castrated and then implanted with testosterone (110 mg/kg) in a Silastic capsule

Female

Control: excluded from capsule implantation and testosterone treatment

Sham: implanted with empty Silastic capsule

Testosterone-treated: implanted with testosterone (110 mg/kg) in a Silastic capsule

Five rats were used per treatment group. Ether anesthesia was utilized during castration and capsule implantation. Blood samples were taken daily for one week and before sacrifice by cardiac puncture under light ether anesthesia, centrifuged at 1200 x g for 5 min, and then frozen in glass test tubes at O°C for analysis. The serum was assayed for testosterone using the Coat-A-Count Testosterone Radioimmunoassay Kit.

Evaporation-Penetration Studies

Skin samples from all of the above groups were treated *in vitro* with ^{14}C-TCE. A System 1 evaporation-penetration cell was used. One week after treatment, rats were sacrificed by an overdose of ether. Each sample was carefully shaved and the subcutaneous fat was carefully scraped away with a razor blade before the sample was mounted in the evaporation-penetration cell. Full-thickness skin samples were used from the flanks of the animals.

At the beginning of each run, skin samples were treated with 5 ul of ^{14}C-TCE containing 0.36 uCi. The exposed surface area of skin was 0.78 cm^2 which resulted in a chemical dose of 9.36 ug of ^{14}C-TCE/cm^2. Receptor solution from the penetration cell chamber was collected at 5, 15, and 30 min and at 1,2,3,4,6 and 10 hr. The receptor solution contained 40 mg/ml bovine albumin dissolved in Tyrode's saline solution. Radioactivity was counted by liquid scintillation spectrometry.[34]

Data Analysis

Plasma time course data was analyzed as in previously reported studies.[25] All other data were reported as the mean $\pm$ SE. Statistical differences between chemical alone and soil treatment groups were determined by analysis of variance (ANOVA) followed by Scheffe's multiple range test or Newman-Kuell's multiple range test. Student's t-test was used to determine differences between males and females. A p value less than 0.05 was considered statistically significant.

RESULTS

Effects of Gender and Soil on the Oral Bioavailability of m-Xylene

The highest peak plasma concentration of radioactivity in females (Table 1) was observed with sandy soil-adsorbed m-xylene (1608 dpm/ml). Clay soil-adsorbed and pure chemical treatments produced approximately equal peak plasma concentrations (975 and 848 dpm/ml, respectively). Neither of the soils altered the peak plasma concentration (900 dpm/ml) in males (Table 13.1). The time to reach peak plasma concentration (20 min) was the same in all treatment groups for both males and females (data not shown).

Table 13.1. Maximum plasma concentration of radioactivity for rats orally exposed to ^{14}C-m-xylene[a].

Treatment	dpm/ml	
	Females	Males
m-Xylene Alone	848	838
+ Sandy Soil	1608	932
+ Clay Soil	975	957

[a] Values represent mean ± SE of five to six rats/group gavaged with an aqueous solution of 5% gum acacia and ^{14}C-m-xylene alone or adsorbed to soil

Sandy and clay soil significantly increased the $t_{1/2}$ of absorption (0.60 and 0.38 hr, respectively) compared to m-xylene alone (0.31 hr) in females (Table 13.2). On the other hand, sandy soil significantly decreased the $t_{1/2}$ of elimination (6.70 hr), while clay soil had no effect versus m-xylene alone (11.42 hr). In males (Table 13.2), soil had no effect on the $t_{1/2}$ of absorption (0.64-0.85 hr) or $t_{1/2}$ of elimination (5.91-6.85 hr). Furthermore, the $t_{1/2}$ of absorption for the m-xylene alone group was significantly faster in females than in males, while $t_{1/2}$ of elimination for the m-xylene alone and clay groups was significantly slower in females than in males.

Adsorption of m-xylene to sandy soil significantly increased the AUC (0.35 $\pm$ 0.04% initial dose/ml per hr) versus m-xylene alone (0.20 $\pm$ 0.01% initial dose/ml per hr) in females. There were no differences in AUC among the male treatment groups. However, the AUC of the female sandy soil group was significantly higher than all male treatment groups (Table 13.3).

Table 13.2. Absorption and elimination half-lives ($t_{1/2}$) of radioactivity in plasma of rats orally exposed to ^{14}C-m-XYLENE[a].

Treatment	$t_{1/2}$ (hr)			
	Absorption		Elimination	
	Females	Males	Females	Males
m-Xylene Alone	0.31 [b]	0.64	11.42 [b]	6.77
+ Sandy Soil	0.60 [c]	0.85	6.70 [c]	5.91
+ Clay Soil	0.38 [c]	0.69	11.50 [b]	6.85

[a] Values obtained from five to six rats/group gavaged with an aqueous solution of 5% gum acacia and ^{14}C-m-xylene alone or adsorbed to soil.
[b] Significantly different from m-xylene alone in males ($p < 0.02$).
[c] Significantly different from m-xylene alone in females ($p < 0.02$).

Fat contained the highest tissue concentration of radioactivity 24 hr post-oral administration of m-xylene, with stomach the second highest in all treatment groups of both sexes (Table 13.4). In male rats, sandy soil-adsorption of m-xylene significantly increased radioactivity in pancreas, while clay soil treatment caused a statistically significant increase in the amount of radioactivity found in the skin (Table 13.4). There were no statistically significant differences between treatment groups for all other tissues analyzed or between female and male rats.

The excretion of radioisotope in male and female groups occurred primarily in the urine (Table 13.5). In females, the majority of activity recovered in the urine following pure (50%) or clay soil (48%) treatment was found within 12 hr of dosing. However, following sandy soil-adsorbed m-xylene treatment in females,
nearly equal amounts of radioactivity were found in urine at the 0-12 hr and 12-24 hr collection periods (34 and 29%, respectively). Moreover, sandy soil

produced a significant decrease in ^{14}C activity during the 0-12 hr urine collection period versus m-xylene alone. During the same time interval, the female sandy soil group excreted significantly less radioactivity than all male treatment groups (Table 13.5). In males, clay soil treatment resulted in excretion of significantly more radioactivity than m-xylene alone during the 24-48 hr collection period.

Radioactivity as parent compound in expired air was a secondary route of excretion in females (14-22%) and males (9-20%) (Table 13.6) with the majority appearing during the first 12 hr of dosing. In females, the sandy soil treatment produced a significantly smaller amount of radioactivity in expired air versus m-xylene alone in the 2-6 hr period following treatment. Furthermore, the amount of radioactivity found in expired air of the female m-xylene alone treatment was significantly higher than male m-xylene alone during the 2-6 and 0-12 hr periods following treatment, while the female clay treatment was higher than m-xylene alone during the 0-12 hr period.

In males, on the other hand, both soils produced a significantly higher amount of radioactivity in expired air versus m-xylene alone in the 0-12 hr period following treatment. Moreover, the clay soil treatment was significantly higher than m-xylene alone during the 2-6 hr period, while the sandy soil treatment was significantly higher during the 6-12 hr period. Carbon dioxide comprised less than 0.1% of the initial dose expired in all male and female treatment groups (data not shown). The total ^{14}C activity recovered in the feces was small (<1%) in all groups of both sexes (data not shown).

The 0-12 hr and 12-24 hr urinary metabolites of m-xylene are shown in Table 13.7. Methylhippuric acid was the major metabolite detected in all male and female treatment groups. Smaller amounts of xylenol and parent compound were also found for the same time period. The type and percentage of m-xylene metabolites were not significantly altered in the presence of soil or between males and females.

Effects of Gender on the *In Vivo* Dermal Bioavailability of Benzene

Gender also influenced the amount of benzene absorbed dermally *in vivo* (Table 13.8). The peak plasma concentration of benzene was higher and was reached more quickly in females (3209 dpm/ml at 8 hr) than in males (2162 dpm/ml at 12 hr).[26] A significantly higher AUC was found in females (0.72 $\pm$ 0.25% initial dose/ml per hr) than in males (0.41 $\pm$ 0.21% inital dose/ml per hr). Moreover, benzene-derived radioactivity was eliminated slower in females (25.6 hr) relative to the males (23 hr) as supported by the longer half-life of elimination in females. Less radioactivity was excreted in urine by females (61.5 $\pm$ 1.7%) than by males (86.2 $\pm$ 2.1%). There were no differences in the amount of radioactivity excreted in expired air between males and females.

Table 13.3. Area under the curve (AUC) for radioactivity in plasma of rats orally exposed to ^{14}C-m-Xylene[a].

Treatment	AUC (% initial dose/ml per hr)	
	Females	Males
m-Xylene Alone	0.20 ± 0.01	0.21 ± 0.02
+ Sandy Soil	0.35 ± 0.04[b,c]	0.22 ± 0.02
+ Clay Soil	0.25 ± 0.02	0.22 ± 0.01

a Values represent mean ± SE of five to six rats/group gavaged with an aqueous solution of 5% gum acacia and ^{14}C-*m*-xylene alone or adsorbed to soil.
b Significantly different from males ($p<0.002$).
c Significantly different from *m*-xylene alone in females ($p<0.005$).

Table 13.4 Tissue distribution of radioactivity in rats orally exposed to ^{14}C-m-Xylene[a].

Fat > Stomach > Pancreas[b] > Skin[c]

a Determined for five rats/group, 24 hr after oral administration of an aqueous solution of 5% gum acacia and ^{14}C-m-xylene alone or adsorbed to soil.

b Significantly increased in the sandy soil adsorbed group versus m-xylene alone in males ($p<0.05$).

c Significantly increased in the clay soil-adsorbed groups versus m-xylene alone in males ($p <0.05$).

Table 13.5. Excretion of radioactivity in urine of rats orally exposed to ^{14}C-m-Xylene[a].

Time (hr)	Females			Males		
	m-Xylene Alone	+ Sandy Soil	+ Clay Soil	m-Xylene Alone	+ Sandy Soil	+ Clay Soil
0 - 12	49.8 ± 2.1	33.6 ± 3.5 [b, d]	48.3 ± 2.9	59.2 ± 2.2	55.6 ± 0.8	54.2 ± 6.3
12 - 24	18.7 ± 3.6	28.8 ± 9.9	19.6 ± 2.2	33.2 ± 7.7	18.8 ± 2.3	15.2 ± 1.4
24 - 48	5.1 ± 1.2	10.8 ± 3.9	10.4 ± 1.1	3.8 ± 0.8	8.9 ± 1.0	10.0 ± 1.9[c]
0 - 48	73.7 ± 4.9	73.2 ± 16.3	78.2 ± 0.6	96.2 ± 8.8	83.3 ± 2.9	79.4 ± 3.3

a Values represent percentage initial dose (mean ± SE) of six rats/group gavaged with an aqueous solution of 5% gum acacia and ^{14}C-m-xylene alone or adsorbed to soil.
b Significantly different from m-xylene alone in females ($p < 0.05$).
c Significantly different from m-xylene alone in males ($p < 0.05$).
d Significantly different from all male treatment groups ($p < 0.0005$).

Table 13.6. ^{14}C-*m*-Xylene in expired air of orally exposed rats[a].

Time (hr)	Females			Males		
	m-Xylene Alone	+ Sandy Soil	+ Clay Soil	m-Xylene Alone	+ Sandy Soil	+ Clay Soil
0 - 2	4.8 ± 0.4	4.6 ± 0.2	5.7 ± 0.7	3.0 ± 0.3	5.0 ± 1.0	5.9 ± 0.3
2 - 6	12.2 ± 2.1 [b]	4.4 ± 1.4 [c]	9.7 ± 0.7	4.0 ± 0.7	8.5 ± 1.2	11.1 ± 1.7 [b]
6 - 12	4.4 ± 1.8	3.7 ± 0.5	5.1 ± 0.9	1.4 ± 0.1	3.4 ± 0.4 [b]	2.6 ± 1.7
0 - 12	21.5 ± 3.3 [b]	12.7 ± 1.8	20.6 ± 0.6 [b]	8.4 ± 1.0	17.3 ± 2.4 [b]	19.8 ±1.5 [b]
12- 24	0.3 ± 0.1	0.7 ± 0.2	0.2 ± 0.1	0.2 ± 0.0	0.1 ± 0.0	0.2 ± 0.0
24 - 48	0.1 ± 0.0	0.1 ± 0.0	0.1 ± 0.0	0.0 ± 0.0	0.1 ± 0.0	0.0 ± 0.0

a Values represent percentage initial dose (mean ± SE) of six rats/group gavaged with an aqueous solution of 5% gum acacia and ^{14}C-m-xylene alone or adsorbed to soil.
b Significantly different from ^{14}C-m-xylene alone in males ($p < 0.02$).
c Significantly different from ^{14}C-m-xylene alone in females ($p < 0.02$).

Table 13.7. Urinary metabolites of ^{14}C-m-Xylene following oral exposure in rats[a,b].

In All Male and Female Treatment Groups:
m-Hippuric Acid > Xylenol > m-Xylene

a Major metabolites were identified by HPLC analysis of urine collected between 0-12 and 12-24 hr from six rats/groups gavaged with an aqueous solution of 5% gum acacia and ^{14}C-m-xylene alone or adsorbed to soil.

b No statistically significant differences were determined within treatments for the same sex or between the sexes.

Table 13.8. Effect of gender on pharmacokinetic parameters for ^{14}C-Benzene administered dermall to rats[a].

Parameter [b]	Males	Females
C_{max} (dpm/ml)	2162	3209
T_{max} (hr)	12	8
$t_{1/2}$ abs (hr)	3.1	4.8
$t_{1/2}$ elim (hr)	23.0	25.6
AUC (% initial dose/ml per hr)	0.41 ± 0.21	0.72 ± 0.25 [c]
Urine (% initial dose)	86.2 ± 2.1	61.5 ± 1.7 [c]
Expired Air (% initial dose)	12.8 ± 1.1	7.3 ± 2.1

a Plasma and excreta were collected from rats treated dermally with 40 µCi of ^{14}C- benzene alone.

b Values for plasma parameters were calculated from five to nine rats/group. The AUC was determined for the 72 hr plasma concentration time curve. Values for excretion (mean ± SE) were obtained from six rats/group 48 hr after treatment.

c Significantly different from males ($p < 0.03$).

Table 13.9. Effect of gender on pharmacokinetic parameters for ^{14}C-TCE administered orally to rats [a].

Parameter[b]	Males	Females
C_{max} (dpm/ml)	2346	3066
T_{max} (hr)	6	16
$t_{1/2}$ abs (hr)	3.5	6.3
Urine (% initial dose)	52.0 ± 4.8	60.3 ± 5.7
Expired Air (% initial dose)	32.3 ± 4.2	29.3 ± 2.2

a Plasma and excreta were collected from rats treated orally with 4.6 µCi of ^{14}C- TCE alone.

b Values for plasma parameters were calculated from five to nine rats/group. Values for excretion (mean ± SE) were obtained from six rats/group 72 hr after treatment.

Effects of Gender on the Oral Bioavailability of TCE

As in the benzene studies, sex differences were observed in the kinetics and bioavailability of TCE after oral exposure.[28,29] This was illustrated by higher values for peak plasma concentration of 3066 dpm/ml in the female group compared to 2346 dpm/ml in the male group. However, the time to attain peak plasma concentration was 2.5-fold faster in males (6 hr) than in females (16 hr). Similarly, the half-life of TCE absorption was almost doubled in females (6.3 hr) compared to males (3.5 hr). The percent of initial dose in urine and expired air were the same for males and females.

Effects of Testosterone on the *In Vitro* Dermal Bioavailability of TCE

Prior to sacrifice, the concentration of testosterone in the serum of the male control and sham groups was approximately 2 ng/ml which is the normal physiological concentration in male rats.[33] The female control and sham groups each had a testos terone level of less than 0.2 ng/ml. Administering testosterone to female rats elevated the testosterone level to 2.8 ng/ml while castration of male animals decreased their concentration to less than 0.2 ng/ml. When testosterone was restored in male rats, concentrations returned to normal (data not shown).

The effect of gender on the *in vitro* penetration of ^{14}C-TCE is shown in Table 13.10. Data are presented as radioactivity accumulated with time. It can be seen that the penetration of TCE in the females was significantly higher compared to that in the males at all times during the 10 hr collection period. Although penetration of radioisotope in both males and females appeared as early as five minutes after treatment (data not shown), no significant differences were observed until 30 min after administration of the chemical.[34] The data in Table 13.11 show the effects of testosterone deprivation in male rats and testosterone administration to female rats. In males, total penetration of ^{14}C-TCE (0-10 hr) was significantly higher in the testosterone-deprived group than in the control, sham, or testosterone-restored groups. In females, total penetration of ^{14}C-TCE (0-10 hr) was significantly lower in the testosterone-treated group than in the control or sham groups.

Thus, the administration of testosterone to female rats decreased dermal penetration of ^{14}C-TCE (1.75 $\pm$ 0.24% initial dose) to concentrations similar to male controls (1.30 $\pm$ 0.13% initial dose), while depriving male rats of testosterone increased the permeability of their skin (2.10 $\pm$ 0.18% initial dose) to concentrations approaching that of female controls (2.53 $\pm$ 0.12% initial dose) (Table 13.11).[34]

Table 13.10. Effect of gender on penetration of ^{14}C-TCE through rat skin *in vitro*.

Time (hr)	Male	Female
0.5	0.3 ± 0.1 [a]	0.5 ± 0.1 *
1.0	0.5 ± 0.1	1.0 ± 0.1 *
2.0	0.7 ± 0.2	1.4 ± 0.1 *
3.0	0.9 ± 0.2	1.7 ± 0.1 *
4.0	1.0 ± 0.2	1.9 ± 0.1 *
6.0	1.1 ± 0.2	2.2 ± 0.1 *
10.0	1.3 ± 0.1	2.5 ± 0.1 *

a Values (mean ± SE) represent the total penetration of ^{14}C-TCE at the indicated time, expressed as a percentage of the applied dose, from five untreated animals/group.

* Significantly different compared to males, ($p < 0.05$).

DISCUSSION

The results of this study indicate that gender as well as the presence of soil produced differences in the kinetics and/or bioavailability of m-xylene following oral exposure. Absorption of m-xylene from the gastrointestinal tract was relatively rapid for all treatments for both sexes with maximum peak plasma concentration occurring within 20 min following gavage. However, female rats exhibited a significantly faster half-life of absorption and a significantly slower half-life of elimination than male rats exposed to m-xylene alone. No differences in bioavailability were observed between the sexes.

Table 13.11. Penetration of ^{14}C-TCE through male and female rat skin *in vitro*.

Treatment	Males	Females
Control	1.30 ± 0.13 [a]	2.53 ± 0.12
Sham	0.98 ± 0.17	2.88 ± 0.19
Testosterone Deprived	2.10 ± 0.18 [b,c]	-
Testosterone Treated	1.18 ± 0.17 [d]	1.75 ± 0.24 [b,c]

a Values (means ± SE) represent the percent of the initial dose collected in the receptor solution from 0-10 hr after treatment. There were five animals/group.

b Significantly different compared to control group ($p<0.05$).

c Significantly different compared to sham group ($p<0.05$).

d Significantly different compared to testosterone-deprived group ($p<0.05$).

Both soils significantly prolonged absorption, while sandy soil significantly shortened elimination of m-xylene associated radioactivity from plasma in females. Further, sandy soil increased the peak plasma concentration as well as produced a significant increase in the oral bioavailability of m-xylene, as evidenced by an increase in the AUC for the 0-24 hr period studied. On the other hand, neither soil altered the absorption, elimination or bioavailability of m-xylene in male rats.

The tissue distribution of ^{14}C-m-xylene associated radioactivity was highest in fat for all treatments for both sexes. This radioactivity more than likely represents unmetabolized m-xylene which has high oil-water and oil-blood partition coefficients.[35] While there were no differences between the sexes in the concentration of radioactivity in fat, the significantly larger amount of fat in female versus male rats has the capacity to store larger amounts of m-xylene.[36] Sato et al. have proposed that for structurally similar, volatile, lipid-soluble chemicals like benzene and toluene the $t_{1/2}$ of elimination is inversely proportional to the amount of chemical stored in fat tissue.[36] This relationship may account, in part, for the longer $t_{1/2}$ of elimination observed in female versus male rats with m-xylene, since additional time would be required to remove larger amounts of chemicals from fat storage sites in females.

Urine as the primary route of excretion in all treatment groups is consistent with the metabolism of m-xylene to water-soluble products, methylhippuric acid (>60%) and xylenol (>3%), which are excreted by the kidney. While the majority of radioactivity in urine was generally excreted during the first 12 hr following treatment, the presence of sandy soil in females resulted in nearly equal amounts excreted in the 0-12 hr and 12-24 hr collection period. A parallel effect was not observed in males.

While there were no significant differences observed between females and males in the total radioactivity excreted in urine during the 48 hr following treatment, there was a trend toward greater urinary excretion in the males versus females particularly following treatment with m-xylene alone. This is supported by significantly smaller amounts of unmetabolized m-xylene excreted in expired air of males versus females during this time. Differences in these excretion patterns suggest greater metabolizing capacity in males versus females, particularly with regard to the formation of methylhippuric acid, the primary metabolite. The higher activity of microsomal mixed function oxidases in male versus female rats[37] and sex-related differences which are known to occur in a number of conjugation enzymes in rats[1] are consistent with these differences.

Therefore, the data presented here demonstrates that ingested soil contaminated with m-xylene produces a higher bioavailability than chemical alone in females versus males. Further, the data implies that the potential health risk in females exposed orally to soil-adsorbed m-xylene is greater than in males.

Although sex-related differences such as we have shown for benzene and TCE bioavailability have been detected for about 200 compounds,[1] the mechanisms by which these differences arise and are maintained are not completely understood. In our *in vivo* dermal benzene studies, more chemical was absorbed in females and the absorbed dose was eliminated more slowly from the body than in males. Although Sato et al. concluded from their work that, because of their large volume of fat tissue, females are more susceptible to a chemical such as benzene which has a high affinity for fat tissue,[36] the sex difference in rats may also be explained by enzymatic differences. Male rats metabolize many xenobiotics by the liver microsomal enzymes considerably more quickly than females.[1,2,37]

Since we also demonstrated that the rate of TCE absorption and peak plasma concentration of radioactivity after oral TCE administration differed between males and females and because testosterone is known to mediate a wide variety of sex differences,[2-4] the *in vitro* dermal bioavailability of TCE as well as the effects of testosterone on bioavailability were investigated. The *in vitro* studies showed that the penetration of TCE was significantly higher in females than in males. However, when male rats were castrated, the TCE absorption rate resembled the absorption rate in females. Conversely, treating females with testosterone produced a similar absorption rate as in males. This data suggests that male-female TCE dermal absorption differences are under hormonal influence.

Since testosterone is known to increase epidermal thickness in male rats,[38] the thickness of the epidermis may play a role in sex differences in the dermal penetration of chemicals. This is supported by the work of Bronaugh et al. who showed a sex-related difference in the percutaneous absorption of water, urea and cortisone.[39] All three of the compounds were absorbed approximately 2- to 3-fold faster through female than through male back skin. Gender differences in the permeability properties of rat back skin were further examined by Bronaugh and his co-workers by a castration experiment in rats.[39] They found that the thickness of the stratum corneum was approximately 2-fold higher in the male back than in females or in castrated males. These values showed an inverse correlation with permeability of benzoic acid. A similarity in lag time measurements between castrated male skin and female skin was the most important indicator of permeability differences in their benzoic acid experiments. Therefore, the gender differences that we observed for benzene and TCE more than likely are due to the effects of testosterone on skin thickness.

ACKNOWLEDGMENT

This research was supported as a project of the National Science Foundation/Industry/University Cooperative Center for Research in Hazardous and Toxic Subtances at New Jersey Institute of Technology, an Advanced Technology Center of the New Jersey Commission on Science and Technology.

REFERENCES

1. Calabrese, E.J., *Toxic Susceptibility, Male/Female Differences*, John Wiley & Sons, New York, 1985, 1, 5, 313.
2. Quinn, G.P., Axelrod, J., and Brodie, B.B., Species, strain and sex differences in metabolism of hexobarbitone, amidopyrine, antipyrine and aniline, *Biochem. Pharmacol.*, 1, 152, 1958.
3. Lucky, A.W., McGuire, J., Nydorf, E., Halpert, G., and Nuck, B.A., Hair follicle response of the golden Syrian hamster flank organ to continuous testosterone stimulation using silastic capsules, *J. Invest. Dermatol.,* 86, 83, 1986.
4. Koyama, Y., Nagao, S., Ohashi, K., Takahashi, H., and Marunouchi, T., Effect of systemic and topical application of testosterone propionate on the density of epidermal Langerhans cells in the mouse, *J. Invest. Dermatol.*, 92, 86, 1986.
5. Paustenbach, D.J., A methodology for evaluating the environmental and public health risks of contaminated soil, in *Petroleum Contaminated Soils*, Volume I, Remediation Techniques, Environmental Fate, Risk Assessment, Kostecki, P.T., and Calabrese, E.J., Eds. Lewis Publishers, Chelsea, Michigan, 1989, 255.

6. Ng, K.M.E., Chu, I., Bronaugh, R.L., Franklin, C.A., and Somers, D.A., Percutaneous absorption/metabolism of phenanthrene in the hairless guinea pig: Comparison of *in vitro* and *in vivo* results, *Fund. Appl. Toxicol.*, 16, 517,1991.
7. Turkall, R.M., Skowronski, G.A., Kadry, A.M., Botrous, M.F., and Abdel-Rahman, M.S., The percutaneous absorption of soil-adsorbed naphthalene in female pigs, *The Toxicologist*, 13, 52, 1993.
8. Abdel-Rahman, M.S., Skowronski, G.A., and Turkall, R.M., Gender differences in the bioavailability of soil-adsorbed phenanthrene after dermal exposure, in *Hydrocarbon Contaminated Soils*, Volume III, Kostecki, P.T. and Calabrese, E.J. Eds.,Lewis Publishers, Chelsea, Michigan, in press.
9. Support Document for the CERCLA 104 Priority List of Hazardous Substances That Will be the Subject of Toxicological Profiles, Agency for Toxic Substances and Disease Registry, U.S. Public Health Service, Department of Health and Human Services, in cooperation with the U.S. Environmental Protection Agency,October, 1992.
10. Sandmeyer, E.E., Aromatic hydrocarbons, in *Patty's Industrial Hygiene and Toxicology*, Volume 2B, Clayton, G.D. and Clayton, F.E., Eds., John Wiley & Sons, New York, 1981, 3253.
11. Marcus, W.L., Chemical of current interest-benzene, *Toxicol. Ind. Hlth,* 3, 205, 1987.
12. Korte, F., and Boedefeld, E., Ecotoxicological review of global impact of petroleum industry and its products. *Ecotoxicol. Environ. Saf.* 2, 55, 1978.
13. Cronkite, E.P., Bullis, J.E., Inoue, T., and Drew, R.T., Benzene inhalation produces leukemia in mice, *Toxicol. Appl. Pharmacol.*, 75, 358, 1984.
14. Maltoni, C., Conti, B., and Cotti, G., Benzene: A multipotential carcinogen. Results of long-term bioassays performed at the Bologna Institute of Oncology, *Amer. J. Ind. Med.*, 4, 589, 1983.
15. Fishbein, L., Xylenes: Uses, occurrence and exposure, *IARC Sci. Publ.*, 85, 109, 1988.
16. Gerarde, H.W., *Toxicology and Biochemistry of Aromatic Hydrocarbons*, Elsevier, London, 1960, 171.
17. Gitelson, S., Aladjemoff, L., Ben-Hador, S., and Katznelson, R., Poisoning by a malathion-xylene mixture, *J. Amer. Med. Assoc.*, 197, 165, 1966.
18. National Cancer Institute, Carcinogenesis Bioassay of Trichloroethylene, CAS No. 79-01-6, DHEW Publ. No. (NIH) 76, 1976.
19. Nakajima, T., Okino, T., Okuyama, S., Kaneko, T., Yonekura, I., and Sato, A., Ethanol-induced enhancement of trichloroethylene metabolism and hepatotoxicity: Differences from the effect of phenobarbital, *Toxicol. Appl. Pharmacol.*, 94, 227, 1988.
20. Inoue, O., Seiji, K., Kawai, T., Jin, C., Liu, Y., Chen, Z., Cai, S., Yin, S., Li, G., Nakatsuka, T.W., and Ikeda, M., Relationship between vapor exposure and urinary metabolite excretion among workers exposed to trichloroethylene, *Amer. J. Ind. Med.*, 15, 103, 1989.

21. Lloyd, J.W., Moore, R.M., Jr., and Breslin, P., Background information on trichloroethylene, *J. Occup. Med.,* 17, 603, 1975.
22. *IARC* Monographs on the evaluation of the carcinogenic risk of chemicals to humans, 20, 545, 1979.
23. National Cooperative Soil Survey: Official Series Description-Atsion Series, prepared by the United States Department of Agriculture-Soil Conservation Service, Washington, D.C., 1977.
24. National Cooperative Soil Survey: Official Series Description-Keyport Series, prepared by the United States Department of Agriculture-Soil Conservation Service, Washington, D.C., 1972.
25. Turkall, R.M., Skowronski, G., Gerges, S., Von Hagen, S., and Abdel-Rahman, M.S., Soil adsorption alters kinetics and bioavailability of benzene in orally exposed male rats, *Arch. Environ. Contam. Toxicol.*, 17, 159, 1988.
26. Skowronski, G.A., Turkall, R.M., and Abdel-Rahman, M.S., Soil adsorption alters bioavailability of benzene in dermally exposed male rats, *Amer. Ind. Hyg. Assoc. J.,* 49, 506, 1988.
27. Turkall, R.M., Skowronski, G.A., Kadry, A.M., and Abdel-Rahman, M.S., Sex differences in the bioavailability of soil-adsorbed m-xylene in orally exposed rats, *Toxicol. Letters*, 63, 57, 1992.
28. Kadry, A.M., Skowronski, G.A., Turkall, R.M., and Abdel-Rahman, M.S., Kinetics and bioavailability of soil-adsorbed trichloroethylene in male rats exposed orally. *Biol. Monitoring.* 1, 75, 1991.
29. Kadry, A.M., Turkall, R.M., Skowronski, G.A., and Abdel-Rahman, M.S., Soil adsorption alters kinetics and bioavailability of trichloroethylene in orally exposed female rats, *Toxicol. Letters*, 58, 337, 1991.
30. Jeffay, H., and Alvarez, J., Liquid scintillation counting of carbon-14; Use of ethanolamine-ethylene glycol monomethyl ether-toluene, *Anal. Chem.* 33, 612, 1961.
31. Skowronski, G.A., Turkall, R.M., Kadry, A.M., and Abdel-Rahman, M.S., Effects of soil on the dermal bioavailability of m-xylene in male rats, *Environ. Res.,* 51, 182, 1990.
32. Legan, S.J., Coon, G.A., and Karsch, F.J., Role of estrogen as initiator of daily LH surge in the ovariectomized rat, *Endocrinol.,* 96, 50, 1975.
33. Steiner, R.A., Bremmer, W.J., Clifton, D.K., and Dorsa, D.M., Reduced pulsatile luteinizing hormone and testosterone secretion with aging in the male rat, *Biol. Reprod.,* 31, 251, 1984.
34. McCormick, K., and Abdel-Rahman, M.S., The role of testosterone in trichloroethylene penetration *in vitro*, *Environ. Res.*, 54, 82, 1991.
35. Sato, A., and Nakajima, T., Partition coefficients of some aromatic hydrocarbons and ketones in water, blood and oil, *Br. J. Ind. Med.*, 36, 231, 1979.
36. Sato, A., Nakajima, T., Fujiwara, Y., and Murayama, N., Kinetic studies on sex differences in susceptibility to chronic benzene intoxication-with special reference to body fat content, *Br. J. Ind. Med.,* 32, 321, 1975.

37. Kato, R., Sex-related differences in drug metabolism, *Drug Metab. Rev.*, 3 (1), 1, 1974.
38. Eartly, H., Grad, B., and Leblond, C.P., The antagonistic relationship between testosterone and thyroxine in maintaining the epidermis of the male rat, *Endocrinol.,* 49, 677, 1951.
39. Bronaugh, R.L., Stewart, R.F., and Congdon, E.R., Differences in permeability of rat skin related to sex and body site, *J. Soc. Cosmet. Chem.,* 34, 127, 1983.

CHAPTER 14

Using Monte Carlo Analysis to Determine Risk Based Cleanup Levels

Teresa S. Bowers, Ph.D. and Amy R. Michelson, M.S., Gradient Corporation, Cambridge, Massachusetts, **Shirley Fu,** Gradient Corporation, Boulder, Colorado

INTRODUCTION

Monte Carlo analysis is a technique for estimating uncertainty and variability in predictive models. The technique differs from traditional use of predictive models in that it does not use single point estimates as values for model input parameters. Rather, Monte Carlo analysis uses probability density functions (or probability distributions) to represent each input parameter. The probability density function is a measure of either variability or uncertainty in the input parameter, and the function reflects the range of possible values and the most probable value for that parameter.

Monte Carlo analysis is carried out for any predictive model by use of a suitable computer software package. The computer program employs random sampling techniques to select values from each input parameter distribution that are used with the predictive model to estimate a value of the outcome variable. Multiple iterations yield an outcome distribution that reflects the range of possible outcome values and a most probable outcome value.

Use of Monte Carlo analysis in risk assessment has become widely discussed and the technique is being used by some agencies to assess site-specific ranges of risk and most probable risk values. This approach is a significant advance over the traditional risk assessment method where risks are assessed by multiplying single values for each input parameter. A risk level derived from single values is not clearly related to any defined segment of the population.

The logical next step to using Monte Carlo analysis in risk assessment is to use Monte Carlo analysis as an aid in deriving cleanup levels. Typically, average acceptable contaminant levels are calculated from the results of a risk assessment, where contaminant levels are related to acceptable health risks. However, the acceptable average contaminant level derived from the risk assessment is not the same as the level to which the soil must be cleaned up in order to achieve this average, and when this value is used as a cleanup level it is not clear what the resulting range of risks, post-remediation, will be. Monte Carlo analysis provides a methodology to relate the range of soil contaminant levels that will occur post-remediation to the expected range of health risks post-remediation, and to thereby calculate a cleanup level that will achieve the desired level of risk and the desired average contaminant level.

USE OF MONTE CARLO ANALYSIS IN RISK ASSESSMENT

Monte Carlo analysis can more accurately characterize and facilitate the interpretation of risks calculated from a traditional risk assessment approach. Currently, within EPA, a number of institutional motivations exist for increasing the use of Monte Carlo analysis.[1] A recent discussion on the use of quantitative uncertainty analysis in risk assessment is provided in a memo issued in February of 1992 by EPA Deputy Administrator F. Henry Habicht.[2] Habicht's memo recommends use of Monte Carlo analysis as an option for providing a more complete description of population exposures and associated risks. EPA's Science Advisory Board (SAB),[3] in a review of EPA's risk assessment guidance, recommended that the agency move toward a full distributional approach in which distributions are developed for each of the terms in the exposure equation and a Monte Carlo analysis be applied to obtain the resulting distribution for exposure. The SAB promotes the use of Monte Carlo analysis as a method for providing a more realistic picture of exposures and risks when various exposure inputs are being combined.

In addition, a number of studies outside of EPA that examine the use of Monte Carlo analysis for calculating risk have recently been published. Several recent studies calculate probability distributions for human health risks at chemically contaminated sites. The Thompson et al.[4] study presents a case study for children playing in soils contaminated with benzene and benzo(a)pyrene. In the Paustenbach et al.[5] study, Monte Carlo analysis is used to assess the distribution of potential health risks to workers exposed to Chromium (VI+) in soils. Numerous additional studies use Monte Carlo analysis as a risk assessment tool.[6-13]

The Traditional Risk Assessment Approach

The traditional risk assessment approach involves calculating a point estimate risk based on a reasonable maximum exposure (RME). EPA defines RME as the highest exposure that is reasonably expected to occur at a site.[2-14] For exposure to carcinogenic chemicals, the point estimate risk is calculated by multiplying the chemical-specific cancer slope factor by an average concentration and an average daily intake, as shown below.

$$\text{Cancer Risk} = \text{Chemical Concentration} \times \text{Intake} \times \text{Slope Factor} \quad (1)$$

where *Cancer Risk* is the unitless probability of an individual developing cancer, *Chemical Concentration* is the 95% upper confidence limit of the arithmetic mean of a set of site sampling results (mg/kg), *Intake* is the average daily intake of a compound, averaged over a lifetime (mg/kg-day) and *Slope Factor* is a toxicity value that defines quantitatively the relationship between dose and response.

The average daily intake of a chemical is calculated by the following equation:

$$\text{Intake} = \frac{\text{IR} \times \text{EF} \times \text{ED}}{\text{BW} \times \text{AT}} \qquad (2)$$

where *IR* is the soil ingestion rate (mg/day), *EF* corresponds to exposure frequency (days/year), *ED* is exposure duration (years), *BW* refers to body weight (kg), and *AT* is the averaging time (days).

To calculate intake, EPA recommends using a combination of some lower values [50th percentile] and some upper values [90 - 95th percentile] for the intake parameters. Recent guidance in the Habicht memo directs risk assessors to use upper values for those intake parameters that possess a higher degree of uncertainty and/or variability.[2]

Traditional Risk Assessment Approach versus the Monte Carlo Approach

Conceptual and practical problems exist with the traditional risk assessment approach. First, EPA's proposed method of combining upper and lower values of parameters for calculating risk can lead to an overly conservative estimate of risk that does not clearly correspond to any defined percentile of the population. The method lacks sophistication because it compounds conservative intake assumptions, and it ignores the distribution of contaminants at a site and the distribution of individual behaviors that lead to variable exposures. The RME point estimate risk can be wrong or misleading because it is often biased away from the mean value of the uncertainty it represents, it provides no indication of the likelihood of the risk occurring, and it provides no indication of the key sources of uncertainty.

In Monte Carlo analysis, instead of single point estimates, probability density functions (or probability distributions) are selected to represent input parameter values. Use of probability density functions allows for consideration of the range of possible values for each parameter and allows for incorporation of the relative frequency with which the values occur. For example, contaminant concentrations at a site and the relative frequency with which receptors may exhibit a particular behavior can both be entered as distributions. The outcome of a Monte Carlo analysis is an exposure or risk distribution that reflects the full distribution of risk, provides an estimate of the likelihood of a given percentile of risk occurring, and allows risk managers to see the risk that is associated with any given percentile of the distribution. A sensitivity analysis performed in conjunction with a Monte Carlo analysis determines the parameters that contribute most to risk.

CALCULATION OF SOIL CONTAMINANT CLEANUP LEVELS

Risk based soil contaminant cleanup levels are traditionally calculated by backwards solution of the risk equation where risk is set equal to a target risk level. For example, using the cancer risk equation (Equation 1), an average acceptable soil contaminant level can be calculated from the expression

$$\text{Acceptable Chemical Concentration} = \frac{\text{Acceptable Cancer Risk}}{\text{Intake} \times \text{Slope Factor}} \qquad (3)$$

where the acceptable cancer risk is set to a target value, e.g., 10^{-6}. The acceptable chemical concentration derived by this procedure is often equated to a soil contaminant cleanup level, where soils containing the contaminant at concentrations exceeding the calculated value are targeted for remediation. Soil contaminant concentrations derived in this manner are average acceptable values, and equating them to a cleanup level specifying remediation at higher concentrations can result in over compliance with target risks for a site.

An alternative to the traditional approach of calculating cleanup levels is to perform the risk assessment using Monte Carlo analysis to describe the distributions of all input parameters including the soil contaminant concentration distribution. Contaminant concentrations in soil, preremediation, can typically be represented by a lognormal distribution.[15] Soil remediation results in a truncation of the lognormal distribution of contaminant concentrations at the prescribed cleanup level, and may involve the addition of clean fill. This process changes the shape of the contaminant distribution (Figure 14.1) and changes the expected range of risk levels that may result from exposure to the soils. It is apparent from Figure 14.1 that the postremediation soil contaminant distribution can be no better represented by a point estimate than can the preremediation distribution.

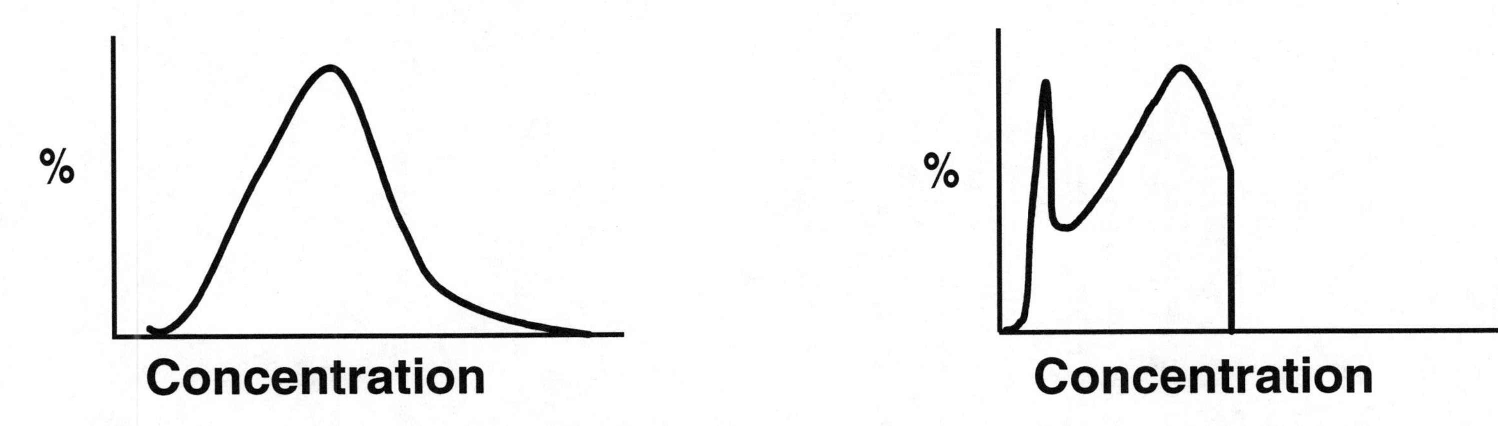

Figure 14.1. Typical soil contaminant distributions. (left) Preremediation, lognormal distribution, (right) Postremediation, the lognormal distribution is truncated at a cleanup level, and a spike is added at low concentration to represent the addition of clean fill.

Monte Carlo analysis is especially well suited to assess the effects of proposed soil remediation because only the soil contaminant distribution need be altered from the initial simulation conditions that are established for the risk assessment. The soil contaminant distribution is truncated at the proposed cleanup level and a second distribution representing the addition of clean fill is added if needed. A postremediation Monte Carlo simulation is run and a range of risks is generated. The 95th percentile risk (or other desired percentile) can then be compared to the target risk. This procedure yields significantly more information than can be gained by the traditional cleanup level approach, where there is no clear way to determine the percentage of a population that will be protected by a cleanup level derived from point estimates of risk.

AN EXAMPLE OF MONTE CARLO ANALYSIS WITH THE U.S. EPA LEAD MODEL TO ASSESS SOIL LEAD CLEANUP LEVELS

The following example describes the use of Monte Carlo analysis together with the U.S. EPA's LEAD Model to predict the range of blood lead levels (a measure of risk) observed in children living in Midvale, Utah and to assess the effects of an example soil lead cleanup level. The predictive model relates the concentration of lead in soil to blood lead levels in children. The effect of a specified soil lead cleanup level on the calculated blood lead distribution is assessed by altering the soil lead concentration distribution that is input to the model so that it reflects post-remediation conditions. The Monte Carlo analysis is then further used to illustrate the effect of cleanup to the proposed level on postremediation blood lead levels.

The LEAD Model

The LEAD Model was developed by EPA[16] to predict blood lead levels in young children (ages 6 to 72 months) exposed to lead in soil, house dust, air, water, food, and maternal blood. The basic equation for predicting a blood lead level is:

$$\text{Blood Lead} = \text{BSF} \times \text{Uptake} \qquad (4)$$

where *Blood Lead* has units of μg Pb/dL blood, *BSF* stands for a biokinetic slope factor* (μg/dL per μg/day), and *Uptake* is the amount of lead (μg/day) that has been absorbed into the body from the gastrointestinal and respiratory tracts. Total lead uptake is a summation of uptake from all potential lead sources, including soil, house dust, air, water, and food. Uptake from each source can be expressed as:

$$\text{Uptake} = A \times I \times C \tag{5}$$

where *A* is the fraction of the daily intake of lead that will be absorbed into the body (unitless), *I* refers to the ingestion rate (*e.g.* g/day of soil and dust), and *C* represents the concentration of lead in the source (*e.g.* mg/kg or μg/g lead in soil).

The LEAD Model must be calibrated to site-specific environmental lead data such that predicted blood lead levels are in accord with observed blood lead levels for the community. The calibration is typically done by adjusting the values of either the absorption or ingestion input parameters for soil and dust. The result of the calibration is a quantification of the effect of given levels of lead in soil on levels of lead in blood, based on the assumptions used in the model.

Monte Carlo Analysis and the LEAD Model

Monte Carlo analysis can be used together with the LEAD Model by specifying the likely range of each LEAD Model input variable. These include the measured range of environmental concentrations of soil, dust, and water, and estimates of the range of behavioral parameters, such as soil and dust ingestion rates. A Monte Carlo analysis using Midvale environmental lead concentrations and standard inputs to the LEAD Model (modified to include ranges) is performed here. The geometric mean soil lead level determined by Bornschein et al.[17] for the Midvale community is 399 mg/kg, with a geometric standard deviation of 2.54. The values of the other probability density functions and the

---

*The biokinetic slope factor used here is an approximation derived from the multicompartment pharmacokinetic parameters that form the basis for the translation of uptake into blood lead in the LEAD Model. Although this portion of the LEAD Model includes numerous parameters and equations, our experience has shown that the resulting relationship between uptake and blood lead is described by a very narrow range of values over the blood lead levels seen in this data set. As a result, and for simplicity in adopting a Monte Carlo approach to the LEAD Model, we have approximated this portion of the model with one variable.

application of Monte Carlo analysis to the LEAD Model is described in detail in Gauthier and Bowers.[18] The simulated range of blood lead levels predicted by the model for this soil lead level range is shown in Figure 14.2, and a comparison of predicted to actual blood lead levels is given in Table 14.1.

A second simulation of blood lead levels, postremediation, is shown in Figure 14.3. This simulation was performed with the soil lead distribution truncated at 500 mg/kg, where replacement soils are assumed to have a concentration ranging from 0 to 50 mg/kg (cleanup and replacement concentration values chosen for illustrative purposes only). All other model inputs are the same as those used to generate Figure 14.2. Table 14.2 shows a summary of the upper percentile blood lead levels calculated before and after soil cleanup for this example. The geometric mean blood lead level of the community drops from 5.6 to 4.3 μg/dL, while the 95th percentile blood lead level drops from 14.0 to 9.4 μg/dL. The geometric standard deviation of predicted blood lead levels drops as well, from 1.67 to 1.56.

Table 14.1. Blood Lead Levels Predicted by Monte Carlo Analysis with the LEAD Model for the Midvale, Utah Community

Percentile	Observed Blood Lead Level, μg/dL	Predicted Blood Lead Level, μg/dL
50	5.5	5.4
60	6.0	6.1
70	7.0	7.1
80	8.5	8.5
90	10.5	11.2
95	14.5	14.0
Geometric Mean	5.1	5.6
Geometric Standard Deviation	1.88	1.67

Soil lead cleanup levels are typically evaluated with the intent of protecting 95% of the population from having blood lead levels above a specified target, typically 10 μg/dL. In this case, the Monte Carlo analysis predicts that a cleanup level of 500 mg/kg will result in 95% of the population below a blood lead level of 9.4 μg/dL, indicating that the cleanup level of 500 mg/kg may be more restrictive than necessary to meet target health goals for the community.

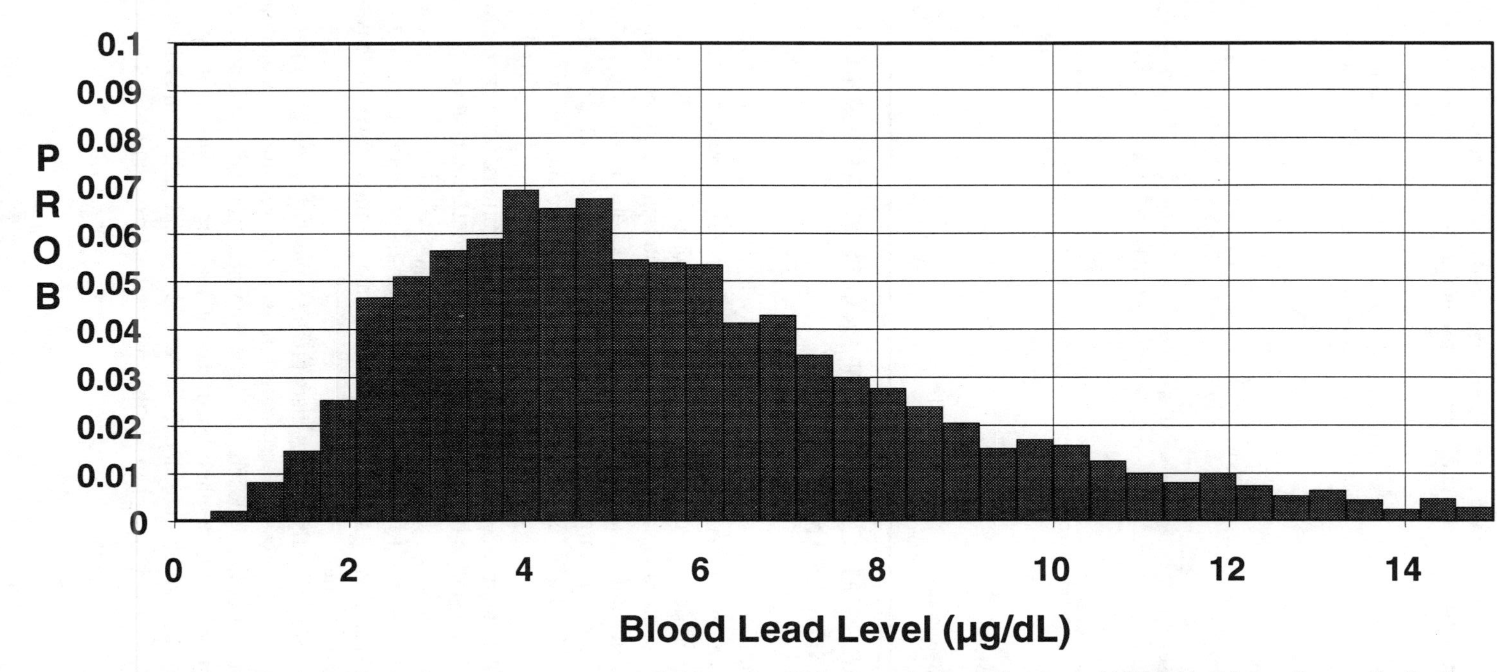

Figure 14.2. Monte Carlo simulation of blood levels, preremediation, using Midvale environmental data and LEAD Model equations and other inputs.

Table 14.2. Blood lead levels predicted by Monte Carlo analysis with the LEAD model: preremediation and postremediation.

Percentile	Preremediation Predicted Blood Lead Level, μg/dL	Postremediation Predicted Blood Lead Level, μg/dL
50	5.4	4.1
60	6.1	4.7
70	7.1	5.3
80	8.5	6.2
90	11.2	7.7
95	14.0	9.4
Geometric Mean	5.6	4.3
Geometric Standard Deviation	1.67	1.56

FURTHER APPLICATIONS OF MONTE CARLO ANALYSIS IN ASSESSING CLEANUP LEVELS

An additional use of Monte Carlo analysis lies in risk analysis and cleanup level calculations for contaminants for which there are multiple sources. For example, suppose a contaminant is found in both soil and water at a site, and each source contributes a significant portion of the total exposure. Furthermore, the sources of contamination of the soil and water are unrelated. A traditional multiple source exposure and risk model would represent both the soil and water contaminant levels by a point estimate. Monte Carlo analysis can be used to consider the range of concentrations of contaminants found in both the soil and water. If the range of water contaminant concentrations is to be changed, for example, by the state enforcing a new maximum contaminant level (MCL), then the soil contaminant cleanup level can be adjusted to reflect the necessary reduction in exposure to soil required in light of the changing exposure to water. Monte Carlo analysis is well suited to estimate cleanup levels where multiple sources are important.

Monte Carlo analysis can also provide the basis for performing a cost benefit type of analysis where multiple sources require remediation. For example, suppose that exposure to a contaminant occurs in both residential soils and in nonresidential, neighborhood recreational areas. Different contaminant cleanup levels can be considered for the residential and nonresidential soils. Assuming that a risk model exists that relates total exposure to both residential

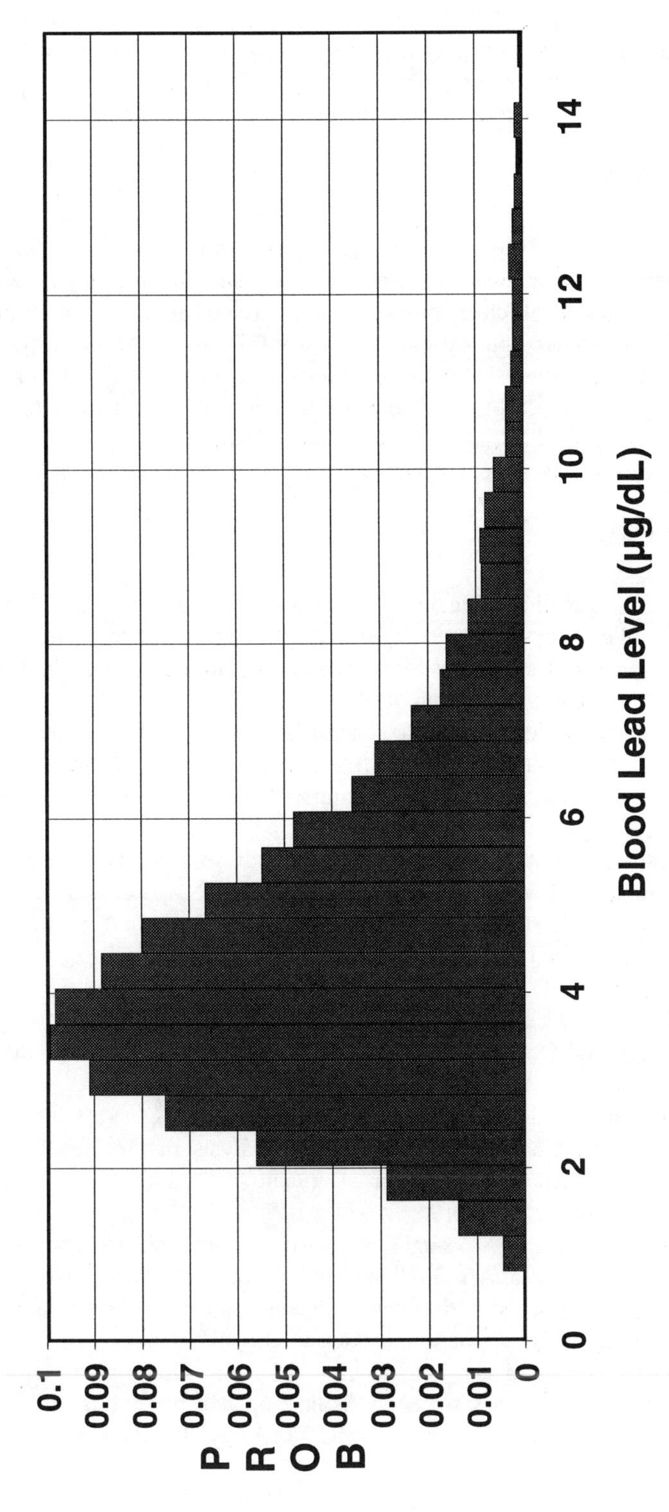

Figure 14.3. Monte Carlo simulation of blood lead levels, postremediation, using Midvale environmental data and LEAD Model equations and other inputs. The Soil lead concentration distribution input into the simulation has been truncated at 500 mg/kg, and a spike added that represents clean fill with concentrations ranging from 0 to 50 mg/kg.

and nonresidential soils, then Monte Carlo analysis can be used to explore the trade-offs between various soil contaminant cleanup levels for the two sources that, together, will yield an acceptable total risk. The cleanup levels can then be related to volume of soil remediation required, and thereby, to costs.

CONCLUSIONS

Monte Carlo analysis is a powerful technique that has applications extending beyond risk assessment into more accurate assessments of the impact of proposed contaminant cleanup levels on postremediation risk distributions. Its use, as in all other applications, is dependent on an adequate predictive model, and adequate representations of the distributions and central tendencies of the input parameters. Lack of such information is not a reason to not use Monte Carlo analysis, but rather in indication of where effort must be spent to improve future risk assessment capabilities.

REFERENCES

1. Frey, H.C., Quantitative analysis of uncertainty and variability in environmental policy making, prepared for the Center for Energy and Environmental Studies, Department of Engineering and Public Policy, Carnegie Mellon University, Pittsburgh, 1992.
2. Habicht, F.H., Guidance on risk characterization for risk managers and risk assessors, memorandum from F.H. Habicht, Deputy Administrator, to Assistant and Regional Administrators, U.S. Environmental Protection Agency, 1992.
3. Environmental Protection Agency Science Advisory Board (EPA SAB), An SAB report: Review of the Office of Solid Waste and Emergency Response's draft risk assessment guidance for Superfund Human Health Evaluation Manual by the Environmental Health Committee, EPA-SAB-EHC-93/007, 1993.
4. Thompson, K. M., Burmaster, D. E., and Crouch, E. A. C., Monte Carlo Techniques for Quantitative Uncertainty Analysis in Public Health Risk Assessment, *Risk Analysis,* 12, 53-63, 1992.
5. Paustenbach, D. J., Meyer, D. M., Sheehan, P. J., and Lau, V., An Assessment of Quantitative Uncertainty Analysis of the Health Risks to Workers Exposed to Chromium Contaminated Soils, *Toxicology and Industrial Health,* 7, 159-196, 1991.
6. Alberts, M.T. and J.D. Rouge, Stochastic health risk assessments: Case studies in California AB 2588 air toxics hot spots alternative analyses, Paper, presented at the 85th Annual Meeting and Exhibition of the Air and Waste Management Association, Kansas City, 1992.
7. Burmaster, D. E. and von Stackelberg, K., Using Monte Carlo simulations in public health risk assessments: Estimating and presenting full distributions of risk, for presentation at HMC-Northeast, Boston, 1991.

8. Constantinou, E., Seigneur, C., and Permutt, T., Uncertainty analysis of health risk estimates - Application to power plant emissions, presented at the 85th Annual Meeting and Exhibition of the Air and Waste Management Association, Kansas City, 1992.
9. Copeland, T. L., Holbrow, A. M., and Connor, K., Use of quantitative uncertainty analysis in air toxics risk assessments, presented at the 85th Annual Meeting and Exhibition of the Air and Waste Management Association, Kansas City, 1992.
10. ENVIRON Corporation, A comparison of Monte Carlo simulation-based exposure estimates with estimates calculated using EPA and suggested Michigan Manufactures Association exposure factors, prepared for Risk Assessment Subcommittee, Act 307 Program Advisory Group, 1993.
11. Keenan, R. E., Price, P. S., Henning, M. H., Goodrum, P. E., Gray, M. N., Sherer, R., and Porter, W. L., A Monte Carlo risk assessment for dioxin in marine fish: Using a MicroExposure^{TM} approach to evaluate the need for fish advisories, submitted to the 1993 TAPPI Environmental Conference, 1993.
12. Price, P. S., Sample, J., and Strieter, R., Determination of Less-Than-Lifetime Exposures to Point Source Estimates, *Risk Analysis,* 12, 367-382, 1992.
13. Wen-Whai, L., Firth, M. J., and Harris, R. H., Health risk reduction based on Monte Carlo simulation and air dispersion modeling at a chemical processing facility, presented at the 85th Annual Meeting and Exhibition of the Air and Waste Management Association, Kansas City, 1992.
14. Environmental Protection Agency (EPA). 1989. *Risk Assessment Guidance for Superfund*, 1, Human Health Evaluation Manual (Part A), interim final, Office of Emergency and Remedial Response, EPA/540-1-89-002.
15. Ott, W. R., A physical explanation of the lognormality of pollutant concentrations, *J. Air Waste Manage. Assoc.*, 40, 1378-1383, 1990.
16. U. S. EPA, *Guidance Manual for Site-Specific Use of the U. S. Environmental Protection Agency Lead Model*, Draft, 1991.
17. Bornschein, R. L., Clark, C. S., Pan, U. W., and Succop, P. A., *Midvale Community Lead Study*, Dept. of Environ. Health, Univ. Cincinnati Medical Center, 1990.
18. Gauthier, T. D. and Bowers, T. S., Monte Carlo simulation of the U.S. EPA LEAD Model, ms. in prep.

CHAPTER 15

Soil Ingestion Issues and Recommendations

Edward J. Calabrese and Edward J. Stanek, School of Public Health, University of Massachusetts, Amherst, Massachusetts

REVIEW OF PUBLISHED STUDIES

It has long been recognized that contaminated soil may present a potential public health concern because of groundwater contamination since groundwater is a significant drinking water source. Recently, regulatory and public health agencies have become concerned that consumption of contaminated soil by children may present a significant public health problem. For example, elevated levels of lead in soil and dust are suspected of contributing to elevated blood lead levels as a result of soil/dust ingestion (Spittler, 1986). Also widely discussed has been the dioxin contamination of Times Beach, Missouri. The Centers for Disease Control (CDC) derived a theoretical cancer risk associated with levels of dioxin in soil (Kimbrough et al., 1984). A major concern in the CDC assessment was the assumed consumption by children of soil containing dioxin.

The knowledge of how much soil and dust children ingest is critical for those involved with the issue of assessing public health risks from environmental contamination. Numerous site-specific clean up decisions especially for those tightly bound to soil contaminants (e.g., dioxin, PCBs, lead, cadmium, others) are often driven by assumptions concerning estimates of soil and more recently dust ingestion.

While early qualitative estimations of childhood soil ingestion have been made by several groups (Lepow et al., 1974; the National Research Council 1980; and Day et al., 1975), these attempts lack sufficient quantitative evaluation to allow confident estimation of actual soil ingestion. Subsequently, scientists at CDC developed an estimation for specific age groups based on unpublished behavioral observations of children aged 1.5 to 3.5 years. These children were estimated to ingest 10 g of soil/day (Kimbrough et al., 1984).

The first attempt to estimate human soil ingestion quantitatively was presented by Binder et al. (1986) using aluminum (Al), silicon (Si), and titanium (Ti) as soil tracer elements. These elements were selected since their concentration is high in soil but low in food products and their gastrointestinal tract absorption is low. The amount of soil ingested was calculated based on the fecal and soil concentrations of the tracer elements and the amount of fecal output. In their study involving 59 diapered children aged one to three years residing in Montana, the calculated mean soil ingestion estimates for the tracers Al and Si were 181 and 184 mg/day and ten times higher (1,834 mg/day) for Ti. The authors were unable to resolve the apparent conflict between estimates based on the various tracers.

Clausing et al. (1987) and Van Wijnen et al. (1990) have estimated the amount of soil consumed by children living in the Netherlands following a method similar to that of Binder et al. (1986). Clausing et al. (1987) reported mean soil ingestion values ranging from 127 mg to 1,084 mg/day, depending on the marker, with Ti yielding the highest estimate. The Binder et al. (1986) and Netherlands studies (Clausing et al., 1987; Van Wijnen et al., 1990) are indirect attempts to estimate soil ingestion and could be improved by measuring the concentration of tracers in food and other ingested products (e.g., medicines), of the participating subjects as well as the presence of tracers in diapers and other materials that contact the feces. Based on these and other limitations (see Calabrese and Stanek (1991) for a critical review), the Binder et al. (1986), Clausing et al. (1987), and Van Wijnen et al. (1990) studies are precluded from providing definitive evidence of soil ingestion.

Two additional soil ingestion studies on children have been published that include substantial improvements on the methodology used by the early investigators. The first study was on children aged one to four in western Massachusetts (Calabrese et al., 1989), while the second study was on children aged two to seven in the state of Washington (Davis et al., 1990).. Both studies accounted for tracer ingestion due to food consumption as part of their study protocol. Estimates of soil ingestion were made for three elements in the Davis et al., study, and eight elements in the Calabrese et al. study (Table 15.1).

Estimates of median soil ingestion were markedly lower in the Calabrese and Davis studies as compared with earlier investigations. Estimates of median soil ingestion based on Al were less than one-fourth the earlier estimates, while estimates based on Si and Ti were less than one-half and one-seventh the earlier estimates, respectively. Still, there was marked variation in the mean and median soil ingestion estimates for the individual studies. Estimates of median soil ingestion based on different tracers differed by over 300% in the Davis study, and by over 800% in the Calabrese study.

Due to the improvements in study design, the Davis and Calabrese studies provide the best estimates of soil ingestion to date. Since their conduct, much effort has been made to understand the reasons for the large variability in tracer specific estimates, and determine the most reliable estimate of soil ingestion (Stanek and Calabrese, 1991; Calabrese and Stanek, 1991). These investigations have identified the food/soil ratio for a tracer as a predictor of soil ingestion reliability. Basically, the larger the ratio, the less reliable the soil ingestion estimate for a given tracer due to a high background noise to signal ratio.

Those tracers (i.e., Ba, Mn) displaying the poorest performance in the adult validation study of Calabrese et al. (1989) in terms of precision of recovery were those with the highest food to soil ratios. Conversely, those tracers displaying very low food to soil ratio displayed considerably improved precision of recovery. Consequently, tracers with low food to soil ratios were estimated to have markedly lower (more sensitive) soil ingestion detection limits (see Stanek and Calabrese 1991; Calabrese and Stanek, 1991). Average daily ingestion of elements in food were larger in the Davis study than the Calabrese study (by 278%, 41% and 110%, for Al, Si, and Ti, respectively), thus implying that soil ingestion estimates are less reliable in the Davis study.

The net impact of high food/soil ratios for a study has been large input-output misalignment errors. These errors have resulted in negative soil ingestion estimates for as many as 45% of study subjects depending on the specific tracer. While the negative misalignment errors can be easily recognized, the positive misalignment errors can only be guessed at due to the limitations in the study designs. Subsequent and on-going research in this area (see Recent Progress on Soil Ingestion) has served to further clarify such limitations.

In summary, estimates of soil ingestion to date are highly variable and of questionable reliability. Mean and median estimates for the study populations are inconsistent in given studies. The limited reliability has made subject-specific soil ingestion estimates, except for soil pica (> 1.0 gm/day) (Calabrese et al. 1991), impossible to construct.

Table 15.1. Soil ingestion estimates in children (mg/day).

	Binder et al.		Van Wijnen et al.		Davies et al.		Calabrese et al.	
	Mean	Median	Mean	Median	Mean	Median	Mean	Median
Al	181	121	--	--	40	25	153	29
Si	184	136	--	--	82	59	154	40
Ti	1834	618	--	--	246	81	218	55
Ba							32	<0
Mn							<0	<0
V							459	96
Y							85	9
Zr							21	16
Limiting Tracer Method (LTM)								
(Day Care Center)			103	111				
(Campers)			213	160				

The current studies also have significant limitations with respect to their generalizability. While the original University of Massachusetts (Calabrese et al., 1989) study provided a higher reliability in soil ingestion estimates of the study participants due to improved precision of recovery estimates and lower soil ingestion detection limits than other reports, it is important to emphasize that the study has significant limitations with respect to its generalizability to other populations of children especially those residing in urban areas and children of other Social Economic Status (SOES) and racial backgrounds. The non-random nature of the selected population affects its capacity to be generalized from an academic community in western Massachusetts to children in other communities. In addition, the study population was observed only between Monday and Thursday for two consecutive weeks. While suggesting a possible magnitude of inter-subject soil ingestion variation, the University of Massachusetts as well as other soil ingestion studies provide no insight for seasonal, regional and ethnic variation in soil estimates nor whether soil ingestion differentially occurs on weekend rather than week days. Another factor inadequately considered in these studies was the relationship of the extent of grass cover and how that was quantitatively related to soil ingestion.

The collective limitations of the present soil ingestion data base to offer generalizations to other populations of children concerning quantitative estimates of soil ingestion presents a serious challenge to regulatory/public health officials performing soil based exposure assessments.

Despite the completion of four studies on soil ingestion in children, most of the initial benefit of these investigations has been in the development of improved understandings of how to design, conduct, analyze and interpret soil ingestion study data. Current methods now permit the development of study protocols that can adequately address critical issues of tracer selection, sample size, duration of study, and sources of positive error (e.g., input misalignment, unknown source input) and negative error (e.g., output misalignment, sample loss during analysis), such that highly reliable estimates of soil ingestion can be derived.

Recent Progress on Soil Ingestion

Since the publication of the original study on soil ingestion in 1989 (Calabrese et al., 1989), the University of Massachusetts (UMass) soil research group has extensively re-evaluated their original findings and have been able to advance understandings in several relevant areas:

(1) Clarification of the Causes of Intertracer Variation in Soil Ingestion Estimates. The major sources of error in the UMass soil ingestion study have recently been identified and quantified on a subject-tracer basis. The principal sources of error are (a) input/output

misalignment[1] error due to both study design limitations and the presence of high background levels of tracers in ingested food relative to ingested soil, (b) unknown source error for several tracers. By comparing soil ingestion estimates on a subject by day basis, it has been possible to quantify the input and output error per element (Table 2). Furthermore, additional sources of element ingestion are evident. For example, Ti and V appeared to have been ingested from sources other than soil and food, thereby falsely inflating soil ingestion estimates for affected tracers. Table 15.2 illustrates the magnitude and type of positive and negative error within the UMass children soil ingestion study. This knowledge can readily be incorporated in the design and conduct of future studies so that more reliable estimates of soil ingestion can be obtained.

Table 15.2. Positive/Negative Error (Bias) In Soil Ingestion Estimates In the UMass Mass-Balance Study.* The Error has been identified by Source (Output/Input misalignment, sample loss, extraneous source) and Quantified by Tracer leading to improved new mean estimates of soil ingestion. (Values are given as mg of soil ingested/day)

	Negative Error (Bias)		Positive Bias		Net Bias	Mean	Adjusted (Improved) Mean
Tracer	Output Error	Sample Loss	Input Error	Extraneous Source Error			
Al	6.3	--	8.0	3.2	+ 4.9	153	148.1
Si	7.8	--	9.5	15.1	+ 16.8	154	137.2
Ti	156.2	--	138.4	97.9	+ 80.1	218	137.5
V	24.9	--	83.3	243.6	+302	459	157
Y	48	--	1.6	1.7	- 44.8	85	129.8
Zr	25.3	69	0.0	0.9	- 93.4	25	118.4

*Values indicate impact on mean of 128-subject-weeks in mg of soil ingested per day.

The new range of 118.42 to 157 is 1.325-fold
The old range of 25 to 459 is 18.36-fold

Variation in the mean is reduced by 93% as a result of the quantification of the different sources of error.

[1] Input misalignment error would occur when an unusually high quantity of tracer is ingested on a day just prior to the start of the soil ingestion study and this quantity is captured in fecal samples during the study. This "extra" amount of fecal tracer would be incorrectly attributed to soil ingestion (i.e., input misalignment error). An output misalignment error occurs when tracers ingested in food are not captured in fecal samples due to slow transit time and the study ending before the passage of food occurs. This is the principal cause of the high number of children in the Calabrese et al. (1989) and Davis et al. (1990) studies displaying negative soil ingestion values. In fact, 44 of 128 subject-weeks did not provide a fecal sample on the final day of the Calabrese et al. (1989) study, thereby contributing to incorrect lower and negative soil ingestion estimates.

(2) Differentiating Soil and Dust: Methodology/Application. The UMass team developed a methodology to estimate whether the source of residual tracers in the feces samples was of soil or dust origin (Stanek and Calabrese, 1991).

The strategy for distinguishing indoor dust from outdoor soil ingested soil is based on element concentration ratios. For illustration, let C(s) denote the concentration of an element in outdoor soil and indoor dust, and Y the total residual amount of an element in urine and feces (after subtracting food) for a subject-week. Then define the quantities:

$$S = \frac{C(s)\text{-element A}}{C(s)\text{-element B}} \quad D = \frac{C(d)\text{-element A}}{C(d)\text{-element B}} \quad \text{and } R = \frac{Y\text{-element A}}{Y\text{-element B}} \tag{1}$$

For example, if element A was four times more plentiful in outdoor soil than element B, but both elements were equally plentiful in indoor dust, then D = 1 and S = 4. We would expect R to fall between 1 and 4, since the residual for each element must be composed of a combination of outdoor soil and indoor dust. In practice, the observed value of R may be larger than 4 or less than 1 due to the imperfect match of collected food ingestion with collected fecal output. With eight tracer elements, 28 element ratios can be constructed. These 28 tracer ratios provide considerable opportunity to distinguish soil from dust ingestion whereas using three tracers (as in the Binding, Davis and Van Wijnen studies) would provide only three possible tracer ratios, thus greatly restricting the potential to differentiate soil from dust but also the opportunity to confirm that any estimated differences in soil vs dust ingestion by other tracer ratios. Overcoming this critical obstacle provided a basis (along with the need to quantify source error [Table 2]) for proposing to measure eight (rather than three) soil tracers in the present scheme.

This methodology was strikingly successful when applied to the soil-pica child identified by Calabrese et al. (1991). Table 3 presents the results for the tracer ratio comparisons for the soil pica child during week two of the study. There was a maximum total of 28 pairs of tracer ratios based on the eight tracers. Of the 28 tracer ratio pairs 19 ratios for the residual fecal sample were available for quantitative evaluation. Of these 19, nine fecal tracer ratios (i.e., Mn/Ti, Si/Ti, Ba/Y, Si/Y, Al/Y, Ba/Ai, Si/Al, Mn/Si, Ba/Si) fell within the boundaries for soil and dust. The remaining ten fecal tracer ratios (Ba/Ti, V/Ti, Al/Ti, Y/Ti, Ma/Y, V/Y, Mn/Al, V/Al, Si/V, Mn/Ba) fell outside of the boundaries for soil and dust. Whenever a value fell outside of the boundaries the source of the residual tracers was concluded to be 100% from the source it was most similar to. For example, tracer ratio No. 16 for Si/V (Table 3) was judged to indicate that 100% of the residual fecal tracers for this ratio were from soil. For tracer ratios where the values were between the boundaries an interpolation was performed to estimate the relative contribution of soil and dust to the residual fecal tracer ratios.

The results indicate that all ten of the ratios that exceeded the boundary did so on the soil side. These ten ratios were interpreted as indicating that 100% of the fecal tracer ratios were from soil origin. The nine residual fecal samples within the boundaries revealed that a high percentage (i.e., 71-99%) of the residual fecal tracers were estimated to be of soil origin.

Table 15.3. Ratios of Soil, Dust, and Residual Fecal Samples in the Soil Pica Child

Tracer Ratios	Soil	Fecal	Dust	Estimated % of Residual Fecal Tracers of Soil Origin as Predicted by Specific Tracer Ratios
1. Mn/Ti	208.368	215.241	260.126	87
2. Ba/Ti	187.448	206.191	115.837	100
3. Si/Ti	148.117	136.662	7.490	92
4. V/Ti	14.603	10.261	17.887	100
5. Ai/Ti	18.410	21.087	13.326	100
6. Y/Ti	8.577	9.621	5.669	100
7. Mn/Y	24.293	22.373	45.882	100
8. Ba/Y	21.854	21.432	20.432	71
9. Si/Y	17.268	14.205	1.321	81
10. V/Y	1.702	1.067	3.155	100
11. Al/Y	2.146	2.192	2.351	88
12. Mn/Al	11.318	10.207	19.520	100
13. Ba/Al	10.182	9.778	8.692	73
14. Si/Al	8.045	6.481	0.562	81
15. V/Al	0.793	0.487	1.342	100
16. Si/V	10.143	13.318	0.419	100
17. Mn/Si	1.407	1.575	34.732	99
18. Ba/Si	1.266	1.509	15.466	83
19. Mn/Ba	1.112	1.044	2.246	100

DUST VS SOIL

Several recent reports (Calabrese and Stanek 1992; Stanek and Calabrese, 1992) have indicated that the source of residual fecal tracers in the Calabrese et al. (1989) study is of both outdoor soil and indoor dust origin. These papers present techniques for how the source of tracers can be quantitatively differentiated. While considerable interspecies variation existed in the source of residual fecal tracers, approximately 50% of the tracers were of indoor origin. A subsequent study by Calabrese et al. (1992) estimated that 30% of the indoor dust was comprised of tracked in soil. Taken collectively, the median child in the Calabrese et al. (1992) study had approximately 65% of their residue fecal tracers of outdoor soil origin.

Statistic Selection

For regulatory/risk assessment purposes, some have recommended using a mean estimate rather than median. The mean has the advantage of being simpler and more easily understood. We feel that this is a weak argument for using the mean, since the mean will be strongly influenced by extreme values. In contrast, the median has been shown to be much more robust than the mean (Calabrese et al., 1991), in the analysis of the Calabrese et al. (1989) data using a variety of assumptions in the formulation of different population estimates. However, the use of other percentiles (such as the 75%) would be a sound measure if some estimate larger than the median were desired. If some estimate of the mean is insisted upon, a better estimate will be the geometric mean since this estimate will account for the skewness of daily soil ingestion values observed among children. In fact, in forming confidence intervals for soil ingestion, better coverage can be obtained by forming confidence intervals based on the geometric mean (using log base e), rather than the simple arithmetic mean. However, the use of the geometric mean argues against simplicity.

If it was necessary to select a single estimate for soil ingestion we would recommend an estimate on a combined soil and dust element concentration, and consider the best estimate to be based on the median. The rejection of the arithmetic mean is based not only on its instability as a measure of central tendency of the population but that it does not have any precise meaning in the assessed population. For example, with variables that have skewed distributions, the mean does not represent any benchmark in terms of a percentile. This is in contrast with the median, which represents the 50th percentile.

AGE RELATED CHANGES

It has been generally assumed by various state/federal regulatory and public health agencies that all human age groups ingest soil. It has been concluded, based principally on professional judgement, that children ingest more soil than adults and that children with high hand to mouth activity (i.e. ages one to four) ingest more soil than children of other ages.

Analysis of the Calabrese et al. (1989) data revealed that soil ingestion increased linearly with age for all tracers. This was particularly evident for Ti while much less for Zr (Stanek et al., 1991). The slopes of these two most reliable tracers differ to such an extent (slope 7.36-Ti, 0.49-Zr) that it cannot be determined for the Calabrese et al. (1989) study population that soil ingestion increases as children increase in age from one to four.

While it is believed that children aged one to four years ingest more soil than other age groups this assumption is not based on empirical data. Incidental or intentional soil ingestion in children five to ten years may be more or less than one to four year old but this study and others provide no quantitative information on the soil ingestion rates that answer this question. An attempt to estimate soil ingestion in the six adults used in the three week tracer recovery validation study indicated an average soil ingestion rate of approximately 40 mg/day (Calabrese, et al., 1990). However, the estimated rate of soil ingestion in this pilot study was considerably below the actual estimated detection limit of that particular study because of the small sample size and high food tracer to soil tracer ratio (see Stanek and Calabrese, 1990). Thus, the reported soil ingestion estimates for adults in Calabrese et al. (1990) could not be seen with sufficient precision of recovery to derive accurate judgements about soil ingestion rates in adults. The data base, therefore, does not include confident values for soil ingestion for adults while no clear evidence exists that age related changes in soil ingestion occurred in the Calabrese et al. (1989) study. The age analysis for children is also further compromised because the sample size for each age group was small (i.e. ~ ten for six month age intervals). Because of the small sample size for age specific soil ingestion values, the soil ingestion detection levels are far higher than values that were estimated.

In light of the inadequacies of the soil ingestion data base how are age adjustments in soil ingestion to be made? It would appear logical that adults should ingest significantly less soil than young children. It would seem reasonable, in the absence of reliable quantitative data, to assume that an "average" adult ingests from 25 to 10% of the "average" child (one to six years old) based on diminished hand to mouth activity and other maturational and social factors.

Based on this rationale it is recommended that children six to twelve years of age be assumed to ingest 25% of the soil ingestion value of a one to six year old child while those > 12 years of age be assumed to ingest 10% of the one to six year old child.

RURAL VS URBAN/SUBURBAN CHILDREN

No quantitative data exist on the comparative soil ingestion rates of children from rural, urban and suburban areas. This remains an important data gap to be filled. At present, any attempt to make a distinction in soil ingestion rates would be speculative. There may be a number of potential factors affecting the differential rate of soil ingestion amongst rural, urban and suburban children such as time spent outdoors, degree of grass cover of outdoor play areas, quantity of dust in home and others. However, in the absence adequate information on these variables, the present emphasis will focus on the extent of grass cover because of the obvious direct access to contact with soil. Under such circumstances it is not unreasonable to suggest the incorporation of an uncertainty factor analogous to those used in risk assessment activities for non-carcinogens. Since this represents concern with inter-individual variation an uncertainty factor of approximately one to ten is selected depending on the degree of grass cover in areas where children play. If grass cover were extensive (>90%) then an UF of 1 would be appropriate. However, if grass cover were more limited (50-90%) in areas of access, then a 5-fold factor would be recommended. While a 10-fold factor would be used if grass cover were <50%. This approach may have site specific application but it is not recommended for national or statewide guidance.

SEASONALITY

The Calabrese et al. (1989) study was conducted in the fall (Sept./Oct) in Massachusetts. It may be speculated that ingestion of soil may be highest in the summertime and lowest in the winter in Massachusetts based on the premise that children play longer hours outdoors in the summer with greater direct contact with soil. However, it may be argued that soil contact may actually be greater in the spring before the growth of grass becomes significantly thickened or during more rainy seasons such as spring and winter depending on geographical locations. Thus, it is possible that seasonal effects may markedly vary according to a variety of factors and that soil ingestion may not be highest in the summer months in all locations. In addition, there may be seasonal variation in the tracking in of dust within the home with perhaps more mud being tracked into the home during the more rainy seasons. In the absence of information to clarify these uncertainties in the data base, no seasonal effect is recommended at this time.

IDENTIFICATION OF PICA CHILDREN

The consumption of non-food items, especially by young children, is a very common activity; when this activity is excessively performed it becomes characterized as pica. The range of non-food items that such children may ingest is extremely variable, including: clothing, books/paper, crayons, soil, cigarettes, household furnishings and other items.

The prevalence of pica behavior appears to be highly variable, being contingent on the definition of pica, the population assessed amongst other factors. Table 15.4 reveals that the prevalence of pica behavior can range from 10% in Caucasian children to 66% in institutionalized psychotic children. It appears, therefore, that children one to six years old display a pica prevalence that is between 15 and 30% with no obvious significant variation between males and females.

The identification of pica children presents a major initial stumbling block since there are no definitive criteria for this behavior. The present literature often represents subjective judgements based on individual perceptions of what comprises pica behavior, with limited standardized behavioral norms concerning whether children display pica behavior.

Some evidence exists suggesting that there is considerable variation amongst pica behaviors especially concerning what items are preferentially ingested (Barltrop, 1966; Harvey et al., 1986). More specifically, a child with pica behavior may ingest only selective items to the exclusion of others. For example, a pica child ingesting books or paper may not ingest other items such as cigarettes or soil. In contrast, a child with a preference for soil may not ingest other non-food items. In fact, Harvey et al. (1986) has observed that soil pica behavior comprises but a small subset of childhood pica behaviors. Their data suggest that there is an age-dependence in object selectivity and that such selectivity increases with age. The potential implications of the Harvey et al. (1986) data are that not all children with pica ingest soil and in fact only a subset of children with pica ingest greater than average amounts of soil. If one quarter (25%) of children display pica behavior it may be reasonable to assume that about 25% of those children as being soil pica children (Harvey et al., 1986). This would result in about 6.25% of the population aged 1-6 years displaying soil pica behavior. Given this theoretical estimate of 6.25% for an estimated soil pica prevalence, it would be important to compare this value with estimates based on soil tracer ingestion studies for children in the 1-6 year age range. The four available soil ingestion studies (Binder et al., Calabrese et al., Davis et al., and Van Wijnen et al.) were examined for evidence of pica soil evidence. These collective studies have provided daily soil ingestion on 517 children. If soil pica were subjectively defined in quantitative terms as consumption of greater than one gm of soil per day, then ten individuals would be identified from these four studies as having displayed this behavior. This would amount to a soil-pica prevalence of 1.9% from the four available soil ingestion studies. This would be lower than the earlier noted theoretical estimate of 6.25% for soil pica in one to six year olds.

Table 15.4. Range of Pica Behavior Prevalence

Group Description	# Subjects	% of Pica	Reference
Retarded Children	30	50	Kanner, 1937
Black Children > 6 mo.	386	27	Cooper, 1957
White Children > 6 mo.	398	17	
Black, 1-6 years	486	32	Millican et al., 1962
White, 1-6 years	294	10	
Children, low income	859	55	Lourie et al., 1963
Children, high income		30	
Children, 1-6 (interview)	439	15	Barltrop, 1966
Children, 1-6 (mail survey)	227	50	
Institutionalized, psychotic 3-13 years	40	66	Oliver, 1966
Spanish American Children (California)	21	32	Bruhn & Pangborn, 1971
Children (Mississippi)	115	16	Vermeer & Frate, 1979

This soil tracer estimation of the prevalence of soil pica children of course rests on very limited data. The nine individuals in the Van Wijnen et al. study displayed the pica-like behavior (> 1000 mg/day) on only a single observation day over a two to five day period. The soil ingestion values of these subjects was not adjusted downward for food ingestion of the tracer elements, thus leading to variable overestimates of soil ingestion. The one child pica subject in the Calabrese et al. study was observed over two separate four day periods and displayed soil-pica behavior only in the second of the two week period of observation. These data suggest that those displaying soil pica behavior do so irregularly and thus would not be predicted to consistently ingest > 1 gram of soil per day. If one accepted that about 2% of children one to six years of age occasionally ingest >1.0 gram of soil per day, what percentage would ingestion > 10 grams per day. The Calabrese et al. (1989) data suggest that only one child of the 517 (0.2%) ingested greater than ten grams of soil per day. It should be noted that soil ingestion estimates for this soil pica child were seen with a precision of 100 $\pm$ 20 or less for Al, Si, and Ti.

Over what duration of normal life span would one display soil pica? While there are no adequate data to resolve this issue, it is generally believed that pica behavior is of limited duration with the prevalence in the population being highest over one to three years of age but declining to 1-5% by the age of six (Barltrop, 1966). If soil pica declined accordingly then the soil pica prevalence at age six might be predicted to be .02-1.0%.

Despite the inadequate data base concerning soil ingestion about soil-pica children, it is becoming necessary to offer tentative guidance in this area. Soil Pica - is a subset of pica behavior and has a prevalence in the one to six age old population of under 8% based on survey methods (Harvey et al., 1986). The quantitative tracer methodology for soil ingestion is believed superior to the qualitative survey information of soil pica prevalence since it offers definably precise estimates of exposure. It is, therefore, more likely that the actual prevalence of soil-pica in children is far below the 8% figure given above. It should be noted that the soil tracer methodology estimates that 2% will occasionally ingest at least one gram of soil on a given day. The 2% figure is likely to have been considerably lower if Van Wijnen et al. (1990) had adjusted for food intake. The soil tracer methodology estimates that 0.19% ingest up to 10-13 grams of soil per day. The duration of exposure for these estimates is most likely restricted to ages one to six (i.e. five years). While it is possible that soil pica may be observed in some children beyond age six, the prevalence of this behavior is expected to rapidly decrease as one ages. Note that the prevalence calculations employed above (i.e. arriving at the 0.19% value) used the ages of greatest prevalence and would be markedly lower for ages five and six.

It is, therefore, generally recognized that an inadequate data base exists with respect to the prevalence of soil pica, the amount of soil such children ingest and over what duration soil-pica behavior occurs. However, the limited data that do exist suggest that soil pica as defined by approximately 1000 mg/day may exist in an upper bound of 2% of children aged one to six. A small subset of this population (~ 0.2%) is speculated to ingest up to 10 gm/day.

With the notable exception of the one child in the Calabrese et al. study no conclusive data exist that any other pica children (> 1000 mg/day) were observed in the above four cited studies since food ingestion was not adjusted by Van Wijnen et al. (1990), nor were these behaviors seen on repeated days.

If one were to err on the side of safety with a speculative-upper bound daily soil ingestion rate one possible course of action may be the following:

(1) Assume that 2% of children aged one to six years exhibit soil pica of 1 gram of soil per day.
(2) Assume that 0.2% children ingest 10 grams of soil day from one to six years of age.

If, however, a more realistic estimate of soil ingestion in soil pica children were desired then the following suggestions may be followed:

(1) Assume that 1% of children exhibit soil pica of 1 gram of soil per day for four days per week and 500 mg/day for three days per week for four years.
(2) Assume that 0.2% children ingest 10 grams of soil for three days per week and 200 mg of soil for four days per week for four years.

DISCUSSION

Selection of the "correct" soil ingestion number is not a very wise goal as much as simple solutions are desired. Soil ingestion is likely to be influenced by a variety of factors that need to be assessed and then quantitatively incorporated within a soil ingestion derivation procedure. This chapter provides a guide for how to proceed along such a soil ingestion derivation process. It attempts to identify the critical issues and to show how such factors may affect soil ingestion values and how they may be quantitatively dealt within the context of available data or in default values. Table 15.5 presents the structure of the decision framework recommended to lead to a rational and defensible soil ingestion rate. This approach is designed to assist but not replace professional judgement by public health/regulatory risk assessment specialists in this site-specific approach to assessing soil ingestion by children.

Table 15.5. Decision Framework For Deriving Soil Ingestion Rate

Tracer	1.	Needs to have acceptable precision of recovery.
	2.	Narrow C.I. for distribution of median.
	3.	High inter-tracer reliability.
Statistic	1.	Stable measure of central tendency (median, geometric mean).
	2.	Select percentile of choice.
Age	1.	Data are inadequate to differentiate age.
	2.	Age related behavioral changes suggest that older children and adults ingest from 1/4 to 1/10 that of children.

Table 15.5. Decision Framework For Deriving Soil Ingestion Rate

Urban/Suburban/ Rural	Use UF approach - use UF of from 5 - 10-fold if grass cover is limited (e.g. 50-90% covered).
Seasonality	This is also unknown; no adjustment is recommended at this time since reasonable cases can be made for different seasons providing greater risk of soil ingestion.
Dust/Soil	Recommend using a combined soil/dust measurement.
Pica	Assume 1/200 children ingest about 1 gm soil 4 days/wk for 4 years during the 1-6 age span.
Soil vs Dust	Limited data indicate that up to 50% of residual fecal tracers can be of indoor origin.

REFERENCES

1. Barltrop, D. (1966). The prevalence of pica. *Am. J. Dis. Child.*, 112:116-123.
2. Binder, S., Sokal, D. and Maughan, D. (1986). Estimating the amount of soil ingested by young children through tracer elements. *Arch. Environ. Health.* 41, 341-345.
3. Bruhn, C.M., and Pangborn, R.M. (1971). *J. Am. Diet. Assoc.*, 58:417-4-20.
4. Calabrese, E.J., Barnes, R., Stanek, E.J., Pastides, H., Gilbert C.E., Veneman, P., Wang, X., Lasztity, A. and Kostecki, P.T. (1989). How Much Soil Do Young Children Ingest: An Epidemiologic Study. *Reg. Toxic. and Pharm.* 10:123-137.
5. Calabrese, E.J., and Stanek, E.J. III. (1991). A guide to interpreting soil ingestion studies. II. Qualitative and quantitative evidence of soil ingestion. *Reg. Toxicol. and Pharm.* 13:278-292.
6. Calabrese, E.J., and Stanek, E.J. III. (1992). Distinguishing outdoor soil ingestion from indoor dust ingestion in a soil pica child. *Regulatory Toxicol. Pharm.*, 15:83-85.
7. Calabrese, E.J., and Stanek, E.J. III, Gilbert, C.E., and Barnes, R.M. (1990). Preliminary adult soil ingestion estimates; Results of a pilot study. *Reg. Toxicol. Pharm.*, 12:88-95.
8. Cooper, M. (1957). Pica. Springfield, IL: Charles C. Thomas. 109 pp.
9. Davis, S., Waller, P., Buschbom, R., Ballou, J., White, P. (1989). Quantitative Estimates of Soil Ingestion in Normal Children Between the Ages of 2 and 7 Years: Popuation-based Estimates Using Aluminum, Silicon, and Titanium as Soil Tracer Elements. *Arch Env. Hlth.*, 45:112-122.

10. Harvey, P.G., Spurgeon, A., Morgan, G., Chance, J. and Moss, E. (1986). A method for quantifying hand-to-mouth activity in young children. *J. Child. Psychol.*
11. Kanner, L. (1937). Child Psychiatry, pp. 340-353. Springfield, IL: Charles C. Thomas.
12. Lourie, R.S., Layman, E.M., and Millican, F.K. (1963). The epidemiology of lead poisoning and children. *Arch. Pediat.*, 79:72-76.
13. Millican, F.K., Layman, E.M., Lourie, R.S., Rakahashi, L.Y., and Dublin, C.C. (1962). The prevalence of ingestion and mouthing of non-edible substances by children. *Clin. Proc. Child. Hosp.* (Wash.), 18:207-214.
14. Oliver, B.E., and O'Gorman, G. (1966). *Develop. Med. Child.* Neurol., 8:704-706.
15. Porter, J.W. U.S. EPA Office of Solid Waste and Emergency Response, Jan. 27, 1989). Memorandum to regional administrator, Region 1-X, regarding interim final guidance on soil ingestion rates.
16. Stanek, E.J. III, Calabrese, E.J., and Gilbert, C.E. (1990). Choosing a best estimate of children's daily soil ingestion. In: *Petroleum Contaminated Soil.* Vol. 3. P.T. Kostecki and E.J. Calabrese, (eds.). Lewis Pub., Chelsea, MI, pp. 341-348.
17. Stanek, E.J., III, and Calabrese, E.J. (1991). A guide to interpreting soil ingestion studies. I. Development of a model to estimate the soil ingestion detection level of soil ingestion studies. *Reg. Toxicol. and Pharm.*, 13:253-277.
18. Stanek, E.J. III, and Calabrese, E.J. (1992). Soil ingestion in children: Outdoor soil or indoor dust. *J. Soil Contamination*, 1(1):1-28.
21. Stanek, E.J. III, Calabrese, E.J., and Zheng, L. (1990). Soil ingestion estimates in children: Influence of age and sex. *Trace Substances In Environ. Health*, 24:43.
22. Van Wijnen, J.H., Clausing, P., and Brunekreef, B. (1989). Estimated Soil Ingestion By Children. *Env. Res.*, 51:147-162.
22. Vermeer, D.E., and Frate, D.A. (1979). Geophagia on rural Mississippi: environmental and cultural contexts and nutritional implications. *Am. J. Clin. Nutr.*, 32:2129-2135.

CHAPTER 16

Development of a Health Risk Assessment Methodology for Mineral Spirits

Lee R. Shull, EMCON, Sacramento, California, **Elizabeth A. Allen**, Jacobs Engineering, Sacramento, California, and **Gary A. Long, Ann Lunt, Keith Marcott,** and **Scott E. Davies,** Safety-Kleen Corp., Elgin, Illinois

INTRODUCTION

The need for a well founded, scientific, and practical approach for deciding "how clean is clean" for addressing hydrocarbon contaminated soil and groundwater has been the subject of much discussion in recent years. Establishing methods for deriving soil cleanup levels is one of the stated goals of the Council for the Health and Environmental Safety of Soils (CHESS)[1]. Clearly, progress toward achieving this goal has been slowed by a wide range of difficult scientific issues, some of which are associated with the science of risk assessment itself and others related to analytical chemistry and toxicity testing. However, perhaps the single most perplexing scientific issue underlying all others is the question of how to deal with complex mixtures consisting of hundreds, if not thousands in some cases, of individual chemicals (e.g., crude oil), each one possessing inherent toxicity and environmental behavior characteristics. An added complication is the substantial batch-to-batch variability in chemical composition for commercial products refined from crude oil. The reason for this variability is that commercial products are refined by distillation with temperature being the primary controlling factor, not chemical composition.

Moreover, not all chemicals have been qualitatively identified in most petroleum-based complex mixtures, particularly products such as fuel oils, grease, and crude oil. Routine qualitative and quantitative analyses of either commercial products or samples of contaminated soil or groundwater for the purpose of establishing a chemical-by-chemical breakdown of hydrocarbon mixtures is currently impractical, primarily because the low potential usefulness of such data does not justify the high cost of routine chemical analysis. Even if such data were routinely available, only a handful of these hydrocarbons have been subjected to the battery of toxicity tests foundational to deriving the necessary toxicity criteria for performing baseline health risk assessments (BHRAs) and deriving health-based cleanup levels (HBCLs). To perform a BHRA or HBCL calculation, specific toxicity criteria are essential to the process, namely chemical-specific reference dosages (RfDs) for assessing non-carcinogenic substances, and cancer potency factors (CPFs) for assessing carcinogenic substances.

Because a consensus methodology for either assessing baseline risk or setting cleanup levels for complex hydrocarbon mixtures has not been forthcoming, a number of different approaches have been recommended by regulatory agencies. These various approaches can be broadly categorized into three types:

1. *Ignore the total petroleum hydrocarbon (TPH) fraction and emphasize only certain discrete compounds with established toxicity criteria.* Typical examples of compounds included are the alkyl benzenes such as benzene, toluene, ethylbenzene, and total xylenes (BTEX) in gasoline, or the polycyclic aromatic hydrocarbons (PAHs) in diesel. The main rationale cited for this approach are: (i) these selected compounds are the predominate contributors to risk; thus, the relative significance of other TPH constituents are insignificant, (ii) analytical procedures are well-established and affordable for individual "higher risk" compounds, and (iii) essential toxicity criteria (RfDs, CPFs) have been established. A frequent argument against this approach is that the overwhelming majority of petroleum hydrocarbons present as the TPH fraction are not quantitatively addressed.
2. *Assume the TPH fraction in soil or groundwater is equivalent to fresh product.* This approach has become feasible with the recent development by the U.S. Environmental Protection Agency (EPA) of provisional RfDs and CPFs for several petroleum products, including gasoline, diesel, kerosene, and jet fuels (JP-4, JP-5)[2]. However, the principal argument against use of this approach is that petroleum products can change significantly after release into soil or groundwater due to the influence of differential rates of degradation and dispersion on individual compounds in the mixture. These influences are commonly referred to as "weathering." Because the aromatic versus the aliphatic constituents in hydrocarbon mixtures are prone to faster rates of degradation and dispersion, the assumption that a TPH fraction in soil or groundwater is equivalent to fresh product is likely to greatly overestimate risk and result in unrealistically low cleanup levels.
3. *Subdivide TPH into categories of chemicals and develop toxicity criteria for each category.* The subject of this paper is the application of this approach to mineral spirits (MS), a complex petroleum hydrocarbon mixture. A similar approach for TPH gasoline was reported as being developed by the State of Massachusetts in conjunction with ABB Environmental Services, Inc. for BHRA and HBCL purposes[3].

In addition to these approaches, regulatory agencies have mandated TPH cleanup levels that are not health-based. Two such approaches are:

1. *Remediate TPH to a concentration equivalent to the practical limit of quantification (PLQ).* This approach is generally considered by most environmental professionals as overly conservative, unnecessary, and cost-prohibitive. However, this approach is required by some states.
2. *Remediate TPH to pre-established cleanup levels.* These levels vary among states, and typically range between 10 and 1,000 parts per million for soil[4]. This approach is frequently criticized for lack of basis.

Safety-Kleen Corp. (S-K), which is a major international recycler of petroleum-based solvents including mineral spirits (MS), commissioned the development of a standardized procedure for conducting BHRAs and deriving site-specific HBCLs at sites with residual MS in soil and/or groundwater. Presented herein is a description of methodology and the data used to derive essential toxicity criteria for chemical fractions in MS, a description of a simple methodology for estimating concentrations of chemical fractions in MS from BTEX and TPH analytical data, and a case example illustrating the methodology.

BACKGROUND INFORMATION ON MINERAL SPIRITS

Uses and Chemical Composition

Mineral spirits (MS) is one of several classes of petroleum-based solvents with wide commercial application. While the term "mineral spirits" is used to define a specific commercial solvent, it is also the generic name assigned to a broad range of refined petroleum solvents, including Stoddard solvent, 140° flash aliphatic solvent, low-aromatic white spirits (LAWS), petroleum naptha, and petroleum distillates. These are but a few examples of the wide variety of different MS preparations available from petroleum companies involved in the general practice of refining crude oil into commercial products. MS is produced from a straight-run distillate of paraffinic or mixed base crude oil. Individual batches of MS are sometimes blended to formulate customized mixtures for specific industrial applications, or for usage in specific environments such as colder climates. MS is also used as a diluent in paints, coatings and, waxes, as a dry cleaning agent, as a degreaser and cleaner, and as a herbicide[5,9].

MS preparations are defined more on the basis of boiling range than chemical composition; boiling range for MS is 150-220°C[6], which places it between gasoline and kerosene. Chemical composition will differ from one preparation to another due to variation in the crude oil being distilled and variation in the processing units of different refineries. The hydrocarbon content of MS typically falls in the C-7 to C-12 range, with the majority of hydrocarbons in the C-9 to C-12 range. A typical chemical composition of an MS preparation is 30-50% straight and branched chain alkanes (paraffins), 30-40% cycloalkanes (naphthenes), 10-14% aromatics (primarily C8+ compounds), and $<$ 1% olefins[6-

[9]. Benzene, if present, is generally detected only in trace amounts[9]. Indans and tetralins, which are classes of substituted benzenes, are also present in small amounts (generally < 1%). Depending on the blend, the aromatic content can be varied during production to provide either low aromatic (typically 10-20%) or high-aromatic grades (45% or more aromatic hydrocarbons) of MS. Blends of MS supplied by S-K are primarily C-9 to C-13, with C-8 hydrocarbons present only in trace amounts[7]. The boiling range is 151–224°C, indicating that the mixture is weighted more towards slightly larger carbon-containing compounds than other products in this classification. Compounds in the C-10 to C-12 range make up approximately 85 to 88% of the total, with C-14 hydrocarbons generally accounting for ≤1%[8]. Toluene, xylene, and ethylbenzene, as part of the aromatic fraction, account for approximately 2% of the total identified compounds[7].

Table 16.1 gives the chemical composition of a typical batch of Stoddard solvent, a type of MS. As shown, many constituents have been identified and quantified, but more than half of the hydrocarbons are unidentified. The unidentified fraction is mainly comprised of aliphatic compounds.

Behavior in the Environment

As previously stated, the relative concentrations of the individual compounds and chemical fractions in MS will change as a function of both time and distance from the point of introduction into the environment. Some MS constituents will be more mobile than others in soil and/or groundwater, some will volatilize more rapidly than others, and some will degrade due to various biological and chemical processes more rapidly than others. Depending on environmental conditions, MS that has weathered for a significant period of time will likely differ significantly in chemical composition from fresh product. Accordingly, the potential for human exposure and the adverse health impacts that may result are directly related to the nature and extent of weathering.

Transport in Soil/Groundwater Systems

The environmental fate of MS is essentially a function of the physical-chemical properties of MS constituents, such as solubility, volatilization potential, soil sorption, and degradation. Table 16.2 lists some key physical-chemical properties for some constituents in MS. In addition to these properties, fate processes are also influenced by the nature and amount of the spill, soil types, and a multitude of other environmental conditions.

Transport processes are initially more important than transformation and degradation processes in determining the initial fate of MS in the environment. For surface spills, volatilization is the primary fate pathway, with subsequent atmospheric photolysis of individual components[10]. Compounds having greater than nine carbons, which predominate in MS, become weathered primarily by evaporation and biodegradation[11]. Reduced temperatures increase persistence by

Table 16.1. Percentage (by weight) of various hydrocarbons in a stoddard solvent sample.

Component	Percentage by Weight
4-Methylheptane	0.01
t-1,4-Dimethylcyclohexane	0.02
n-Octane	0.08
2,5+3,5-Dimethylheptane	0.20
1,3,5-Trimethylcyclohexane	0.05
Ethylbenzene	0.03
2,3-Dimethylheptane	0.19
m-Xylene	0.20
p-Xylene	0.05
3,4-Dimethylheptane	0.04
4-Methyloctane	0.32
2-Methyloctane	0.53
3-Ethylheptane	0.09
3-Methyloctane	0.53
3,3-Diethylpentane	0.07
o-Xylene	0.24
1,1,2-Trimethylcyclohexane	0.10
Isobutylcyclopentane	0.02
n-Nonane	5.27
Cumene	0.10
2,2-Dimethyloctane + Isopropylcyclohexane	1.24
2,6-Dimethyloctane	1.58
3,6-Dimethyloctane	0.40
3,3-Dimethyloctane + C_{10} Dinaphthene	0.67
n-Propylbenzene	0.27
1-Methyl-3-Ethylbenzene	1.03
1-Methyl-4-Ethylbenzene	0.42
1,3,5-Trimethylbenzene	1.13
4-Methylnonane	1.93
2-Methylnonane	2.12
1-Methyl-2-Ethylbenzene	0.41
3-Methylnonane	1.92
t-Butylbenzene + 1,2,4-Trimethylbenzene	2.50

Table 16.1 (cont.)

Component	Percentage by Weight
Isobutylcyclohexane	0.90
Isobutylbenzene	0.18
n-Decane	11.85
sec-Butylbenzene	0.12
1,2,3-Trimethylbenzene	0.46
1-Methyl-3-Isopropylbenzene	0.80
1-Methyl-4-Isopropylbenzene	0.21
Indan	0.08
1-Methyl-2-Isopropylbenzene	0.07
1,3-Diethylbenzene	0.19
1-Methyl-3-*n*-Propylbenzene	0.57
1-Methyl-4-*n*-Propylbenzene	0.26
n-Butylbenzene	0.16
1,2-Diethylbenzene	0.57
1,4-Diethylbenzene + 1,3-Dimethyl-5-Ethylbenzene	0.06
1-Methyl-2-*n*-Propylbenzene	1.47
1,4-Dimethyl-2-Ethylbenzene	0.28
1,3-Dimethyl-4-Ethylbenzene	0.38
1,3-Dimethyl-2-Ethylbenzene	0.14
n-Undecane	8.36
1,2,3,4-Tetramethylbenzene	0.24
Naphthalene	0.61
n-Dodecane	1.99
2-Methylnaphthalene	0.04
n-Tridecane	0.06
1-Methylnaphthalene	0.02
Total Identified Hydrocarbons	53.87
Unidentified Aliphatic Hydrocarbons	38.53
Unidentified Aromatic Hydrocarbons	7.62
Total	**100.02**

retarding the rates of volatilization and biodegradation. Under such conditions, downward migration into the soil and to groundwater may be expected to predominate following surface releases. Elevated temperatures, lateral spreading, and adsorption onto surface vegetation may facilitate evaporation. If the hydrocarbon phase is distributed to a soil zone where constituents can volatilize into soil pore space air, MS may diffuse in all directions, including upward [12-14].

Rate of migration through soils is a function of the extent of sorption to soil particles. For the individual components of MS, the magnitude of soil sorption is dependent on the size of the molecule and inversely related to aqueous solubility. Environmental factors, such as temperature, salinity, and pH do not appear to have as important an influence on sorption as molecular size and solubility[11,12,15].

The water solubility (log kow) of most of the chemical components in MS is quite low (Table 16.2). The aromatic constituents possess greater water solubility than paraffinic compounds but are similar to the naphthenic compounds constituents. Therefore, these compounds pose the greater threat of leaching from soil into groundwater. Aliphatic hydrocarbons > C12 are essentially insoluble in water[11,12,16-18].

MS as a mixture is not considered highly volatile; the overall vapor pressure is three millimeters of mercury at 20°C[5]. However, volatilization of the lighter constituents of MS from subsurface soils may be a significant fate process. The extent and rate of volatilization is dependent on multiple environmental factors such as soil porosity, ambient temperature, and wind patterns. Physico-chemical properties such as the Henry's Law constant and the vapor-soil sorption coefficient will also influence the rate of volatilization[5]. While the rate of volatilization of MS from soil has not been studied to a significant degree, the behavior of similar complex hydrocarbon mixtures serves as an indicator of the probable behavior of MS in the environment. For example, volatilization of gasoline components from residual concentrations in soil and at the groundwater interface was implicated in the detection of gasoline vapors in nearby basements[5].

As illustrated in Table 16.3, partitioning of low soil concentrations (below aqueous solubility) of selected hydrocarbons in MS among soil particles, soil water, and soil air can be predicted using Mackay's equilibrium partitioning model[5]. The fractions associated with the water and air phases are expected to have higher mobility than the fractions adsorbed to soil particles. As shown, in unsaturated topsoil, sorption predominates for all three categories of hydrocarbons. Partitioning in soil-air is relatively low for most categories, but is highest for the naphthenic compounds. Both the aromatic and naphthenic compounds partition to a much greater extent into soil water, and as such would be expected to migrate with infiltrating water. However, in saturated, deep soils (no air and negligible soil organic carbon), the percentage of aromatic hydrocarbons partitioned in the water phase is much higher than for the naphthenic compounds. From this simple partitioning model, it is clear that the behavior of individual hydrocarbons in MS is quite variable. However, it is also clear that there are apparent behavioral trends within each of the three chemical categories; the paraffinic fraction, the naphthenic fraction, and the aromatic fraction.

Table 16.2. Physical-chemical properties of various mineral spirits hydrocarbons[a]

Compound	Physical-Chemical Properties		
	Log K_{ow}	K_{oc}	H^b
Paraffinic Compounds			
Octane	5.18	73,000	2.96
n-Nonane	4.67[c]	23,400[c,d]	4.93[e]
Dodecane	7.06	5.5×10^6	7.4
Naphthenic Compounds			
Methylcyclopentane	3.47	1,400	0.36
Cyclohexane	3.44	1,330	0.18
Methylcyclohexane	4.10	6,070	0.039
Aromatic Compounds			
Toluene	2.69	240	0.0066
Xylenes	3.16	700	0.007
Trimethylbenzenes	3.65	2,150	0.005
Naphthalene	3.30	962	0.00048
Methylnaphthalene	3.87	3,570	0.00044

[a] Modified from reference 5.
[b] Henry's Law constant. Units equal atm-m^3/mol.
[c] Montgomery, J.H., Ed. (1991) Groundwater Chemical Desk Reference, Volume 2, Lewis Publishers, Chelsea, MI.
[d] Calculated using K_{ow} from Montgomery and Equation 4-9 in Handbook of Chemical property Equation Methods: Environmental Behavior of Organic Compounds. Lyman, W.J., et al., Eds. McGraw-Hill Book Co., N.Y.
[e] Mackay, D., and Shiu, W.Y. (1981). A Critical Review of Henry's Law Constants for Chemical of Environmental Interest. J. Phys. Chem. Ref. Data. 10(4):1175-1199.

Transformation Processes in Soil/Groundwater Systems

MS can undergo both abiotic (e.g., photooxidation) and biotic degradation in the environment[5]. As with partitioning and transport, the nature of the release and the extent of exposure to sunlight will have a significant impact on the rate of degradation. Specific environmental factors such as temperature, moisture, aerobic versus anaerobic conditions, the presence of microorganisms capable of utilizing hydrocarbons as a substrate, and the availability of nutrients all play important roles in determining the rate and extent of degradation.

Photooxidation is the primary chemical transformation process involved in degrading petroleum hydrocarbons in the environment[10,14,19]. Alkanes and monosubstituted benzenes are relatively resistant to photolysis in aqueous systems; trisubstituted benzenes and naphthalenes photolyze at rates comparable to volatilization[14]. Penetration of MS constituents in soil below the limits of exposure to solar radiation limits photooxidation. The oxygenated products of photooxidation are generally more water soluble than the parent hydrocarbons and thus are more likely to be leached from soil[14,15].

In regards to biological degradation, natural ecosystems contain a wide range of various hydrocarbon-degrading bacteria and fungi. In general, microorganisms exhibit decreasing ability to degrade n-alkanes with increasing hydrocarbon chain length, but have been shown to degrade n-alkanes up to C44[20]. n-Alkanes are more easily biodegraded than branched or cycloalkanes and aromatics are generally more rapidly biodegraded than alkanes. n-Alkanes, n-alkylaromatics, and aromatics in the C10 - C22 range are the most readily biodegradable. Those ≤ C9 are primarily removed by volatilization when possible, and hydrocarbons with condensed ring structures, such as PAHs, are relatively resistant to biodegradation[14].

Overview of the Toxicology of Mineral Spirits

i. Animal Studies

Carcinogenicity

MS has not been evaluated for carcinogenicity[5,6,9], primarily because carcinogenesis testing of complex chemical mixtures such as MS is typically not done. Rather, such testing is routinely performed on individual chemical components. However, there is no definitive evidence suggesting that exposure to MS results in an increased risk of cancer in either humans or laboratory animals.

Genotoxicity

Stoddard solvent, a specific type of MS has been shown to not be mutagenic in both in vitro and in vivo systems. In the Ames microbial assay, a common microbial mutagenesis test system, MS has tested negative both with and without microsomal activation. Negative results have also been reported in both the mouse lymphoma and dominant lethal assays[5,21].

Short-term Toxicity

As with most petroleum solvents, high concentrations of MS vapors can have an irritating effect on skin, eyes, and mucous membranes, and can cause narcosis (sleep). Several studies have evaluated the short-term exposure effects to various petroleum solvent hydrocarbon mixtures, most of which confirm the occurrence of central nervous system (CNS) depression and respiratory tract irritancy. The major factor determining the acute inhalation hazard is the volatility. Mixtures containing compounds with nine or more carbons tend to not be sufficiently volatile to produce air concentrations high enough to be lethal over short exposure periods (4–6 hrs)[6]. In general, petroleum solvents such as MS are not considered highly toxic unless aspirated or inhaled in concentrations sufficient to result in narcosis. In general, MS containing larger fractions of aromatic constituents are more acutely toxic than mixtures containing lower aromatic concentrations. Similarly, both skin and eye irritation are also greater with aromatic solvents[22].

Riley et al.[23] exposed rats to white spirit vapors (boiling range 150-190°C). The sample contained 61% paraffins, 20% naphthenes, and 19% aromatics, mainly C9-C12 hydrocarbons. The animals were exposed for four hours per day (hr/day) for four consecutive days to average concentrations of 291 milligrams per cubic meter (mg/m^3) on the first day and 188 mg/m^3 on the remaining three days. No differences in body weights or respiratory rates were noted between the exposed animals and the control (untreated) animals. However, histological evaluation revealed the presence of inflammatory cell infiltrate in the nasal cavity, trachea, and larynx. The epithelial lining of the nasal cavity and the larynx showed loss of cilia, hyperplasia of the mucous or basal cells, and squamous metaplasia.

In a similar study, Carpenter et al[24]. conducted an extensive investigation into the effects of various petroleum hydrocarbon solvents, including a Stoddard solvent. Rats showed no adverse effects after eight hours at 4220 ppm while the No-Observed-Effect-Level (NOEL) for dogs was 510 ppm in the same time period. Exposure to 1,400 ppm for eight hours was not lethal to rats[24]. Toxic symptoms included eye irritation, loss of coordination, and bleeding from the nostrils. Similar symptoms were observed after exposure to 800 ppm for eight hours except there was no loss of coordination. Female beagles were exposed to 1400 ppm; one dog exhibited eye irritation, salivation, tremors and convulsions within a five-hour period while the other dog was asymptomatic during and after eight hours of exposure. Cats exposed to 43 ppm for six hours showed no adverse effects[25]. Rector et. al.[26] exposed rats, guinea pigs, rabbits, dogs, and monkeys to MS for eight hours daily, five day per week for 30 exposures to vapor levels of 290 ppm. The only adverse effects noted were minor congestion and emphysema of guinea pig lungs.

Chronic Toxicity

Long-term exposure to petroleum hydrocarbons has been shown to have toxic effects on the kidneys of male rats. These changes are characterized by hyaline-droplet formation in the epithelium of the proximal convoluted tubules, degenerative changes in the proximal convoluted tubules of the renal cortex, and tubular dilation and necrosis at the corticomedullary junction[27]. These changes are distinctive to the male rat and are not observed in castrated rats, female rats, or any other species. Recent studies have shown that the male rat exhibits a metabolic peculiarity, and that these renal effects are due to a decrease in the urinary clearance of a unique protein called α-2-micro-globulin[27,28].

When Sprague-Dawley and Fischer 344 rats of both sexes were exposed to Stoddard solvent vapor at concentrations of 100 and 800 ppm, six hours per day, five days per week for eight weeks, kidney changes were seen in male rats only[27]. Similar nephrotoxic effects were observed in male rats exposed to dearomized white spirits at vapor levels of 300 or 900 ppm for six hours daily, five days per week up to 12 weeks. The incidence and severity increased with increasing concentrations and exposure duration. No other significant toxic effects were noted[29].

In a 12-month study, male Sprague-Dawley rats exposed to vapor levels of 6,500 mg/m^3 white spirits, eight hours daily, five days per week, had a decreased urinary concentrating ability, a decreased net acid excretion following a mild ammonium chloride load, and an increased urinary lactate dehydrogenase (LDH) activity[28]. No toxic effects were reported in male Harlan-Wistar rats exposed to 140° flash aliphatic solvent at vapor levels up to 37 ppm, six hours daily, five days per week for 72 days, or in dogs exposed similarly for 73 days[25].

Rector et. al.[26] conducted a series of inhalation studies with MS containing 80-86% aliphatic hydrocarbons, 1% olefins, and 13-19% aromatics, and composed mostly of C9-C12 aliphatic hydrocarbons. Five species were exposed: rats, guinea pigs, rabbits, beagle, and squirrel monkeys. Two exposure schedules were employed: 90-day trials in which the animals were exposed 23.5 hours per day; and six-week studies of eight hours per day, five days per week for 30 exposures, two weeks without exposure, and an additional 30 exposures. In the 90-day trials, concentration of 18-200 ppm were tested; in the 30-day studies, concentrations of 93 and 212 ppm were used. In the 90-day trials, 27% of the guinea pigs died at 57 ppm, and 79% died at 200 ppm. Three percent of the rats (in exposed and control groups) died. No deaths were reported in other species. No deaths occurred in either the 30 day and 60 day trials. In the 90-day studies, slight decreases in body-weight gain were noted in guinea pigs and monkeys at higher concentrations. Evidence of irritation and congestion of the lungs was noted in all species, no changes were seen in the hematological and biochemical variables that could be attributed to the exposure to MS vapor.

Human and Epidemiological Studies

Short-term Toxicologic Effects

MS can cause eye, nose, and throat irritation in humans. Acute exposures to high vapor concentrations can cause narcotic effects and headaches. Exposure for six hours to vapor levels of 50-200 ppm white spirits produced dryness of the mucous membranes, anorexia, nausea, vomiting, diarrhea, and fatigue[30]. One of six volunteers exposed to a vapor level of 150 ppm for 15 minutes reported eye irritation; all six reported eye irritation after 15 minutes at 470 ppm[24]. Acute exposure to MS for up to 50 minutes at 4,000 mg/m^3 had no effect on perceptual speed, numerical ability, and manual dexterity. The exposure did result in the prolongation of reaction time and a possible impairment of short-term memory[31]. Dermal exposure to the liquid can cause dermatitis.

Chronic Toxicologic Effects

Numerous cases of prolonged dermal and inhalation exposure to different petroleum hydrocarbon solvents such as MS have been reported and reviewed[5,9,-31]. Exposures over extended periods to unknown concentrations have resulted in headaches, irritation of the eye, nose and throat, fatigue, bone marrow hyperplasia, and in extreme cases, death. Because of the complex nature of these mixtures and the difficulty in ascertaining exposure to specific chemical components, it has been virtually impossible to assess the exact etiology of many of these toxic effects. However, there is no evidence of either the long-term neuropathic effects caused by hexane (a trace component in MS) or the bone marrow and myelotoxic effects caused by benzene (also a trace component in MS) in humans exposed to MS.

Summary

The toxicology database is much more extensive on individual chemical compounds than for MS, particularly some of the aromatic constituents including naphthalene, xylenes, toluene and ethylbenzene. Based on evidence from both human and laboratory animal studies, it is clear that MS constituents are readily absorbed in the three portals of entry (gastrointestinal tract, lungs, skin). In general, acute toxicosis requires very high levels of exposure, such as those necessary to cause narcosis. Chronic toxicity and toxic effects vary among different chemical constituents, but the most frequently impacted organ/systems are the liver, lungs and kidneys. The aromatic fraction contains the most toxic constituents in MS. However, there is no evidence that either MS (the mixture) or any of the individual compounds in MS are carcinogenic.

RISK ASSESSMENT METHODOLOGY

General Approach

The overall goal of the project commissioned by S-K was to develop a risk assessment methodology that is practical, cost-effective, based on good science, and acceptable to regulatory agencies. Specifically, it was important that the methodology satisfy certain conditions, including; (a) it must be adaptable to virtually any environment, (b) it must incorporate generally-accepted risk assessment methodologies, (c) it should not be overly complex and should be viewed as a "screening" type approach, and (d) it must be capable of accommodating the limited analytical data typically used in characterizing residual hydrocarbons in soil and groundwater, namely TPH as MS and the usual volatile organic compounds (e.g., ethylbenzene, toluene, xylene) and semi-volatile compounds (e.g., naphthalene) typically analyzed for during site investigation programs. With these conditions in mind, a risk assessment methodology was developed that consisted of six basic steps:

Step 1. Subdivision of MS into chemical fractions;
Step 2. Selection of individual marker compounds for each chemical fraction;
Step 3. Development of toxicity criteria for each marker compound or group of marker compounds;
Step 4. Derivation of media-specific screening values (MSV's);
Step 5: Estimation of concentrations of each chemical fraction;
Step 6. Risk characterization.

The first three steps involve the development of essential toxicity criteria for assessing risk associated with MS residual MS hydrocarbons in environmental media. Steps 3, 4, and 5 are sequential steps in assessing risk associated with residual MS hydrocarbons on a site-specific basis.

Step 1: Subdivision of mineral spirits into chemical fractions. The decision was made to subdivide MS into three chemical fractions, namely

- the *paraffinic fraction* predominated by both straight and branched alkanes,
- the *naphthenic fraction* predominated by cycloalkanes
- the *aromatic fraction* predominated by alkylbenzenes.

For reasons discussed in Step 3 below, the paraffinic and naphthenic fractions were combined into one fraction. Our rationale for selecting these three fractions was based on both scientific data and professional judgement. A key assumption was made that compounds within each of the fractions would behave similarly in a soil or water matrix. Based on the discussion of environmental fate and transport closure, and data given in Table 16.3, this is clearly an overly simplistic assumption that will result in some unknown degree of uncertainty in the process. In addition, a review of the toxicology literature revealed the lack of critical toxicity data for virtually all compounds in both the paraffinic and naphthenic fractions, indicating the impropriety of expanding the number of fractions beyond three. Also, we determined that whereas it may be feasible to estimate content of these three fractions from TPH and aromatic analytical results (Step 4), such estimations would likely not be feasible for additional fractions.

Step 2: Selection of Marker Compounds for each Chemical Fraction. Six marker compounds were selected as representatives of each of the three fractions. These compounds are:

- *n-nonane*, the marker compound for the paraffinic fraction;
- *cyclohexane*, the marker compound for the naphthenic fraction;
- *ethylbenzene, naphthalene, toluene,* and *xylene*, the marker compounds for the aromatic fraction.

Table 16.3. Equilibrium partioning of various mineral spirits hydrocarbons in a model environment[a]

Compounds	Unsaturated Top Soil (%)			Saturated Deep Soil (%)	
	Soil	Water	Air	Soil	Water
Paraffinic Compounds					
Octane	97.4	0.01	2.6	99.7	0.3
n-Nonane					
Dodecane	99.9	0.0001	2.6		
Naphthenic Compounds					
Methylcyclopentane	85.4	0.3	14.3	85.5	14.5
Cyclohexane	91.6	0.4	8.0	84.8	15.2
Methylcyclohexane	95.9	0.08	4.0	96.2	3.8
Aromatic Compounds					
Toluene	96.5	1.9	1.6	52.1	47.9
Xylenes	98.8	0.7	0.5	74.4	25.6
Trimethylbenzenes	99.6	0.2	0.2	90.0	10.0
Naphthalene	99.4	0.5	0.05	80.2	19.8
Methylnaphthalene	99.8	0.1	0.01	93.7	6.3

[a] Adapted from reference 5. Calculated percentages should be considered rough estimates.

These six compounds were selected primarily on the basis of four criteria: (1) frequency of detection in MS preparations; (2) relative concentrations in MS preparations; (3) availability of compound-specific toxicologic data essential to developing risk assessment toxicity criteria, specifically dose-response data (e.g., NOAEL or LOAEL data); and (4) practical ability to quantify concentrations in environmental samples.

Cyclohexane. A large fraction of mineral spirits (approximately 30-40%) consists of naphthenic compounds, which are primarily saturated cycloaliphatic hydrocarbons. Several alkylated isomers of cyclohexane can exist in MS (Table 16.1. Toxicologic evidence from chronic inhalation studies suggest that alkylated cyclohexanes are generally of lower toxicity than unsubstituted cyclohexane[32]. Additionally, the cycloparaffins as a group exhibit narcotic properties, are CNS depressants, and can cause nephrotoxic effects. As a conservative measure, we concluded cyclohexane is a plausible marker compound for the naphthenic fraction in MS on the basis of similar toxicologic endpoints, toxicity, and environmental behavior.

n-Nonane. Although n-decane may be present in a somewhat greater quantity in MS than n-nonane (Table 16.1), our review of the toxicology literature indicated that whereas essential toxicity data are available for n-nonane, such data are lacking for n-decane.

Aromatic compounds. Available chemical information indicates that the aromatic fraction in MS is comprised predominantly of numerous alkyl benzenes of which ethylbenzene, toluene, and xylene are the most familiar. Lesser amounts of a wide range of both alkylated and non-alkylated naphthalenes are also present (Table 16.1). The percentage of the aromatic fraction contributed by these four marker compounds can range up to 15%. The remaining 85% consists of a wide variety of other aromatic compounds, many of which have not been identified (Table 16.1). Therefore, these four compounds were chosen because they are consistently present at relatively high concentrations in MS, the toxicology database is well-established for each one, and all four compounds are routinely measured by commercial analytical laboratories using established EPA methodologies.

Step 3: Toxicity Criteria for Chemical Fraction. Whereas toxicity criteria (RfDs) have been established by U.S. EPA for the four aromatic compounds (ethylbenzene, naphthalene, toluene and xylenes; Table 16.4), no such criteria are available for cyclohexane or n-nonane. In the following section, inhalation and oral RfD-equivalent values are calculated for the aliphatic constituents in MS using standard EPA procedures. In addition, weighted RfD-equivalent values are derived for both the total aromatic fraction and the total aliphatic fraction in MS.

Aliphatic Fraction

n-Nonane. A NOAEL for n-nonane of 3,086 mg/m^3, was determined in an inhalation study conducted in rats[24]. The animals were administered n-nonane six hours per day, five days per week for 13 weeks. Micropathological evaluation of the tissues at the termination of the study revealed no lesions attributable to vapor inhalation. A NOAEL for application to health risk assessment in humans is derived from the animal NOAEL by adjusting for exposure frequency and uncertainty as follows:

$$NOAEL\ (human) = \frac{NOAEL\ (animal)\ x\ CF_1\ x\ CF_2}{UF} = 5.5\ mg/m^3 \tag{1}$$

Table 16.4. RfD values for total aliphatic hydrocarbons, total aromatic hydrocarbons and aromatic compounds in mineral spirits.

Component Fraction	RfD		Toxicological Manifestation
	Inhalation (mg/kg/day)	Oral (mg/kg/day)	
Ethylbenzene	0.29[a]	0.10[a]	Liver, Kidney, Reproductive
Naphthalene	0.009[c]	0.004[b]	Liver, Blood
Toluene	0.11[a]	0.2[a]	Liver, Kidney, CNS
Xylene	0.09[c]	2[a]	Decreased Body Weight, CNS
Aliphatic hydrocarbons[e]	1.30[d]	0.70[d]	Liver, Kidney
Aromatic hydrocarbons[f]	0.3[d]	0.2[d]	Liver, Lungs, Kidney

[a]EPA[33,35,36].
[b]EPA[34].
[c]EPA[34] (The RfD for this chemical is currently under review by an EPA work group. The previous RfD is there fore used as the interim RfD).
[d]Calculated from a NOAEL using the methodology established in EPA[34].
[e]Based on n-nonane and cyclohexane
[f]Based on ethylbenzene, naphthalene, toluene, and xylene

where:

CF_1 = Exposure duration correction factor (6/24 hours/day)
CF_2 = Exposure duration correction factor (5/7 days/week)
UF = Uncertainty factor (10 for interspecies extrapolation, 10 for sensitive individuals) = 100

RfD values in units of mg/kg/day can then be calculated using the following equation:

$$RfD\text{-}equivalent = \frac{CA \times IR \times AB}{BW} \quad \textbf{(2)}$$

where:

CA = RfC (mg/m^3);
IR = Inhalation rate (20 m^3/day);
AB = Absorption efficiency (for calculating an oral RfD using inhalation data or an inhalation RfC, AB = 0.5, based on the assumption that

gastrointestinal absorption is twice the steady state alveolar absorption rate; for calculating an inhalation RfD from an inhalation RfC, AB = 1.0);

BW = Average adult body weight (70 kg).

Using this equation, the inhalation RfD is calculated to be 1.6 mg/kg/day and the oral RfD is 0.8 mg/kg/day.

Cyclohexane. A NOAEL for cyclohexane of 1,745 mg/m^3 was determined in an inhalation study conducted in rabbits[32]. The animals were administered cyclohexane 6 hr/day, 5 days/week for 10 weeks. Using Equation 1, a NOAEL of 1,745 mg/m^3, adjusting for exposure frequency (i.e., 6/24 hr/day, 5/7 days/week) and dividing by an uncertainty factor of 100, the human NOAEL is calculated to be 3.1 mg/m^3 or 0.9 mg/kg/day (Equation 2). The equivalent oral RfD is 0.4 mg/kg/day (Equation 2).

Toxicity criteria for the total aliphatic fraction. Because it is currently not feasible to quantify the paraffinic and naphthenic fractions separately in environmental samples, a weighted-average reference dose-equivalent (RfD_{eq}) for the two fractions was calculated using toxicity criteria developed for n-nonane and cyclohexane above and the relative amounts of each fraction (i.e., paraffins represented by n-nonane, and naphthenes represented by cyclohexane) in typical MS preparations. Of the total aliphatic fraction, available information indicates that paraffins represent 47-59% and naphthenes represent 35-40% of MS. Therefore, assuming a paraffin and naphthene ratio of 60:40, the weighted-average RfC_i for the aliphatic fraction of MS is calculated to be:

$$RfD_i = (1.6 \text{ mg/kg/d}^3 \times 0.6) + (0.9 \text{ mg/kg/d}^3 \times 0.4) = \mathbf{1.3\ mg/kg/d} \quad \mathbf{(3)}$$

where:

1.6 mg/kg/d = RfD_i for the paraffinic fraction;
0.8 mg/kg/d = RfD_i for the naphthenic fraction;
0.6 mg/kg/d = relative proportion of the paraffinic fraction;
0.4 mg/kg/d = relative proportion of the naphthenic fraction.

Similarly, the oral RfD for the aliphatic fraction is:

$$RfD_o = (0.8 \text{ mg/kg/day} \times 0.6) + (0.4 \text{ mg/kg/day} \times 0.4) = \mathbf{0.7\ mg/kg/day}$$

where:

0.8 mg/kg/d = RfD_o for the paraffinic fraction;
0.4 mg/kg/d = RfD_o for the naphthenic fraction;
0.6 mg/kg/d = relative proportion of the paraffinic fraction;
0.4 mg/kg/d = relative proportion of the naphthenic fraction.

Aromatic Fraction

Since only about 87% of the total aromatic fraction is generally described as containing compounds with more than eight carbons[5], and since it is not practical to measure these compounds individually, in environmental samples, it is necessary to select a marker compound that is representative of the C8+ fraction. Accordingly, we selected ethylbenzene as the surrogate compound for this fraction (i.e., 87% of the total aromatic fraction is assumed to be toxicologically equivalent to ethylbenzene). This is a conservative assumption because ethylbenzene has a lower oral RfD than either toluene or xylene (Table 16.4). Therefore, assigning 87% weight to ethylbenzene and apportioning the other three compounds equally (i.e., 4.33% each), the weighted RfD_i is calculated to be:

$$RfD_i = (0.11 \text{ mg/kg/d} \times 0.043) + (0.009 \text{ mg/kg/d} \times 0.043) + (0.09 \text{ mg/kg/d} \times 0.043) + (0.29 \text{ mg/kg/d} \times 0.87) = \mathbf{0.26\ (0.3\ mg/kg/d)}$$

where:

0.11 mg/kg/d = EPA inhalation RfD for toluene (Table 16.4);
0.09 mg/kg/d = EPA inhalation RfD for xylene (Table 16.4);
0.009 mg/kg/d = EPA inhalation RfD for naphthalene;extrapolated from the oral RfD (Table 16.4);
0.29 mg/kg/d = EPA inhalation RfD for ethylbenzene (Table 16.4).

The weighted oral RfD as determined by Equation 3 is:

$$RfD_o = (0.20 \text{ mg/kg/d} \times 0.043) + (2.00 \text{ mg/kg/d} \times 0.043 + (0.004 \text{ mg/kg/d} \times 0.043) + (0.10 \text{ mg/kg/d} \times 0.87) = \mathbf{0.2\ mg/kg/d}$$

where:

0.20 mg/kg/d = EPA oral RfD for toluene (Table 16.4);
2.00 mg/kg/d = EPA oral RfD for xylene (Table 16.4);
0.004 mg/kg/d = EPA oral RfD for naphthalene (Table 16.4);
0.10 mg/kg/d = EPA oral RfD for ethylbenzene (Table 16.4).

Step 4. Calculate Media-Specific Screening Values

Media-specific screening values (MSV's) can be calculated using equations modified from EPA[37-40]. Whereas these equations are considered sufficient for calculating MSV's, it should be stressed that they are based on standard default assumptions that may or may not reflect site-specific conditions. Professional discretion must be exercised in determining if more site-specific data are more appropriate for assessing risk. Several important points about the following equations should be noted: (a) most of the default values are based on *upperbound* assumptions, (b) the equations are based on a *residential* land-use condition, which is a worst-case assumption, and (c) use of toxicity criteria in the equations assumes *100% absorption* efficiency.

Soil

Potential health impacts under an assumed onsite residential scenario from MS constituents in soil can occur from one or more exposure pathways, including direct contact with the soil, or inhalation of constituents volatilized from soil into ambient or indoor air, or inhalation of fugitive dust generated from impacted soil. However, for the purposes of this report, only direct contact with soil will be illustrated here.

$$MSV_{soil}\ (mg/kg) = \frac{RfD_o \ x\ ED\ x\ BW\ x\ 365\ days/yr}{[(IR_{soil}) + (S\ x\ SA\ x\ ABS)]\ x\ EF\ x\ ED\ x\ 10^{-6}\ kg/mg} \tag{4}$$

where:

RfD_o = oral reference dose (mg/kg/day); Table 4
BW = body weight (70 kg)
ED = exposure duration (30 yrs)
EF = exposure frequency (350 days/yr)
IR_{soil} = soil ingestion factor (114 mg-kg/day-yr), which is age adjusted for 0-30 years and based on the assumption of 200 mg/day for ages 1-6 years and 15 kg body weight, and 100 mg/day for ages 7-30 and 70 kg body weight.
S = dermal contact rate (1.45 $mg/cm^2/day$ for potting soil; 2.77 for clay soil)
SA = surface area of exposed skin (4211 cm^2), which is age-adjusted and assumes exposure of arms, legs, and hands.
ABS = dermal adsorption factor (unitless), which is chemical-specific and assumes 50% for organic MS constituents.

The simplified equation, which is based on default values listed above including an S value of 2.77 $mg/cm^2/day$, is:

$$MSV_{soil}\ (mg/kg) = (2.2\ x\ 10^4)\ x\ RfD_o \tag{5}$$

Water

Under the residential land-use scenario, theoretical exposure to MS constituents in groundwater can occur as a result of inhalation of volatiles in conjunction with typical household usage (bathing, dish washing, clothes washing, toilet bowls) as well as direct ingestion. Whereas dermal absorption is a potentially complete exposure pathway, it is not incorporated into the MSV. Instead, it is assumed that theoretical exposure from ingestion and inhalation is sufficiently conservative to cover any risk resulting from dermal exposure. MSVs can be estimated with following equation:

$$MSV_{soil}\ (mg/L) = \frac{BW \ x \ AT \ x \ 365 \ days/yr}{EF \ x \ ED \ x \ [1/RfD_i \ x \ K \ x \ IR_a) + (1/RfD_o \ x \ IR_w)]} \tag{6}$$

where:

RfD_o = oral reference dose (mg/kg-day); Table 16.4
RfD_i = inhalation reference dose (mg/kg-day); Table 16.4
BW = body weight (70 kg)
AT = averaging time (30 yrs)
ED = exposure duration (30 yrs)
EF = exposure frequency (350 days/yr)
IR_{water} = water ingestion rate (2 L/day)
IR_{air} = daily indoor inhalation rate (15 m^3/day)
K = volatilization factor (0.0005 x 1000 L/m^3)

The simplified equation, which is based on the default values listed above, is:

$$MSV_{water}\ (mg/L) = \frac{73}{(7.5/RfD_i + 2/RfD_o)} \tag{7}$$

Step 5: Estimation of Concentrations of Chemical Fractions in Environmental Samples. During site characterization programs involving MS, soil and/or groundwater samples are typically analyzed for TPH using a modified EPA Method 8015, or a modified ASTM Method D3328 as an alternative. TPH is the total quantity of all hydrocarbons including paraffinic, naphthenic and aromatic compounds. Aromatic compounds are frequently analyzed separately using such procedures as EPA

Method 602 (water) or EPA 8020 (soil). However, it is usual practice to identify and quantify only certain aromatic compounds because of methodological and cost limitations. The concentration of the *total* aromatic fraction is not quantified for similar reasons. The objective in step five was to estimate the concentrations of both the total aliphatic and total aromatic fractions, each of which corresponds to the toxicity criteria developed in step 3.

First, the total aromatic concentration in soil and/or groundwater samples is estimated from site data for ethylbenzene, naphthalene, toluene and xylene. In MS preparations, the percentage of these four compounds is assumed to range up to 15% of the total aromatic fraction. The remaining 85% consists of a wide variety of other aromatic compounds, many of which have not been identified (Table 16.1). In cases when the laboratory reports a finding of an aromatic chemical other than one of the four marker compounds (e.g., benzene), such chemicals should be addressed in a health risk assessment independently of MS. The total aromatic fraction in individual environmental samples can be estimated from the four marker compounds using the following equations:

1. Sum the total concentrations of the four marker compounds:

$$\text{Total concentration of aromatic marker compounds (e.g., mg/kg-soil, mg/L water)} = [\text{ethylbenzene}] + [\text{toluene}] + [\text{xylenes}] + [\text{naphthalene}] \quad (8)$$

2. Estimate the total aromatic concentration:

$$\text{Total aromatic concentration (e.g., mg/kg-soil, mg/L water)} = \frac{\text{Total concentration of marker compounds (Eq. 8)}}{0.15} \quad (9)$$

3. Estimate the total aliphatic concentration:

(10)

Total aliphatic hydrocarbon concentration	= TPH concentration as determined by the modified EPA 8015	- Total aromatic concentration (Eq. 9)

Step 6. Risk characterization

A screening-level risk characterization of a site can be accomplished by comparing chemical and media-specific MSV's derived in step 4 with media-specific concentrations of chemical fractions determined in step 5. Consistent with EPA a series of three tests can be performed.

Test 1: Determination of a chemical-specific and media-specific hazard quotient (HQ)

The first test evaluates the potential health significance of a single chemical and a single medium (or exposure pathway). The resulting Hazard Quotient (HQ) is the ratio of the concentration of a substance in a medium (C_{medium}) with the health-based MSV for that substance in the same medium. If the value of the HQ is greater than one, then the concentration of the substance in the medium in question is considered potentially hazardous.

$$HQ = \frac{C_{medium}}{MSV_{medium}} \tag{11}$$

Test 2: Determination of chemical-specific total HQ

The second test evaluates the potential health significance of multiple media (exposure pathways) for a single chemical constituent. Exposures associated with various media are assumed to be cumulative. If the value of HQ_{total} is greater than one, then the combined concentrations of a single chemical constituent in various media are considered potentially hazardous.

$$HQ_{total} = HQ_{medium\ 1} + HQ_{medium\ 2} + \dots\ HQ_{medium\ n} \tag{12}$$

Test 3: Determination of a Hazard Index (HI)

The third test evaluates the potential significance of multiple chemicals and multiple media (or exposure pathways). Consistent with EPA methodology[37], only chemicals with similar toxicologic manifestations should be summed. As shown in Table 16.4, the six marker compounds have similar toxicologic manifestations in mammalian systems; liver impacts are common to all substances. Therefore, it is appropriate to sum all HQ values of all six constituents, which is a Hazard Index (HI). If the HI exceeds one, then the collective concentrations of substances either measured or estimated as present in media at a site are considered to constitute a potentially significant health impact. Similarly, if the sum of the HI does not exceed unity, then the site is considered safe.

Discussion

Health risk assessments performed as part of site remedial investigation programs can serve several different practical purposes, such as (a) determining whether the type and extent of contamination is significant enough to warrant further investigation, (b) determining whether mitigative measures should be instituted to protect human receptors from immediate danger, (c) identifying and evaluating the relative contribution to overall risk of multiple exposure pathways, or multiple chemicals, or multiple exposure routes, or (d) eventually deriving media specific, chemical specific, health based cleanup levels. Furthermore, health risk assessments can range in complexity from relatively simple, worst case, deterministic analyses to very comprehensive, reasonable case, probabilistic analyses. Practical benefit can be derived from risk assessments at both ends of the spectrum as long as all parties, including principal responsible parties (PRP's), risk assessors and regulators, understand the specific purpose of each type of analysis.

Although intentionally simplistic in approach, the risk assessment methodology presented herein makes it possible to evaluate a complex hydrocarbon mixture taking into account site-specific environmental weathering influences. Alternatives to this approach are either restricted by the impracticality of characterizing the residual hydrocarbons present at a site, or the impropriety of assuming the residual hydrocarbon in soil, groundwater or air is equivalent in toxicity to fresh (unweathered) product.

We believe an approach based on separating complex mixtures into chemical fractions for assessing risk and deriving health based cleanup levels, as we have done, for MS is logical. We also recognize that this methodology possesses some unknown degree of uncertainty, the amount of which is difficult to judge because of the numerous data gaps that exist primarily in the areas of chemical analysis and toxicity testing. However, to compensate for these data gaps, several conservative elements have been incorporated, such as selecting cyclohexane as the surrogate compound for the naphthenic fraction, and selecting ethylbenzene as the surrogate compound for the >C8+ aromatic fraction.

Successful development of an improved risk assessment methodology depends on alleviating these data gaps. The logical sequence of studies needed to accomplish this goal, we believe, is as follows. First, science needs to better characterize the behavior of individual hydrocarbons in environmental media, focusing specifically on structure-activity relationships. For example, comparative analysis of the extent of alkylation of different kinds of hydrocarbons on the degree of sorption to soil particles, or on rates of biological degradation, or on rates of volatilization. Based on environmental behavior characteristics and chemical structure, hydrocarbon compounds can then be subdivided into logical chemical groups. Second, chemists should develop analytical methodologies for routinely detecting and quantifying these chemical fractions in environmental samples. Third, toxicologists should conduct appropriate toxicity testing on each chemical fraction. Clearly, this effort is multidisciplinary and would require coordination among both government and industry.

CASE EXAMPLE

Introduction

The example presented herein illustrates an application of the MS risk assessment methodology described in this chapter. In this example, the principal objectives of the analysis were: (a) to determine whether the site in question poses an immediate danger to human health, (b) to compare the relative risks associated with various hydrocarbon residues associated with MS in soil and groundwater, (c) to determine the relative risk associated with soil versus groundwater for the purpose of orienting the development of further site investigation studies and evaluation of potential remediation approaches.

General Description of the Site

The site, which is located in the midwest United States, is situated on 2.45 acres. It is a distribution point for MS, plus a collection point for spent solvents generated by S-K customers. Two 10,000 gallon USTs were previously used to store product and spent MS at the site.

The site is located in a relatively flat area, with an elevation approximately 1,300 feet above sea level on an alluvial terrace, approximately three miles west of a major river. The alluvium is of unknown depth and primarily contains silty sand with occasional layers, and minor coarse-grained silty sand and gravel layers. The uppermost aquifer occurs within the terrace alluvium. Groundwater with a hydraulic gradient $< 0.4\%$ is located at a depth of 11 to 13 feet. The sand and gravel layers hold the majority of the groundwater, and are interconnected, thus acting as a single aquifer in response to long-term withdrawals of water. The average hydraulic conductivity has been estimated at 234.5 feet per day or 8.26×10^{-2} cm/sec.

The region is characterized by short, cold winters and long, hot summers. The annual precipitation is 28.93 inches, with an average annual snowfall of 15.4 inches. Seventy-five percent of the precipitation in the region falls between April and September.

Land and Water

The area surrounding the site is used exclusively for small businesses, industrial, and commercial facilities and is zoned for industrial use. The site is bordered by a vacant lot to the north, and industrial enterprises on all other sides. No wetlands or critical habitats, residences, parks, schools, day-care centers, hospitals or convalescent homes are located within 0.5 miles of the site. There is no evidence that the area within 0.5 miles of the site will change from being used as an industrial area in the foreseeable future.

Groundwater use is currently limited to commercial or non-drinking domestic purposes. All businesses in the area are served by a municipal water supply system. The nearest down-gradient public water supply well is located four to five miles from the site. Current use of wells near the facility suggest that additional well drilling could occur in the future.

Surface runoff from the site enters the storm sewer system near the southeast corner of the property. An approximately four acre open detention pond collects the drainage 600 feet to the south of the site. Outfall from the pond is returned to the sewer system and flows into a floodway where it eventually empties into a major river.

Description of Residual Hydrocarbons in Soil and Groundwater

Table 16.5 provides a summary of analytical results from three subsurface soil and groundwater investigations conducted over a three year period. Soil quality was evaluated from the ground surface to the groundwater table, which is approximately 13 feet below grade. Soil samples were collected and analyzed for MS using either Modified EPA Method 8015 or Modified ASTM Method D3328, 40 CFR Part 264 Appendix IX volatile organic compounds (VOCs) using EPA Method 8240, and semivolatile organic compounds (SVOCs) using EPA Methods 8270. The investigations revealed the presence of residual MS (TPH as MS), ethylbenzene, naphthalene, toluene, and xylenes, all of which are components of MS. Figure 16.1 shows the areal distribution of residual MS in soil.

Groundwater monitoring data were collected from five onsite monitoring wells and one onsite water supply well. One of the monitoring wells was installed up-gradient and the remaining four wells were installed at down-gradient locations. Wells were sited based on expected groundwater flows, the location of the former USTs, and the results of soil investigations. It was determined that groundwater degradation occurred due to introduction of MS into soil at a depth of approximately 9.5 feet below grade. Groundwater quality data are summarized in Table 5.

Table 16.5. Summary of chemicals detected on-site.

Chemical	No. samples analyzes/total no. samples	No. detects-/no. samples analyzed	Frequency of detection (%)	Range of detected concentrations	Detection limits
				(mg/kg)	(mg/kg)
Soil					
Ethylbenzene	35/35	2/35	5.7	0.140-0.530	0.0054-5
Mineral Spirits	35/35	8/35	29	52-4,000	3-150
Naphthalene	23/35	8/23	35	0.076-4.9	0.05-0.330
Toluene	32/32	2/32	5.7	0.0088-0.250	0.0054-5
Xylenes (total)	32/32	4/32	11	0.750-4.6	0.0054-5
				(mg/L)	(mg/L)
Groundwater					
Ethylbenzene	15/17	1/15	20	0.013-0.060	0.005
Mineral Spirits	15/17	2/15	15	0.120-600	0.009-1.8
Toluene	15/17	1/15	13	0.041-0.045	0.005
Xylenes (total)	15/17	1/15	27	0.011-0.450	0.005

Screening Analysis

For the purposes of this illustration and using the MS risk assessment methodology, the steps involved in the analysis were: (a) evaluation and identification of potentially significant exposure pathways (standard risk assessment methodology), (b) derivation of MSV's corresponding with each potentially significant exposure pathway (Step 4), (c) estimation of the total aliphatic and total aromatic fractions (i.e., exposure point concentrations) from site monitoring data (Step 5), and (d) risk characterization for each chemical constituent and each potentially significant exposure pathway (Step 6).

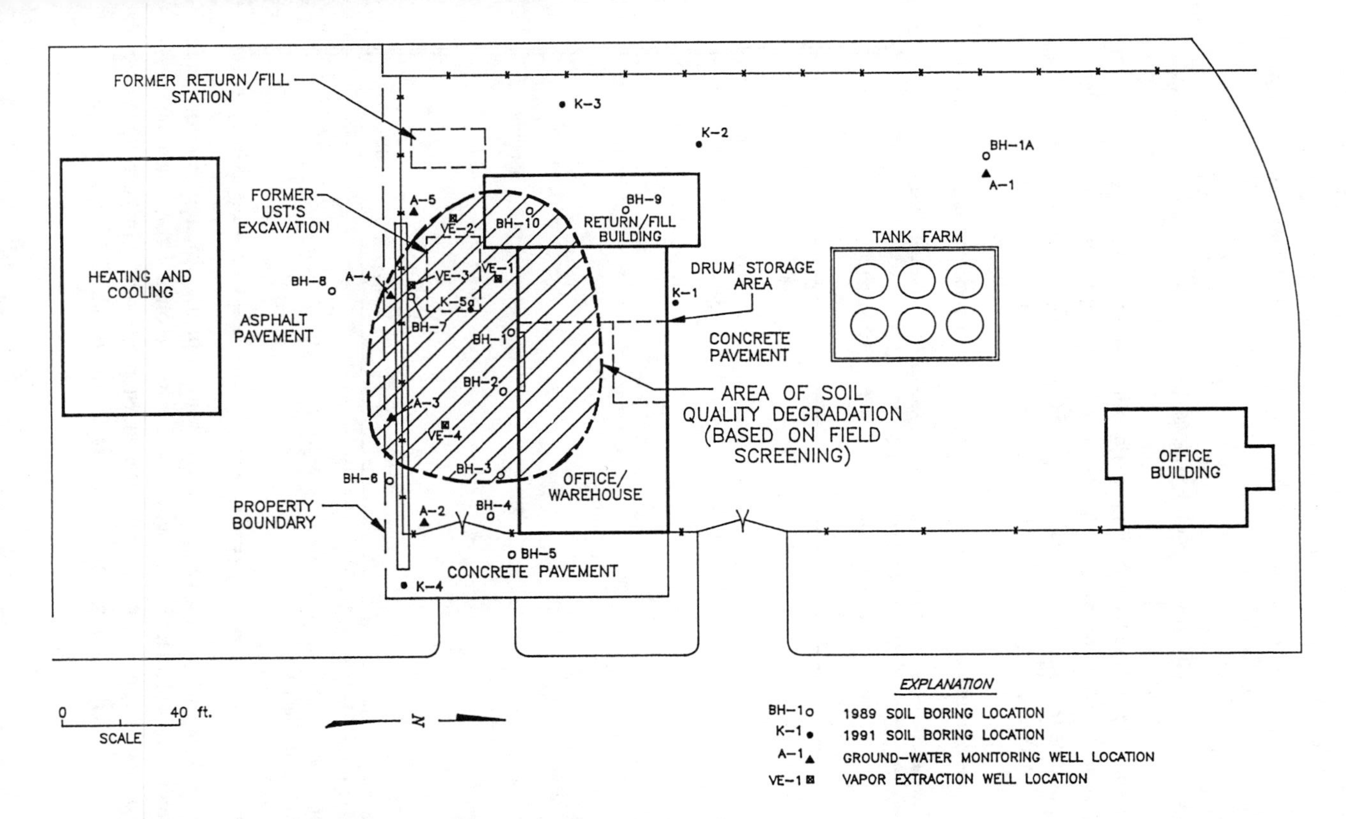

Figure 16.1. Site map showing area of soil impacted by mineral spirits.

Chemicals and Exposure Pathways Evaluated

For the purposes of this case example, chemicals of potential concern (COC's) at the site were determined to be MS, ethylbenzene, naphthalene, toluene, and xylene. Residual concentrations of these compounds in soil and groundwater at the site were based on results from the three site investigation programs (Table 16.5). Also for purposes of this example, exposure pathways and routes evaluated are: (a) soil (ingestion, and dermal contact routes), and (b) groundwater (ingestion and inhalation routes).

Derivation of media specific screening values (MSV's)

MSV's were determined for soil using Equations 4 and 5 and RfD_0 values for each constituent given in Table 16.4. MSV's for groundwater were calculated using Equations 6 and 7 and RFD_0 and RfD_i values listed in Table 16.4. Calculated MSV's for both soil and groundwater are given in Table 16.6.

Table 16.6. Relative risk of mineral spirits and associated aromatic constituents in soil.

Chemical	Maximum Concentration in Soil (mg/kg)	MSV (mg/kg)[a]	HQ[b]
Mineral Spirits			
Aliphatic Fraction	3,931[c]	15,400	0.30
Aromatic Fraction	68.53[d]	3,960	0.02
		HQ_{MS}	0.32
Measured Constituents			
Ethylbenzene	0.53[c]	2,200	0.0002
Naphthalene	4.90[c]	88	0.06
Toluene	0.25[c]	4,400	0.00006
Xylene	4.60	44,000	0.0001
		$HQ_{Aromatics}$	0.06
		HQ_{Total}	0.4

[a] Calculated using EPA[37-40]
[b] Ratio of maximum concentration to screening value
[c] Calculated using Equation 10
[d] Calculated using Equations 8 and 9

The concentrations of the total aromatic and aliphatic fractions in soil and groundwater were calculated using Equations 9 (total aromatic concentration) and 10 (total aliphatic concentration) presented in Step 5 above. In keeping with a screening type analysis, maximum concentrations of all COC's were used in these calculations. The relative proportions of these two fractions are tabulated for soil and groundwater in Tables 16.6 and 16.7, respectively.

Risk Characterization

To estimate the relative risk of individual COC's for the exposure pathways evaluated, media specific HQ's can be easily calculated. HQ's for individual COC's are presented in Tables 16.6 and 16.7 for soil and groundwater, respectively. A Hazard Index (HI) was calculated by summing the two media HQ_{total} values. The HI was calculated to be 71.8 (71.4 + 0.4).

Table 16.7. Relative risk of mineral spirits and associated aromatic constituents in groundwater.

Chemical	Maximum Concentration in Groundwater (mg/L)	MSV (mg/L)[a]	HQ[b]
Mineral Spirits			
Aliphatic Fraction	599.4[c]	8.5	70.5
Aromatic Fraction	0.56[d]	2.1	0.3
		HQ_{MS} =	70.8
Measured Constituents			
Ethylbenzene	0.06[c]	1.6	0.04
Toluene	0.045[c]	3.2	0.01
Xylene	0.45[c]	0.9	0.50
		$HQ_{Aromatics}$ =	0.6
		HQ_{Total} =	71.4

[a] Calculated using EPA[37-40].
[b] Ratio of maximum concentration to screening value.
[c] Calculated using Equation 10.
[d] Calculated using Equation 8 and 9.

As shown in Table 16.6, direct contact with soil (ingestion, dermal contact) does not pose a significant risk. With an HQ of 0.32, the aliphatic fraction poses the highest relative risk compared to other COC's. Conversely, the groundwater is unacceptable for domestic usage by humans (Table 16.7). The HQ_{total} was calculated to be 71.4 (Table 16.7), which is well above unity. As with soil, the aliphatic fraction is the predominate contributor to theoretical risk. Although xylene is less than an HQ of one, because it approaches unity, some additional consideration may be warranted.

Other pathways not presented in this example, but ones that were evaluated in the risk assessment performed for this site included: leaching of MS constituents from onsite soil into groundwater, and volatilization of MS constituents from onsite soil into ambient air and accumulation in indoor air. Determination of exposure point concentrations for these pathways required the use appropriate analytical modeling (e.g., SESOIL and AT123D for estimating leaching rates and groundwater concentrations over time).

Summary and Conclusions

The results of this screening risk assessment demonstrate that the aliphatic components of MS pose the greatest relative risk at the site, at least for the two exposure pathways evaluated. Additionally, the total aromatic fraction as well as the four aromatic marker compounds in both soil and groundwater are negligible in potential impact. Weathering is the likely explanation for this result (i.e., the residual aromatic constituents have decreased more rapidly in concentration over time compared to the aliphatic constituents). This information provides valuable information to PRPs, regulators and consultants in planning further site investigation work, evaluating the degree of imminent danger at the site, and conducting preliminary feasibility studies on remedial alternatives.

ACKNOWLEDGEMENTS

The authors wish to acknowledge Ms. Kathy Yost, Mr. Mark Bowland, Ms. Lynette Cockrum, and Mr. Mark Jones, all of EMCON, for their technical assistance and review of the manuscript.

REFERENCES

1. Calabrese, E.J., Kostecki, P.T., The Council for Health and Environmental Safety of Soils, *Reg. Toxicol. Pharmacol.* 16:273, 1992.
2. U.S. Environmental Protection Agency, Memorandum from Joan Dollarhide, Environmental Criteria and Assessment Office, to Carol Sweeney, EPA Region X. Oral reference doses and oral slope factors for JP-4, JP-5, diesel fuel, and gasoline, Cincinnati OH, 1992.
3. Pederson, D., ABB Environmental Services, Inc., Wakefield MA, Huthceson, M., Anastas, N., MADEP, ORS, Boston MA. A risk-based alternative to the TPH parameter, Presentation at the Society for Risk Analysis Annual Meeting. 1992.
4. Oliver, T. and Kosteck; P.T. 1992. *State-by-State Summary of Cleanup Standards*. Dec. 1992.
5. Oak Ridge National Laboratory. *The Installation and Restoration Program Toxicology Guide.* Aerospace Medical Division, Wright-Patterson Air Force Base, OH. 1989. Volume 4, Chapter 67.
6. World Health Organization (WHO). Selected Petroleum Products Environmental Health Criteria 20, WHO, Geneva, 1982.
7. Safety-Kleen Material Safety Data Sheet. Safety-Kleen 105, Part No's 6614 and 6617. 1990.
8. Chemical analysis by Safety-Kleen laboratory, 1980.

9. National Institute for Occupational Safety and Health (NIOSH). Criteria for a recommended standard...Refined Petroleum Solvents. NIOSH 77-192. 1992.
10. Smith, J.H., Harper, J.C., Jaber, H., Analysis and environmental fate of Air Force distillate and high density fuels, Report no ESL-TR-81-54. Tyndall Air Force Base, FL: Engineering and Services Laboratory, 1981.
11. Spain, J.C., Somerville, C.C., Lee, T.J., Butler, L.C., Bourquin, A.W., Degradation of jet fuel hydrocarbons by aquatic microbial communities, Report no. EPA-600/S-83-059, Air Force/EPA interagency agreement. AR-57-F-2-A-016. U.S. Environmental Protection Agency, Office of Research and Development, Gulf Breeze, FL, 1983.
12. Svoma, J., Houzman, V., Protection of groundwater from oil pollution in vicinity of airports, *Environ. Geol. Water Sci.* 6:21, 1984.
13. Corapcioglu, M., and A. Baehr. 1985. Immiscible contaminant transport in soils and groundwater with emphasis on petroleum hydrocarbons: System of differential equation versus single cell model. *Water Sci. Tech.* 17:23, 1985.
14. Bossert, I., Bartha, R., The Fate of Petroleum in Soil Ecosystems, *Petroleum Microbiology,* Atlas, R.M., ed., MacMillan Pub, New York, 1984.
15. McIntyre, W.G., Smith, C.L., deFur, P.O., Su, C.W., *Hydrocarbon fuel chemistry: Sediment water interaction.* Tyndall Air Force Base, FL, Engineering and Services Laboratory Report No. ESL-TR-82-06, November, 1981.
16. Murray, D.A.J., Loskhar, W.L., Webster, G.R.B., Analysis of the water soluble fraction of crude oils and petroleum products by gas chromatography, *Oil and Petrochemical Pollution.* 2:39, 1984.
17. Brammer, P., Identification and quantification of the water soluble components of JP-4 and a determination of their biological effects upon selected freshwater organisms. Report no. AFOSR-TR-82-0108, Annual Technical report (11/81). Bolling Air Force Base, DC: USAF Office of Scientific Research, 1982.
18. Coleman, W.E., Munch, J.W., Streicher, R.P., Ringhand, H.P., Kopfler, F.C., The identification and measurement of compounds in gasoline, kerosene,a nd no. 2 fuel oil that partition into the aqueous phase after mixing. *Arch. Environ. Contam. Toxicol.* 13:171, 1984.
19. Atlas, R.M., Microbial degradation of petroleum hydrocarbons: An environmental perspective." *Microbiol. Rev.* 45:180, 1981.
20. Haines, J.R., Alexander, M., Microbial degradation of high molecular weight alkanes." *Appl. Microbiol.* 28:1084, 1975.
21. Rothman, N., Emmentt, E., The carcinogenic potential of selected petroleum derived products, *Occup. Med.* 3:475, 1988.
22. Hine, C.H., Zuidema, H.H., The toxicological properties of hydrocarbon solvents." *Ind. Med.* 39:215, 1970.

23. Riley, A.J., Collins, A.J., Browne, N.A., Grasso, P., Response of the upper respiratory tract of the rat to white spirit vapor, *Toxicol. Lett.* 22:125, 1984.
24. Carpenter, C.P., Kinkead, E.R., Geary, D.L., Jr., Sullivan, L.J., and J.M. King. Petroleum hydrocarbon studies III. Animal and human response to vapors of Stoddard solvent, *Toxicol. Appl. Pharmacol.* 32:282, 1985.
25. Carpenter, C.P., Kinkead, E.R., Geary, D.L., Jr., Sullivan, L.J., King, J.M., Petroleum hydrocarbon studies VIII. Animal and human response to vapors of 140° flash aliphatic solvent, *Toxicol. Appl. Pharmacol.* 34:413, 1975.
26. Rector, D.E., Steadmen, B.L., Jones, R.A., Siegal, J., Effects on experimental animals of long term exposure to mineral spirits." *Toxicol. Appl. Pharmacol.* 9:257, 1966.
27. Phillips, R.D., Cockrell, B.Y., Effects of certain light hydrocarbons on kidney function and structure in male rats, *Advances in Modern Environmental Toxicology. Volume VII. Renal Effects of Petroleum Hydrocarbons.* Mehlman, M.A. et al. eds. Princeton Scientific Publishers, Princeton, 1984.
28. Viau, C., Bernard, A., Gueret, F., Maldague, P., Gengoux, P., Isoparaffinic solvent-induced nephrotoxic in the rat, *Toxicology.* 38:227, 1986.
29. Phillips, R.D., Egan, G.F., Subchronic inhalation exposure of dearomized white spirits in C10-C11 isoparaffinic hydrocarbon in Sprague-Dawley rats, *Fundam. Appl. Toxicol* 4:808-818, 1984.
30. Pederson, L.M., Cohr, K.H., Biochemical pattern in experimental exposure of humans to white spirits. I. the effects of a 6 hour single dose, *Acta. Pharmacol. Toxicol.* 55:317-324, 1984.
31. Gamberale, F., Annwall, G., Hultengren, M., Exposure to white spirit. II. Psychological functions, *Scan. J. Work Environ. Health.* 1:31, 1975.
32. Crutchfield, W.E., Kitzmiller, K.V., Treon, J.F., The physiological response of the rabbits to cyclohexane, methylcyclohexane, and certain derivatives of these compounds. II. Inhalation, *J. Ind. Hyg. Toxicol.* 25:323, 1943.
33. Integrated Risk Information System, on-line database. Toluene. U.S. Environmental Protection Agency, Washington DC, 1993.
34. Health Effects Assessment Summary Tables (HEAST). U.S. Environmental Protection Agency, Washington, D.C., 1990.
35. Integrated Risk Information System (IRIS) on line database Ethylbenzene. U.S. Environmental Protection Agency, Washington, DC, 1993.
36. Integrated Risk Information System (IRIS), on-line database, Xylene. U.S. Environmental Protection Agency, Washington, DC, 1993.
37. U.S. Environmental Protection Agency. *Risk Assessment Guidance for Superfund--Volume 1, Part A; Human Health Evaluation Manual.* Office of Emergency and Remedial Response, Washington D.C. OSWER Directive 9285.7-01a. Sept. 29, 1989.

38. U.S. Environmental Protection Agency. *Risk Assessment Guidance for Superfund--Volume 1, Part B; Development of Risk-Based Preliminary Remediation Goals,* Office of Emergency and Remedial Response, Washington D.C. 1991.

39. U.S. Environmental Protection Agency. *Exposure Factors Handbook.* Office of Health and Environmental Assessment, Washington D.C. EPA/600/8-89/043. 1989.

40. U.S. Environmental Protection Agency. *Risk Assessment Guidance for Superfund--Volume 1; Human Health Evaluation Manual, Supplement.* Office of Emergency and Remedial Response, Washington, D.C. PB91-921314. March 1991.

CHAPTER 17

Risk Assessment: A Risk Management Tool in Corrective Actions and Closures at Underground Storage Tank Sites

Pedro J. Zavala, Ph.D., William A. Tucker, Ph.D., Eric B. Deaver, PG, Environmental Science and Engineering, Inc. (ESE), Gainesville, Florida, and **Ken Gaylord,** Tesoro Alaska Petroleum Colorado, Anchorage, Alaska

INTRODUCTION

Risk assessment (RA) applications for underground storage tank (UST) corrective action and site closures are gaining wider acceptance and applicability in many states. In 1992, Environmental Science & Engineering, Inc. (ESE) revised its technical and marketing strategies for RA applications for this market sector. Key elements of these plans were communication with state regulatory agencies throughout the nation, identification of states where regulatory agencies were more familiar with RA approaches, and synchronization of fate and transport (F&T) issues with important toxicological factors.

These approaches to the UST RA market were successful in some states. Immediate results materialized in a series of projects in the states of Virginia and Maryland. The Virginia Water Control Board communicated the most interest at the time in RA applications. The most intensely targeted states at the time were Alaska, California, Delaware, Florida, Maryland, and Virginia.

Since 1992, ESE's Gainesville, FL office has performed more than 20 quantitative RAs in Virginia, Maryland, Georgia, Ohio, Alaska, and Michigan. Risk based closures have been obtained for at least 25% of these sites, with the remaining sites still undergoing regulatory review. Currently, closures have been obtained in Ohio, Virginia, and Maryland. The associated costs and time required for report preparation were considered reasonable for this market. RA report preparation costs were less than 5% of typical remediation costs incurred at UST sites. Reports were finalized six to eight weeks after completion of contamination assessments and corresponding authorizations.

The associated costs and time requirements for RAs at UST sites are significantly smaller than RAs for hazardous waste sites under statutes such as Resource Conservation and Recovery Act (RCRA) or Comprehensive Environmental Response, Compensation, and Liability Act (CERCLA). Various factors contribute to this situation: smaller databases, limited chemicals of concern (COCs), and typical receptor pathways. Databases are usually reduced to groundwater and soil samples, and the number of samples usually amounts to a few dozen.

A limited number of COCs is usually observed at UST sites. Usually, benzene, toluene, ethylbenzene, and xylenes (BTEX), and sometimes polynuclear aromatics (PNAs) and methyl tert-butyl ether (MTBE) are COCs that pose health risks as a consequence of petroleum products spills or releases to the environment. Thus, F&T aspects and toxicological issues are simplified when compared with CERCLA or RCRA sites.

Typical pathways of concern at UST sites during an RA evaluation are inhalation of COCs by workers and residents (onsite and offsite), exposure to COCs during recreational activities at nearby streams and rivers, domestic water consumption, and exposure of nearby environmental receptors to COCs in nearby surface water bodies and sediments. Less frequent pathways of concern are human ingestion of contaminated soil, exposure to contaminated fruits and plants, and exposure of terrestrial animals.

The RAs ESE performed were conducted at two levels of detail. The first level included very conservative to conservative assumptions and simple analytical F&T models with exposure concentrations usually based on current COC concentrations in the media of concern. This level of accuracy is usually sufficient for sites with a large number of incomplete pathways and/or COC concentrations close to federal and state guidance levels. The second level included the use of more sophisticated models such as BIOPLUME II[1] to estimate a more realistic exposure concentration. The addition of more sophisticated models to the first level of accuracy proved to be of great advantage in assessing the risks more realistically and devising less costly and more focused remedial approaches when necessary. F&T issues were synchronized more intimately with toxicological considerations. This second level of detail is useful in screening no further action (NFA) candidates, estimating more realistic health based cleanup goals, and supplementing remedial assessment plans. Experience has shown that the health based cleanup levels are usually higher than state or federal guidance levels, and remediation can be effective over a restricted area (e.g., the hot spot of a groundwater BTEX plume). The estimation of site-specific health based levels is akin to the alternate concentration limit (ACL) approach under RCRA hazardous waste regulations [U.S. Environmental Protection Agency (EPA), 1987].[2] ESE has obtained risk based closures using both levels of detail.

Information that is typically collected during a contamination assessment phase at UST sites is usually sufficient for the preparation of an RA. For more realistic results, it is recommended that hydraulic conductivity, organic carbon content, and background groundwater dissolved oxygen be measured in the field. The latter two are rarely measured, but the cost of these extra tests is modest.

In this chapter, an RA application in corrective action at a currently operating gasoline retail station in Chantilly, VA, will be presented in detail. The application of the RA at the Chantilly site has resulted in an NFA with monitoring only (MO) closure at the site. This case study will be followed by some general observations on our experience in the application of RAs at other

UST sites where environmental media have been impacted by a petroleum leak/release. Of special importance will be the description of ongoing RA applications at UST sites in Fairbanks, Alaska.

CHANTILLY SITE

Site Characteristics

The gasoline station is located in Chantilly, Fairfax County, VA. Groundwater flow direction is northward under a major thoroughfare towards a perennial creek located about 700 feet north of a former tank pit (FTP) area at the site. Adjacent land use includes residences and commercial establishments. These establishments use the county water and sewer system. No private wells were reported within a 0.5-mile radius from the site, with the exception of a residential neighborhood located northwest of the site, on the other side of the creek.

During upgrading operations of the retail gasoline station, it was found that petroleum hydrocarbons had impacted soil and groundwater. The upgrading of the station included removing four steel tanks [two 6,000-gallon (gal) and two 4,000-gal] and associated lines from the FTP area and installing a new tank pit in another area of the station. Contamination assessment studies indicated that soil and groundwater had been impacted by gasoline overfills at the FTP area. The impact was significant at depths close to the water table. Reported soil total petroleum hydrocarbon (TPH) levels ranged from 550 to 6,100 parts per million (ppm), and BTEX levels from 224 to 1,142 ppm at the FTP area. Groundwater was impacted over a larger area. The highest reported BTEX levels, found at the FTP area, were about 20 ppm. The plume extended beyond the site premises under a major highway. Background dissolved groundwater oxygen concentrations were estimated to be 3 ppm. Volatilization and aerobic microbial degradation are considered to be the major elimination routes of BTEX in groundwater.

Exposure Assessment

Based on the chemical analyses of soil and groundwater media, BTEX were selected as COCs. Onsite/offsite workers, offsite residents (adults and children), and environmental receptors at the nearby creek were considered as receptors potentially exposed to onsite generated COCs. Domestic water consumption, soil ingestion, inhalation of fugitive dusts, inhalation of volatile COCs, and direct contact were considered as exposure pathways. Through evaluation of the site conditions and receptor activities, various pathways were considered incomplete and were eliminated. Soil ingestion, direct contact, and inhalation to fugitive dusts were considered incomplete because significant soil impact was found at depths greater than five ft. Domestic water consumption was of particular concern because some private wells were reported within a 0.5-mile radius.

Based on F&T observations about the groundwater BTEX plume, it was concluded that the plume is moving in a northerly direction toward the nearby creek and is not discharging significant amounts of COCs in the creek. As the plume leaves the site property, it is expected to move under a major highway, followed by a small wooded area, prior to surface water discharge. Because the only reported private wells are on the other side of the creek, domestic water exposure was considered an incomplete pathway.

Direct contact of humans and aquatic organisms at the creek were considered incomplete pathways. From the F&T studies, the estimated levels of COCs in surface water as a result of onsite groundwater discharge were found to be negligible.

Inhalation of volatile COCs accumulated in offsite commercial establishments and residences by human receptors was considered an incomplete pathway because no such structures exist (or are expected to exist in the future) between the site and the nearby creek. Inhalation of volatile COCs from impacted soil onsite was considered an incomplete pathway. Inhalation of volatile COCs from underlying impacted groundwater and accumulated in the onsite building was considered a complete pathway.

Fate and Transport of COCs

This section consists of four parts. The first is an attempt to understand the current state of contamination since the initial release. The second is a prediction of the fate of the BTEX plume if no remedial action is conducted in any of the impacted environmental media. The third is a prediction of the plume if remedial action is conducted only for soil (source removal). The fourth is a summary of the three cases.

Pre-Existing Conditions Case

It is possible that for perhaps as much as 50 years BTEX have been leaching from impacted unsaturated soil and/or free floating phase at the FTP area. At the time of the site investigation, a small amount of free phase was found at the FTP area (0.02 to 0.08 ft), which disappeared a few months later. The history of the release is not well documented, and the mechanisms of BTEX leaching into groundwater are not well understood. A conceptual approach was developed to account for the behavior of the groundwater BTEX plume up to the present and to predict the future behavior to estimate potential future exposure concentrations. This approach is referred to as the steady state plume and is understood to be only a first level of approximation.

It is postulated that from the start of the release up to the present an average leaching rate of BTEX into groundwater led to the formation of a steady state plume. The source of BTEX was the impacted unsaturated soil close to the water table and the free floating hydrocarbon phase. The BTEX plume reached a steady state at some point in time such that the average rate of leaching equaled the rate of BTEX elimination in the plume. The major elimination routes are expected to be microbial degradation and volatilization.

The average leaching rate was estimated using Darcy's Law (Freeze and Cherry, 1979)[3] and estimates of site-specific parameters. A rate of approximately 1,000 cubic feet per year (ft^3/year) was calculated. The BTEX concentration in groundwater in equilibrium with phase-separated hydrocarbons (PSH) was estimated to be 100 ppm [American Petroleum Institute (API), 1985].[4]

The program BIOPLUME II[1] was used to imitate the conditions that might have led to the existing plume. Table 17.1 shows the input parameters. After reproducing water levels in the area of interest (between the site and nearby creek), a source was simulated at the FTP for a 70-year period. The BTEX leachate concentration was set at 100 ppm, and the initial groundwater BTEX levels were set at zero (Year 0, upper left graph, Figure 17.1). A leaching rate of 1,000 ft^3/yr reproduced the existing state of contamination after approximately 20 to 45 years.

Table 17.1. Bioplume II[1] input parameters[a], Chantilly site.

POROS	(Effective Porosity)	= 0.40
BETA	(Longitudinal Dispersivity)	= 50 ft
DLTRAT	(Ratio of Transverse to Longitudinal Dispersivity)	= 0.45
ANFCTR	(Anisotropy, Ratio of T-yy to T-xx)	= 1.00
DK	(Distribution Coefficient)	= 0.29 L/kg
RHOB	(Bulk Density of Solids)	= 1.59 kg/L
RF	(Retardation Factor)	= 2.15
DEC2	(Reaeration Decay Coefficient)	= 2.60 E-4 day^{-1}

[a] These parameters were used in all Chantilly cases: pre-existing conditions, NFA, and soil removal.

Figure 17.1. is a summary of various results showing the BTEX plume as a function of time for the pre-existing case. The site is shown as a square at about the center of each graph, and the creek is at the top. The groundwater flow is northerly. Year 0 in this figure is the assumed time when gasoline release started. During the following years, the BTEX plume is predicted to have grown until it reached a steady state somewhere between years 20 and 45. The current BTEX plume is shown at the right bottom corner of Figure 17.1 for comparison purposes. This plume is based on current groundwater chemical analysis and appears to be equivalent to the steady state plume.

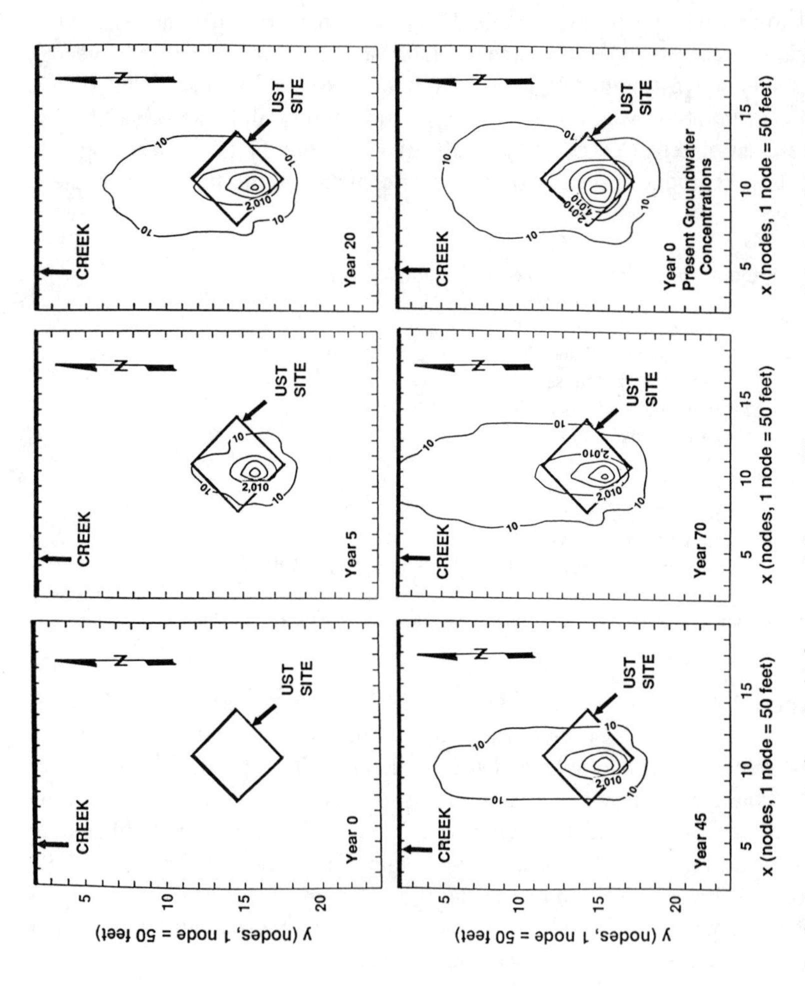

Figure 17.1. BTEX groundwater concentrations (ppb) for pre-existing conditions case as a function of time (Chantilly UST Site).

NFA Case

It is postulated that as the free floating phase disappeared, the leaching rate of BTEX into groundwater decreased. The rate is proportional to phenomena such as the rate of infiltrating rain and water table fluctuations which remove BTEX from the impacted unsaturated zone. A steady state plume is formed at some point in time. This situation is expected to describe the current situation of the site if no soil and no groundwater remediation were to be conducted in the future.

To estimate the leachate rate, some simple assumptions were made. The yield of upland watersheds in the site vicinity was estimated to average 15 inches per year (in/yr). Of this yield, it was conservatively assumed that 20% (three in/yr) runs through the FTP area, which is paved with asphalt and concrete. Thus, the leachate generation rate for a 40 x 40ft tank is estimated to be 400 ft^3/yr (= 40 ft x 40 ft x 3 in/yr ÷ 12 in/ft). The BTEX leachate concentration is assumed to be 100 ppm as in the previous section. The source is assumed to be constant for an indefinitely long period (more than 30 years).

BIOPLUME II[1] was used to model the fate of the BTEX plume under a constant soil loading scenario where free floating phase had recently disappeared. The input parameters are shown in Table 17.1. After reproducing water levels in the area of interest (between the site and nearby creek), a source at the FTP was simulated for a 70-year period at 400 ft^3/yr with a BTEX concentration of 100 ppm. The BTEX leachate concentration was set at 100 ppm, and the initial groundwater BTEX levels were set at currently observed levels (Year 0, Figure 17.2. The results of the BIOPLUME II[1] run predicted that for about 20 years the plume had the same area but levels would decrease during this period. After 20 years, the plume is predicted to shrink significantly to cover an area mostly onsite. The plume did not significantly affect the perennial creek at any time.

Figure 17.2 is a summary of various results showing the BTEX plume as a function of time for the NFA case. The site is shown as a square at about the center of each graph, and the creek is found at the top. The groundwater flow is northerly. Year 0 in this figure is the present groundwater plume based on present groundwater chemical analysis. During the following 20 years, the BTEX plume was predicted to maintain the same size but with decreasing BTEX levels. After 20 to 25 years, the BTEX plume decreases in size and remains mostly onsite. The size and levels reached during Years 20 through 25 remain constant for a long period of time (under the assumption of a constant BTEX soil source), i.e., a steady state plume.

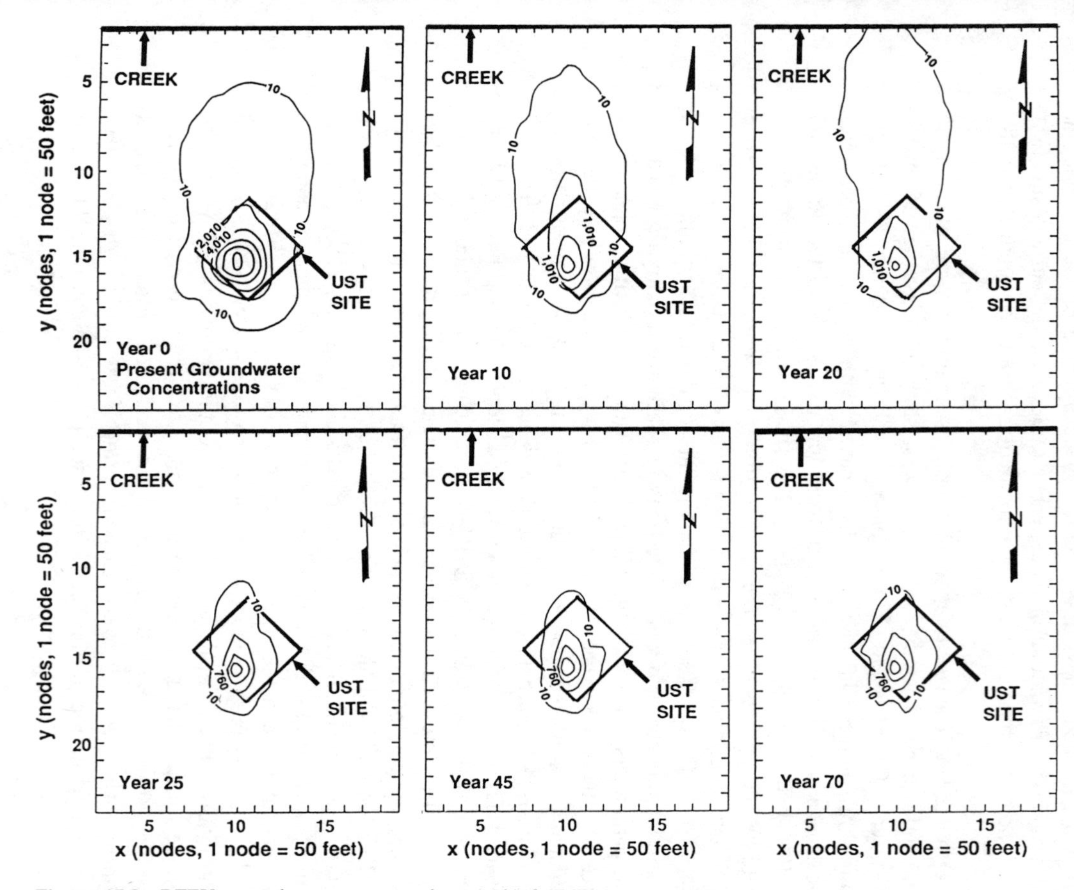

Figure 17.2. BTEX groundwater concentrations (ppb) for NFA case as a function of time (Chantilly UST Site).

Soil Removal Case

This situation is expected to describe the current site situation if only soil remediation is conducted in the future. The constant soil source at the FTP area is removed, and thus the fate of the BTEX plume is predicted as a function of time. This situation would be applicable to corrective action that includes soil remediation but NFA for groundwater media.

BIOPLUME II[1] was used to model the fate of the BTEX plume without a soil loading source. The input parameters are shown in Table 17.1. After reproducing water levels in the area of interest (between the site and nearby creek), the initial groundwater BTEX levels were set at currently observed levels (Year Zero, Figure 17.3). The results of the BIOPLUME II[1] run indicated that, for about 20 years, the plume had about the same size but levels had decreased during this period. After 20 years, the plume shrank significantly and disappeared sometime after 20 to 25 years. The plume did not significantly affect the perennial creek at any time.

This plume behavior is similar to the transient cloud model presented by Tucker and Zavala (1992).[5] The hot spot of the plume was observed to undergo dilution as it moved downgradient. The BTEX plume had essentially left the site somewhere between 10 and 20 years. The predicted lifetime of the plume was 20 years, after which time the hot spot of the plume was about 500 ft from the source. The plume did not reach the creek at any time.

Figure 17.3 is a summary of various results showing the BTEX plume as a function of time for the soil removal case. The site is shown as a square at about the center of each graph, and the creek is found at the top. The groundwater flow is northerly. Year 0 in this figure is the present groundwater plume based on present groundwater chemical analysis. During the following 20 years, the BTEX plume was predicted to shrink and dilute itself as it moved northerly. After 20 to 25 years, the BTEX plume disappeared.

Summary of Cases

Three cases have been considered. The pre-existing case is an attempt to describe the former conditions that might have led to the current state of contamination. The demonstrated ability of this model to reproduce current site conditions provides confidence in the ability to predict future conditions using similar model approaches. The other two cases correspond to the consequences of two different risk management decisions during the corrective action planning stage. For the first, NFA, it is decided that no further remedial action is necessary. The second case, soil removal predicts the effects of source removal (soil remediation) with no direct groundwater remediation.

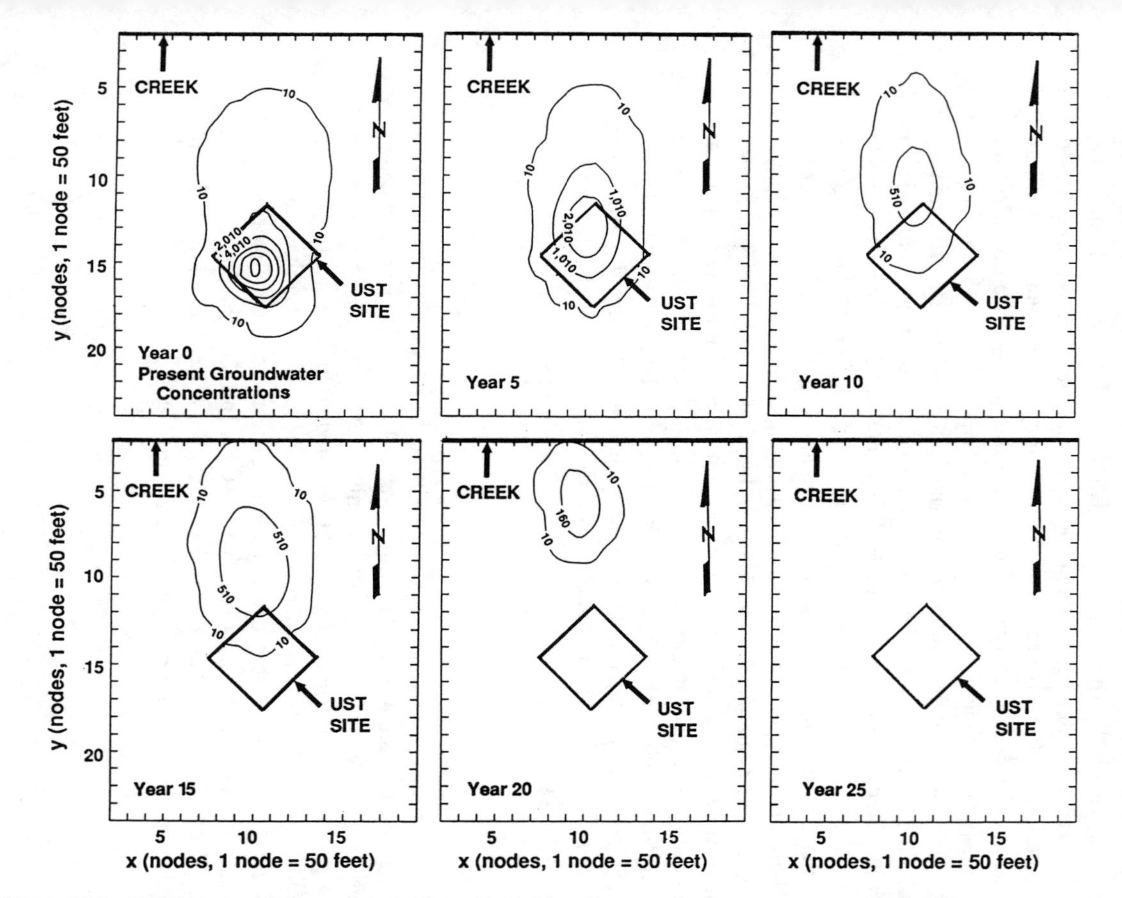

Figure 17.3. BTEX groundwater concentrations (ppb) for soil removal case as a function of time (Chantilly UST Site).

Figures 17.4a and 17.4b are two different comparisons of the NFA and the soil removal cases. Figure 17.4a is a plot of the plume area in acres as a function of time. Figure 17.4b is a plot of Cmax, the maximum concentration predicted at a node [50 x 50 square feet (ft^2)] of the plume hot spot, as a function of time. Figure 17.4c shows the three cases in the same graph. The pre-existing conditions case is overlaid over the other two cases for comparison purposes. Cmax, is plotted as a function of time for all three cases. It is estimated that somewhere between 20 to 45 years of the pre-existing case, the present state of contamination is replicated. Although plots using plume area have more variability than Cmax plots, in general they are useful graphical representations that aid in the interpretation of F&T results. Figure 17.5 is a summary interpretation of the pre-existing case, followed by the two alternative remedial decisions (NFA and soil removal).

Risk Characterization

Based on predictions of the F&T of the BTEX plume under both cases (NFA and soil removal), pathways such as receptor exposure to COCs in surface water bodies were considered to be incomplete. Other pathways had been already eliminated on other grounds. The only pathway of concern was the exposure of onsite workers to BTEX via inhalation of COCs volatilizing from underlying groundwater and accumulating in onsite structures. To estimate the risk of workers at the onsite building, exposure concentrations (indoor BTEX air levels) needed to be calculated, followed by an estimate of BTEX intakes as a result of indoor BTEX inhalation and the corresponding comparison to toxicity parameters (cancer slope factors and reference doses). These calculations are explained in the following sections.

Indoor BTEX Exposure Concentrations

The COCs are expected to volatilize from underlying groundwater and accumulate in the site office building where workers may be exposed. To calculate COC exposure concentrations, the following relationship were used. From Jury *et al.*[6] and Tucker and Hearne[7]

$$F = \frac{na^{10/3} \ x \ Da \ x \ H \ x \ C_{gw} \ x \ 10^{-3}}{n^2 \ x \ h_{gw}} \qquad (1)$$

where:

F = flux ($mg/yr\text{-}cm^2$),
na = soil air porosity = 0.25 (Bonazountas *et al.*),[8]
Da = diffusion coefficient in air [square centimeters per year (cm^2/yr)],
H = Henry's Law constant (dimensionless),

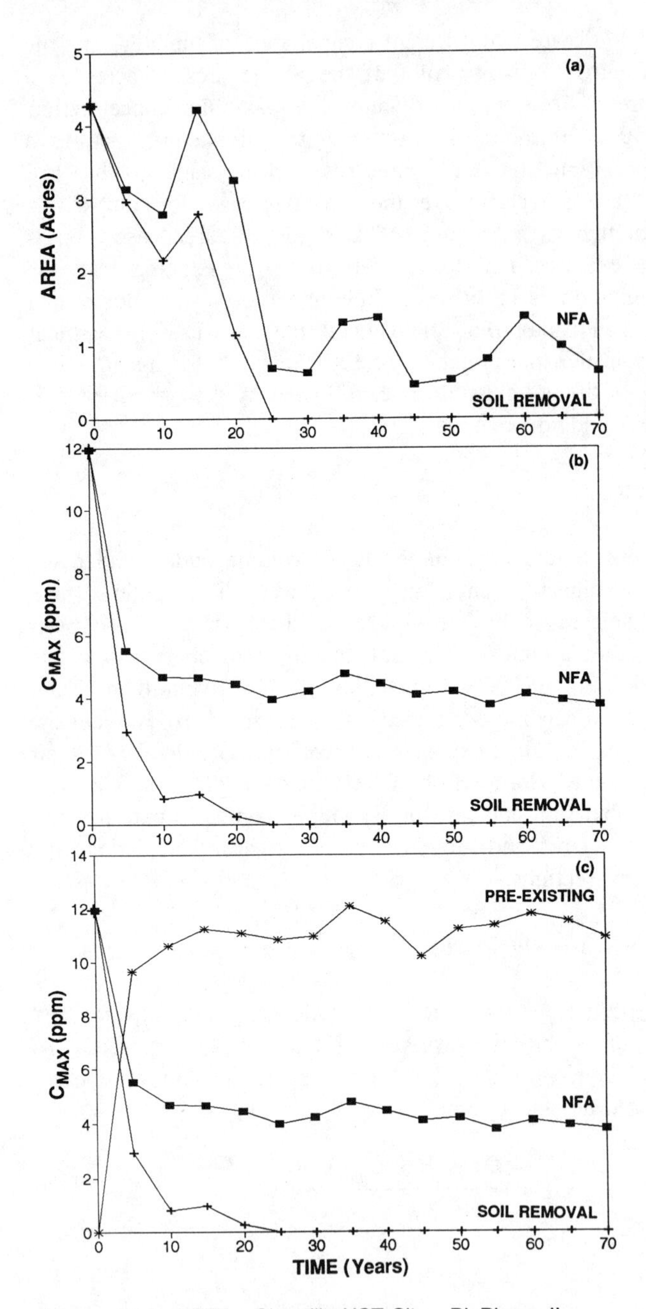

Figure 17.4: BTEX - Chantilly UST Site - BioPlume II

a) Plume area as a function of time for NFA and soil removal cases;

b) Maximum concentration at hot spot of plume as a function of time for NFA and soil removal cases;

c) Maximum concentration at hot spot of plume as a function of time for NFA, soil removal and pre-existing condition cases.

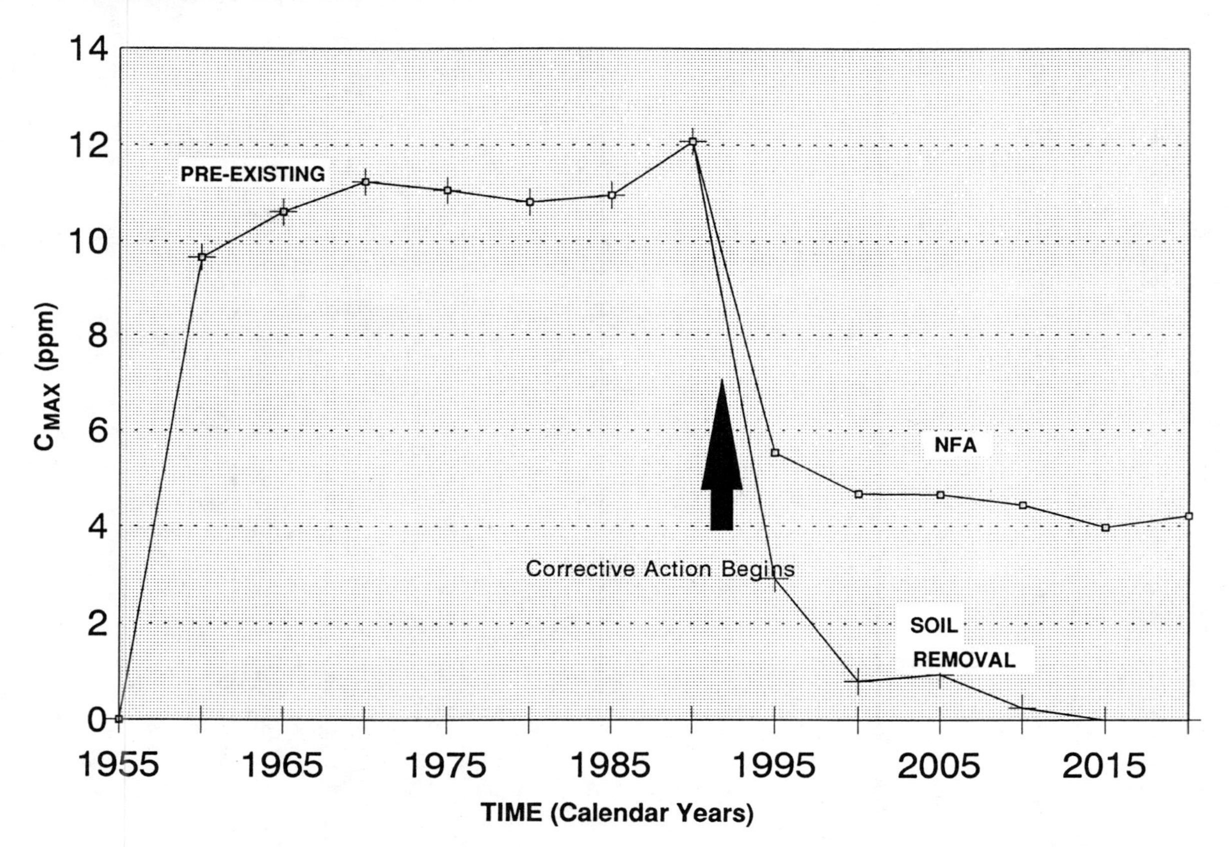

Figure 17.5. Maximum BTEX concentration at hot spot (as predicted by BIOPLUME II) as a function of time: A summary interpretation.

C_{gw} = groundwater exposure concentration (mg/L),
n = vadose soil porosity = 0.40 (Bonazountas et al.),[8]
h_{gw} = depth to water table = 366 centimeters (cm) (12 ft) (site data), and
10^{-3} = conversion factor [liters per cubic centimeter (L/cm^3)].

Then, air exposure concentrations are calculated:

$$C_{air} = F \times (TAC/VAR) \times 10^6 \qquad (2)$$

where:

C_{air} = air exposure concentration [milligrams per cubic meter (mg/m^3)],
TAC = time of exchange for air in building = 0.04 days/exchange (1.10×10^{-4} years/exchange) for commercial/industrial buildings (Ronnberg et al.),[9]
VAR = ratio of building volume to surface area in contact with soil = 305 cm (10 ft) (estimate), and
10^6 = conversion factor [cubic centimeters per cubic meter (cm^3/m^3)].

Indoor BTEX Intake

Intakes were calculated following EPA[10] guidance:

$$Intake = \frac{C_{air} \times IR \times EF \times ED}{BW \times AT} \qquad (3)$$

where:

IR = inhalation rate = 15 cubic meters per day (m^3/day),
EF = 250 days/yr,
ED = 25 years, carcinogenic case,
= 7 years, noncarcinogenic case,
BW = 70 kilograms (kg), and
AT = 25,550 days (70 years), carcinogenic case,
= 2,555 days (7 years), noncarcinogenic case.

Carcinogenic Risks and Hazard Quotients

Using the previously mentioned intakes, carcinogenic risks and hazard quotients (HQs) were evaluated from the following relationships (EPA):[10]

$$CR_i = Intake \times CSF_i \tag{4}$$

$$HQ_i = \frac{Intake}{RfD_i} \tag{5}$$

$$HI = \Sigma_i\, HQ_i \tag{6}$$

where:

CR_i	=	cancer risk for chemical i,
CSF_i	=	inhalation cancer slope factor for chemical i,
HQ_i	=	hazard quotient for chemical i,
RFD_i	=	inhalation reference dose for chemical i, and
HI	=	sum of HQs.

Carcinogenic and noncarcinogenic risks were calculated for both NFA and soil removal cases. Table 17.2 shows the calculated HQs and carcinogenic risks (CRs). The overall CRs were below the EPA acceptable upperbound risk range of 10^{-4} to 10^{-6} (National Contingency Plan),[11] and HIs were below acceptable noncarcinogenic threshold values of unity (EPA).[10] The health risks were calculated following EPA guidance.[10-13]

Table 17.2. BTEX parameters of interest, Chantilly site.

	Benzene	Toluene	Ethylbenzene	Xylenes
CSF	2.9E-2	NA	NA	NA
RFD	2E-2	6E-1	3E-1	9E-2
CR1	1E-5	NA	NA	NA
CR2	2E-5	NA	NA	NA
HQ1	0.16	0.01	0.01	0.12
HQ2	0.16	0.01	0.01	0.12

CSF = inhalation cancer slope factor $(mg/kg/day)^{-1}$.
RFD = inhalation reference dose (mg/kg/day).
CR1 = cancer risk for soil removal case.
CR2 = cancer risk for NFA soil case.
HQ1 = hazard quotient for soil removal case.
HQ2 = hazard quotient for NFA soil case.

Note: Sources for CSF and RFDs were Integrated Risk Information System (IRIS),[15] Health Effects Assessment Summary Tables (HEAST),[16] and EPA.[17]

GENERAL OBSERVATIONS

ESE has obtained risk-based closures in Maryland, Virginia, and Ohio with RAs conducted at both levels of F&T detail. In three of about 12 studied cases, NFA/MO were obtained. For some of the other sites, regulators are considering the RA results before deciding between NFA/MO or groundwater cleanup down to site-specific health-based levels, or drinking water standards. Regulatory review is still underway at other sites. ESE has observed a growing interest of RA applications at UST sites in Virginia, Maryland, Ohio, Michigan, Alaska, Georgia, and Texas. ESE's current statistics are rough, but as RA applications increase at UST sites, better statistics will help project managers and state regulators in corrective action decisions.

Of particular importance are RA applications conducted by ESE and TESORO ALASKA at Fairbanks, AK UST sites. The RAs will be presented in detail in another paper because regulatory review is still pending. RAs at these sites were formulated following the previously mentioned EPA guidances plus procedural guidelines from the Alaska Department of Environmental Conservation (ADEC).[14] The sites were former gasoline stations and are currently used for other commercial purposes. Soil and groundwater were impacted by gasoline. Tanks and related pipelines were removed and the site was undergoing corrective action when the RAs were performed. Corrective action included removal of contaminated soil and air sparging of the impacted groundwater. The sparging was coupled with microbial enhancement at pertinent times by inoculation of hydrocarbon degrading microbial populations and appropriate microbial nutrients.

The Alaska RAs concentrate on the exposures and risks due to BTEX in groundwater if the corrective action were to be halted. No significant BTEX soil loading is expected. Exposure assessment studies, including groundwater modeling with BIOPLUME II,[1] were used in calculating health risks to humans and the environment. No significant impact to downgradient nearby streams were expected by plumes calculated to have lifetimes in the order of a few years.

These RAs are of importance as cooperation proceeds with ADEC in investigating the role of RAs at UST sites in Alaska. These RAs are different from the Chantilly case in the sense that the RA results are used in decisions aimed at ceasing or limiting further corrective action at a site. Because the remedial groundwater approach included microbial degradation, a large number of dissolved groundwater oxygen levels were conducted at the sites of interest. Halting corrective action at sites where hydrocarbon degrading bacterial induction has been performed will be of benefit in future corrective action decisions.

Applications of RA approaches have been presented at UST sites under two different circumstances. The Chantilly site shows RA applications prior to any remedial decision for a station that is undergoing a tank closure project and that will continue to operate as a gasoline retail unit. The Alaska sites show exploratory approaches to former UST sites (currently commercial units) that have been already undergoing corrective actions.

The RAs take into account the present and future use of the sites. The Chantilly station is expected to continue operating as a gasoline retail outlet. The Alaska sites were former gasoline stations now being used for nonpetroleum-related commercial activities. None of the sites are expected to be residential in the future. Present/future land use at sites is an important element in the preparation of RAs, potentially leading to different risk estimates and risk management decisions. As RA applications during corrective action decisions at UST sites evolve, state agencies may have to follow future changes in land use and associated monitoring (post closure issues) to protect human health and the environment. RAs are not devoid of uncertainties in the estimation of risks, but, as in any branch of science, they are expected to improve with time. Advantages of RA applications include a reduction in cost to the sites while being protective of human health and the environment. RAs are understood as predictive tools that provides state regulators and site project managers with an element of balance in their risk management decisions. The applications presented in this chapter have been used in larger petroleum facilities (e.g., terminals) and in general can be extended to sites containing aboveground storage tanks, as well as other hazardous waste sites with more complicated environmental impacts and regulatory compliance aspects.

REFERENCES

1. BIOPLUME II, Version 1.1, Computer model of two-dimensional contaminant transport under the influence of oxygen limited biodegradation in ground water, National Center for Ground Water Research, Rice University, Houston, TX, 1989.
2. U.S. Environmental Protection Agency (EPA), *Alternate concentration limit guidance, Part I, ACL policy and information requirements,interim final,* OSWER Directive 9481.00-6C, EPA/530-SW-87-017, Office of Solid Waste, Waste Management Division, Washington, D.C., 1987.
3. Freeze, R.A. and Cherry, J.A., *Groundwater*, Prentice Hall, Englewood Cliffs, NJ, 1979.
4. American Petroleum Institute (API), Laboratory studies on solubilities of petroleum hydrocarbons in groundwater, Health and Environmental Sciences Department, API Publication No. 4395, 1985.
5. Tucker, W.A. and Zavala, P.J., A practical model for evaluating passive bioremediation of groundwater, in *Proc. of the 1992 Petroleum Hydrocarbons and Organic Chemicals in Ground Water Conference*, API/NGWA, Houston, TX, 1992, 555.
6. Jury, W.A., Spencer, W.F., and Farmer, W.J., Behavior assessment model for trace organics in soil: I. Model description, *J. Environ. Qual.*, 12(4), 558, 1983.

7. Tucker. W.A. and Hearne, F.L., Risk assessment: Tools for reducing liability from underground storage tanks, in 1989 *Oil Spill Conference Proceedings*, San Antonio, TX, 20th Anniversary Conference, 1989.
8. Bonazountas, M., Wagner, J., and Goodwin, B., *Evaluation of seasonal soil/groundwater pollutant pathways,* EPA Contract No. 68-01-5949, Task 9, Monitoring and Data Support Division, U.S. Environmental Protection Agency, Washington, D.C., 1981.
9. Ronnberg, R., Ruotsahainen, R., Sateri, J., Majaneen, A., and Seppanen, O., Indoor climate and the performance of ventilation in 251 residences, in *Proc. of the 5th International Conference on Indoor Air Quality and climate,* Toronto, Canada, 1990.
10. U.S. Environmental Protection Agency (EPA), *Risk assessment guidance for Superfund (RAGS),* Volume 1: Human health evaluation manual, Part A, Office of Emergency and Remedial Response, EPA/540/1-89/002, Washington, D.C., 1989.
11. National Contingency Plan, 55 FR 46:8848, 1990.
12. U.S. Environmental Protection Agency (EPA), *Guidelines for carcinogenic risk assessment,* FR51(185):33992-34003, 1986.
13. U.S. Environmental Protection Agency (EPA), *Guidelines for the health risk assessment of chemical mixtures*, FR 51(185):34014-34025, 1986.
14. State of Alaska, Underground Storage Tanks, Department of Environmental Conservation, 18AAC78. As amended through Aug. 21, 1991.
15. *Integrated Risk Information System (IRIS)*, (NCM/TOXNET), U.S. Environmental Protection Agency, Bethesda, MD, 1991.
16. *Health Effects Assessment Summary Tables (HEAST)*, U.S. Environmental Protection Agency, OERR 9200 6-303 (90-4), NTIS No. PB90-921104.
17. U.S. Environmental Protection Agency (EPA). *Health Advisory for 45 Organics,* Office of Drinking Water, NTIS No. PB87-135578, 1987.

PART IV

REMEDIATION

CHAPTER 18

PCS Disposal and Recycling Database - An Essential Storage Tank Manager's Remediation Tool

Eric B. Deaver, PG, Herndon, Virginia, **Gretchen A. Sauerman,** EIT, Gainesville, Florida, **Jess J. Weiss**, Gainesville, Florida

INTRODUCTION

This chapter discusses the development and uses of a specialized Petroleum Containing Soils (PCS) database system which is designed to address the selection of treatment, recycling or disposal facilities for PCS and sludges. This system is not available for purchase but is available for use through Environmental Science & Engineering, Inc. The searches will be conducted on behalf of active clients for no fee. Other requests will be addressed on a project by project basis. The following sections discuss the purpose and development of the database system. The integration MapInfo™ desktop mapping and specialized application programming for the system are outlined in the next sections. The chapter is closed with a discussion on the use and application of the database during release remediation along with a discussion of related and future implication of geographical computer applications on spill response situations.

PURPOSE OF DATABASE RESPONSE SYSTEM

Environmental Science & Engineering, Inc (ESE) with a nationwide partner communications client developed a progressive site remediation management tool to address the selection of Petroleum Containing Soils (PCS) treatment, recycling and disposal facilities. There are literally millions of tons of PCS generated yearly in the United States. Facility managers and consultants consistently select treatment, recycling and disposal facilities based on past experience/relationships and reputation. This is especially true in emergency situations when the manager does not have the time or ability to competitively bid the soil treatment/disposal facilities. Typically, the facility manager has two to three major national disposal companies with which he does business; assuming as time goes by that these facilities are providing the best cost for the maximum protection of liability. This is not always true. The cost for thermally treating and disposing of PCS in the Washington DC area alone has drastically dropped just in the last three years from $55-60/ton to $30-35/ton. New treatment alternatives are constantly being developed and accepted by the regulatory community.

Centralized landfarming operations previously thought of as high liability facilities useful only for oil field wastes are gaining ground as acceptable (and often preferable) facilities for storage tank related PCS. In order for the facility manager to keep up with these growing resources, he was required to locate each licensed facility with 200 miles of the specific site, interview and inspect the facility, acquire and evaluate competitive bids and finally select and contract the facility. It therefore is perfectly normal for facility managers to establish relations and stick with a few individuals. This has the drawback, however, of increased disposal cost over time, increased transportation cost and liability and antiquated treatment methods being used (possibly increasing longterm owner liability).

It is obvious that a database system is required to greatly reduce the time required to select and evaluate contractors. This is especially true for those managers who are dealing with facilities located throughout the country and at varying distances from their most frequently used disposal sites. In order to provide such a tool to a national communications corporation, ESE devised a method of locating, interviewing and evaluating essentially all of the potential PCS treatment/disposal sites available within the United States. This data, once collected, would require a database system for organization and finally a mapping system to allow for easy deployment in rapid response situations. The cost for development was divided between ESE and its client thereby allowing both parties long term, unrestricted use of the product.

DATABASE DEVELOPMENT

A four-phased approach was used in completing the database: (1) Facility identification, (2) Facility survey of recycling, treatment, or disposal firms, (3) Facility survey of petroleum contaminated rinse water recycling firms, and (4) software integration.

In phase I, several sources were used to identify potentially qualified facilities to handle PCS and associated rinse waters and sludges. In some states, the agency that oversees underground storage tank (UST) regulations had a list of licensed facilities in the state or in neighboring states. Other state agencies utilized included the Solid Waste Divisions (used for obtaining listings of sanitary and industrial landfills), Hazardous Waste Divisions (used for obtaining listings of hazardous waste incinerators and hazardous waste landfills), and Air Permitting Divisions (used for finding licensed mobile incinerators, and brick and rotary kilns).

Not all states had agencies that maintained such databases, however, so additional resources were employed. Licensed waste haulers were also contacted for input on disposal and treatment alternatives in their area. Some "brokering" firms, who provide turn-key disposal services were also helpful in making recommendations in remote areas. On a limited basis, directories from trade associations were also used to complete this phase of the project. In all, more than 600 phone calls were made in phase I.

In the second phase, each soil disposal/treatment facility identified in phase I was contacted by a member of the survey team. The surveyor first determined whether the firm was appropriate for the database (i.e., whether they actually accepted PCS). Survey forms were then filled out either over the phone, or via telefax, depending on time constraints and availability of the information.

Survey forms requested basic information necessary to make an informed decision on whether to use the facility for a given project. The type of facility and vital statistics (address, point of contact, owner, phone and fax number) were obtained. Also, information on maximum (or minimum) petroleum levels accepted (total petroleum hydrocarbons (TPH) and benzene, toluene, ethyl benzene, and xylenes (BTEX) in parts per million(ppm)) were obtained. Some facilities, such as blending operations and some kilns used the soil as a fuel, so they required a minimum British Thermal Unit (BTU) value on the soils.

Other information collected included limitations on the types of soil accepted (clay, silty, sandy, or construction debris) as well as limitations on the origin of materials (some accepted from in the state or in the county only). Costs per ton for hazardous and non-hazardous materials was also collected, since costs are often a major factor in the decision on which facility to use.

Additional details that a site owner would need before making this selection were also collected. Analyses required for approval, manifesting procedures and permit compliance status for the facility would likely be needed, so this information was included on the survey form. With facilities that employed soil cleaning or recycling techniques, the final destination of the "clean soil" was also determined. It is preferable that the soil would be used as roadbase material, as opposed to being disposed in a landfill, since the future liability of the generator would be reduced.

Roughly 2500 facilities nationwide were contacted in phase II and III. Approximately 725 of these facilities actually made it through the screening process and are included in the final database. Many of the state listings were out of date, accounting for calls to facilities that were either out of business, or no longer accepting PCS.

In the third phase, information was collected from facilities that accepted petroleum contaminated waters, and sludges. A number of facilities were found through the National Oil Recyclers Association and the EPA. Also, the major national companies (Chemical Waste Management, Clean Harbors, Safety Kleen, etc) were contacted through their corporate offices. Given the competitive nature of this business, several of the major national firms were hesitant to give out firm unit prices. To compensate for this, a field delimiter was used in the database development phase (discussed later) to note that the unit cost varies, and to call for a firm quote at the time of shortlisting firms.

In phase IV, the information gathered in phases I, II, and III was input into a manageable database to allow for user-friendly manipulation of the data. The phone surveyors used one of five different forms when questioning the facilities, depending on whether the firm was a landfill, soil cleaning/recycling facility, cement kiln, asphalt kiln, portable rotary kiln, or liquid petroleum recycling facility.

Many "yes/no" (Y/N) fields were created in the database development stage to maximize the number of "filters" that could be run on the data. For example, asphalt kiln operators were asked to list which types of soil were acceptable (sand? Y/N, silt? Y/N, etc.) so that it would be possible to run a sort on, for example, all kilns in KANSAS that accept SILT, and DEBRIS, and then rank those entries based on COST PER TON/NON-HAZARDOUS. This procedure was applied in all survey forms, so, as another example, the project manager could run a report of all INDUSTRIAL landfills, in MICHIGAN, owned by a company with 20 OR MORE facilities, and that are LESS THAN 15 YEARS OLD, and again rank these facilities by COST.

Some fields had an additional choice added to the Y/N option. The regulatory compliance field was altered for Y/N/I (I-interim) depending on whether the facility was in full compliance, out of compliance, or in interim status, respectively. A Y/N field was added on whether analyses were required on the soils prior to acceptance. It would be inadvisable to use firms that do not test materials at the gate, since the site owner's soils would be mixed in with untested soils (potentially hazardous) which would increase potential future liability.

As mentioned earlier a field was added to compensate for the larger facilities that did not give out unit costs. Since leaving this field blank or putting in a zero would unfairly rank the facility at the top in cost comparisons, a field entitled "____ vary" (Y/N) was added. The Y option would be used when either the information was not provided due to proprietary constraints, or when the value was determined on a case-by-case basis (perhaps based on concentration levels). Another use of the "___ vary" field was in the maximum levels of BTEX or TPH accepted. Many landfills and kilns will accept PCS up to the state guidelines. Since guidelines are continually subject to change, a firm number in this field could be outdated quickly.

Two other fields, the "TPH_STAT" and "BTEX_STAT" were added to the output forms. These represent greater than (>) or less than (<), depending on which is appropriate for the facility. As mentioned earlier, fuel blenders and kilns require TPH levels greater than a given limit, in order to meet BTU requirements. On the other hand, landfills can only accept TPH levels less than certain limits, in order to meet state regulations. If there are no set maximums, the "STAT" field is left blank, and the "TPH" and "BTEX" fields are placed at one million (parts per million) to indicate no maximum. If the minimum levels vary, or if acceptance is case by case, as evaluated by the state agencies, the "STAT" field is left blank, and the "TPH" and "BTEX" levels are set at 0, and the "___varies" field is set at Y.

With all of these considerations, the data was then entered into a Dbase III+^{TM} data management package. A general understanding of Dbase^{TM} is assumed here, so no specific operating instructions on use of Dbase^{TM} are discussed in this chapter. This database was then integrated with MapInfo^{TM}

a "desktop-mapping" software package, to allow for geographic manipulation of the data. More information on this process follows.

MAPPING OVERVIEW

For the display and query of the PCS database, ESE developed an application program utilizing the MapInfo^{TM} desktop mapping software for DOS. This program would allow users to make inquiries based on location such as closest disposal facility or all facilities in a given radius. The program would also allow Boolean inquiries of the tabular information in a user friendly, menu driven environment.

The development of the mapping component for the PCS database was comprised of two sections: data preparation, and software development.

DATA PREPARATION

During the planning of the mapping program, operational constraints were identified to promote portability and performance. To limit the total disk storage needed to run the program, the level of reference information was limited to state boundaries and city locations. The amount of disk space needed to store the road network for the U.S. would have been prohibitively large for most casual users. This decision to limit the spatial reference to a state or regional level meant that locating and displaying each PCS site with a high level of precision would be an unnecessary effort.

Rather than undertake the arduous & expensive task of assigning specific locations for each individual PCS site, the location was approximated based on each site's ZIP Code. A file of all ZIP Codes for the continental United States containing the latitude and longitude for the centerpoint or centroid of each ZIP Code was matched to the ZIP Code for each PCS site. The coordinates for the ZIP Code centroid were then assigned to that PCS site.

For those few PCS sites located outside the continental U.S. such as Hawaii or Puerto Rico, the latitude and longitude coordinates were derived by locating the site on conventional hardcopy maps, then placing the site point within the MapInfo^{TM} computer map file using relative positioning to known references.

SOFTWARE DEVELOPMENT

In the planning phase the project staff defined several functions to be included in the mapping software. These included: pan and zoom capabilities for map display, radius and proximity searches, distance measurement, and Boolean (conditional if, and, or, not) searches of the tabular database. These functions were then organized into a main menu and a series of sub-menus; the programming modules were organized corresponding to the menu hierarchy.

The mapping program itself was written in MapCode^{TM}, the applications language used by the MapInfo^{TM} for DOS software. Using MapCode^{TM}, only run-time modules of MapInfo™ would be distributed to users with the applications program. By limiting users to the application specifically written for the PCS database ESE could better support the users needs by tailoring menus and help screens to the functions and terminology the PCS users would find familiar. In addition, there was a reduced cost to the users for the run-time module versus the full license of MapInfo™.

Individual program modules were written and tested independently. Once the individual modules were completed, they were assembled into the final application program and on-line help screens were developed for each function and general topics. This program was then distributed to project team members for evaluation and modifications were made as necessary. The application program, PCS datafiles, reference mapfiles and helpfiles were then compressed and integrated into an installation program with the MapInfo™ run-time modules for shipment to the users.

USE OF PCS DATABASE SYSTEM

The PCS database system is both user friendly and limited in input requirements. Once the project manager enters the MapInfo™ environment, a startup file called PCS is called and all database files are loaded. The MapInfo™ system loads state border files, US city files, ESE office location files and all five database files. The initial map (Figure 28.1) will be a full scale map of the US with only the state boundaries showing. From this screen the user can window into a specific site area. The scales change will cause all facility locations as well as major US cities within that area to be displayed. Figure 18.2 would be displayed for this step of a facility search for a site outside of Durham, NC. At this point the search can take two paths: point file search or radius search.

The point file search will locate the closest facility in a particular database file from the PCS site. In the case of the example NC site, the closest landfill, recycler, kiln, cleaner or sludge disposal facility can be identified. To search for cleaning facilities, the closest facilitiy would be displayed with a single key stroke and the database file for that facility would be displayed (and printed) as shown in Table 18.1. The total elapsed time of finding this facility and printing all known information is less than five minutes (including program load time).

The radius search, as the name implies, identifies all facilities in all of the databases within a given mile radius of the site. In the above example, the operator will be searching the Durham NC area within 100 miles of the site. After the radius is input and all databases are searched, Figure 18.3 will be displayed. In this example, six cleaning facilities, no stationary kilns, three recyclers, no landfills, three portable kilns,and three sludge facilities have been identified within the shown radius. A report of each database list (Table 18.2) can then be requested. By selecting each of the facilities in this list, the database file for each facility (Table 18.3) will be displayed for review or printing.

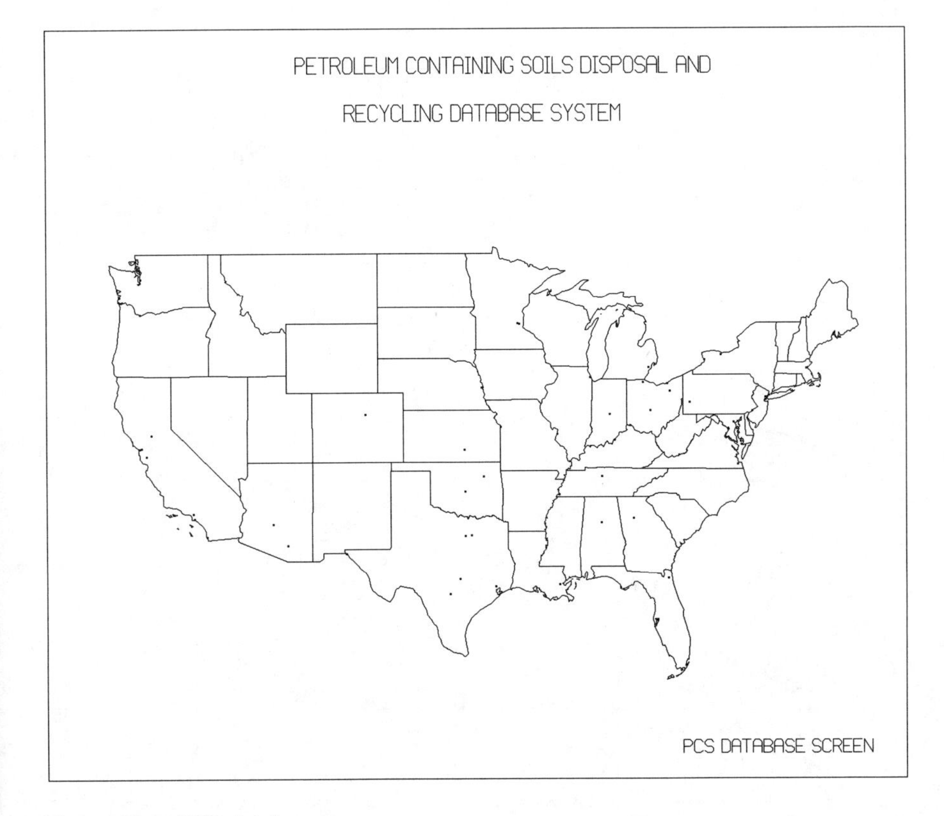

Figure 18.1. PCS database screen.

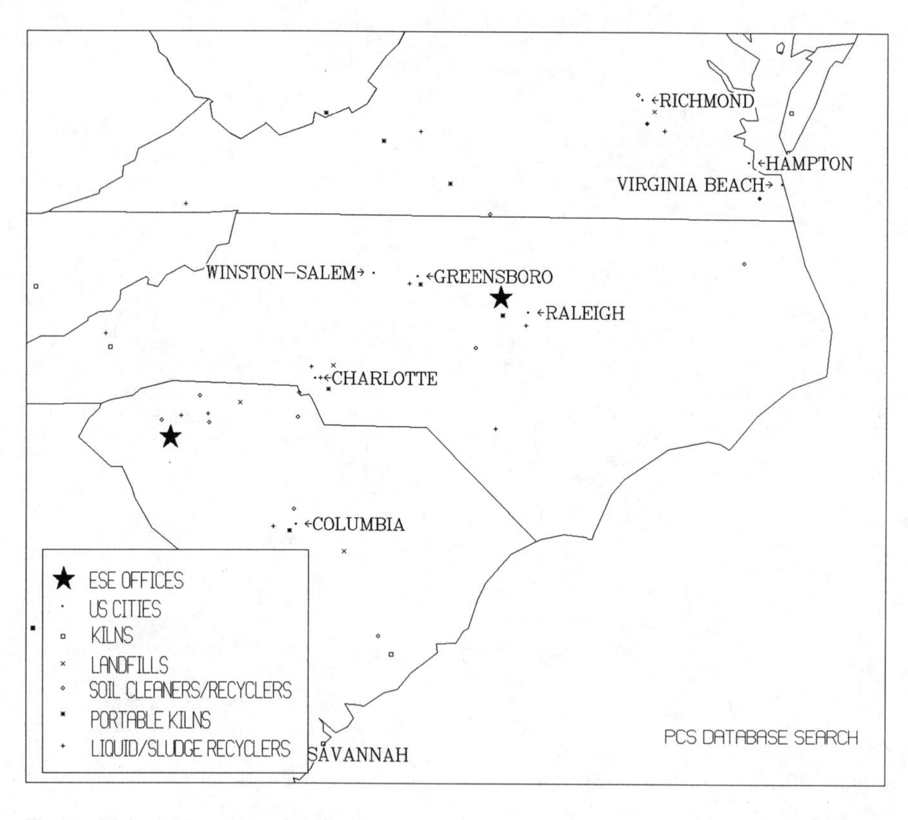

Figure 18.2. PCS database search.

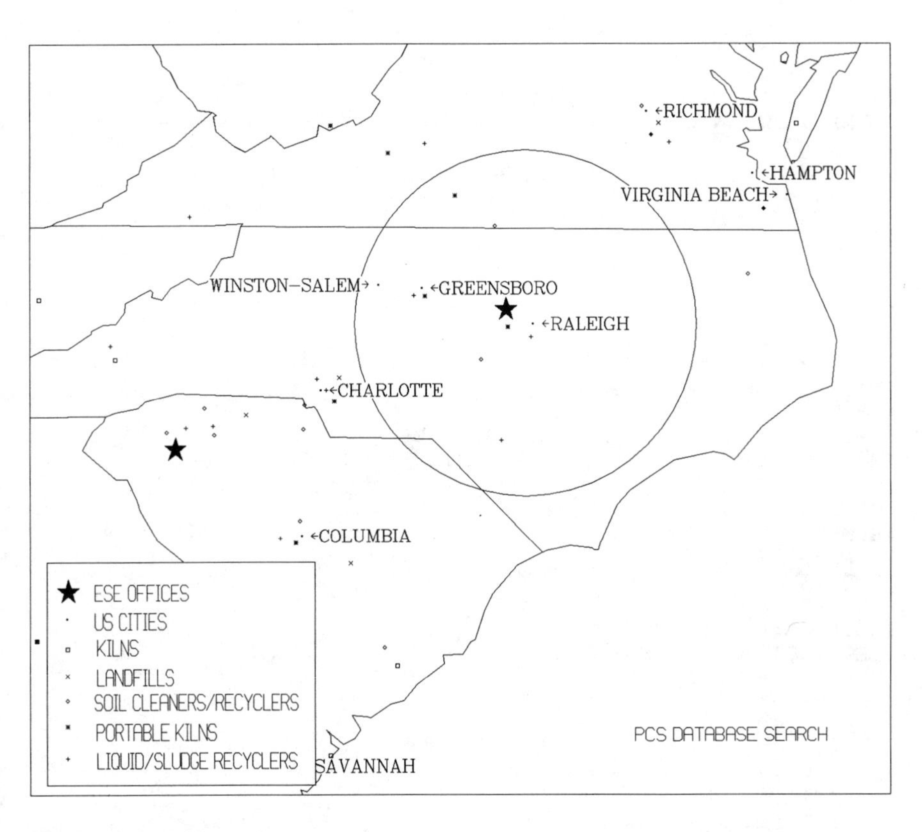

Figure 18.3. PCS database search.

Table 18.1.

FCLTY_TYPE:	BIOREMEDIATION
FCLTY_NAME:	ENVIRO-CHEM
ADDRESS1:	1005 INVESTMENT BLVD.
ADDRESS2:	
CITY:	APEX
COUNTY:	WAKE
STATE:	NC
ZIP1:	27502
ZIP2:	0.0000
OWNER:	ENVIRO-CHEM
CONTACT:	JERRY DEAKLE
TELEPHONE:	9193629010
TELEFAX:	9193629005
NUM_FCLTY:	1.0000
FCLTY_AGE:	2.0000
MAX_INVENT:	100 TONS (PRE-TREATED)
PRIVATE:	Y
PUBLIC:	N
TPH_STAT:	<
TPH:	500.0000
TPH_VARY:	N
BTEX_STAT:	
BTEX:	1000000.0000
BTEX_VARY:	N
NONHAZ_Y_N:	Y
TON_NH:	75.00
TON_NHVARY:	N
HAZWASTE:	N
TON_HAZ:	0.00
TON_HZVARY:	N
CLAY:	Y
SILT:	Y
SAND:	Y
DEBRIS:	Y
ANALYS_Y_N:	Y
LIMITA_Y_N:	Y
LIMITATION:	NO IGNITABLE SUBSTANCES
PROCEDURES:	TCLP METALS, TPH, BTEX, PCB SCAN, % WATER
RSTR_Y_N:	N
RSTR_ORIG:	
PERMIT_Y_N:	N
PERMITS:	
COMPLIANCE:	Y
SITE_ASSES:	N
SOIL_DATA:	TPH, BTEX
CLEAN_SOIL:	FILL FOR SALE
LF_OWNER:	N/A
LFADDRESS1:	
LFADDRESS2:	
LFCITY:	
LFCOUNTY:	
LFSTATE:	
LFZIP1:	0.0000
LFZIP2:	0.0000
CERCLA:	
LFSITEASS:	
INDUSTRIAL:	
SANITARY:	

Table 18.2.

```
MapInfo Search Report for Database M_CLEAN
Thu Aug 05 15:53:39 1993

Search Criteria:
    within 100 miles of (78.731776,35.745792) (6 found)

Points found:

  CHEROKEE SANFORD GROUP
  EARTHTEC SOIL SYSTEMS
  ENVIRO-CHEM
  ENVIROTECH MID-ATLANTIC
  LEE TILE & BRICK
  NOBLE OIL SERVICES


MapInfo Search Report for Database M_PORTAB
Thu Aug 05 15:53:02 1993

Search Criteria:
    within 100 miles of (78.731776,35.745792) (3 found)

Points found:

  ENVIRO-CHEM
  ENVIROTECH MID-ATLANTIC
  FOUR SEASONS IND. SERV.


MapInfo Search Report for Database M_RECYCL
Thu Aug 05 15:53:10 1993

Search Criteria:
    within 100 miles of (78.731776,35.745792) (3 found)

Points found:

  ECOFOLD
  SAFETY-KLEEN/3-031-72
  SAFETY-KLEEN/3-171-71
```

Table 18.3

```
      OWNER: FOUR SEASONS IND. SERV.
   ADDRESS1: POST OFFICE BOX 16590
   ADDRESS2:
       CITY: GREENSBORO
     COUNTY: GUILFORD
      STATE: NC
       ZIP1: 27416
       ZIP2:             0.0000
    CONTACT: JIM NOLES
  TELEPHONE: 9192732718
    TELEFAX: 9192745798
  NUM_KILNS:             2.0000
         NE: Y
         SE: Y
         MA: Y
         SW: Y
         MW: Y
         NW: Y
       CLAY: Y
       SILT: Y
       SAND: Y
     DEBRIS: Y
   TPH_STAT:
        TPH:       1000000.0000
   TPH_VARY: N
  BTEX_STAT:
       BTEX:       1000000.0000
  BTEX_VARY: N
     TON_NH:              50.00
 TON_NHVARY: N
   HAZWASTE: Y
    TON_HAZ:             100.00
 TON_HZVARY: Y
  COST_MILE:               4.00
  COST_VARY: Y
 ANALYS_Y_N: Y
 LIMITA_Y_N: Y
 LIMITATION: NO GREEN CONCRETE DUST
 PROCEDURES: 8240, 8270, BTEX, TPH, TCLP METALS, PROFILE SHEET, ANALYSIS
   RSTR_Y_N: N
  RSTR_ORIG:
 PERMIT_Y_N: Y
    PERMITS: AIR QUALITY PERMIT
     XCOORD:      79762675.0000
     YCOORD:      36001848.0000
```

The total elapsed time to complete the radius search and print all of the identified facilities with a database usually is less than 15-20 minutes.

Each of the above searches can be combined and completed with standard DBase^{TM} filters on any of the database fields. For example, we may like to search for all of the landfills within 500 miles of the site referenced above but only evaluate those sites that accept BTEX levels greater than 30,000 ppm and at a cost of less than $50/ton. In this case a filter of BTEX>50,000 "and" TONSNH<50 would be put on a radius search with a radius of 500 miles from the site. The result of this search is the identification of the 12 facilities identified in Table 18.4. Of course, the database file for each facility will be displayed upon its selection from this list. Any of the fields can be filtered for searches although it is most effective to filter on numeric field since character fields must match exactly in order to pass the filter. The added time for a filter to be added to the searches above is approximately five extra minutes.

Table 18.4.

```
MapInfo Search Report for Database M_LANDFL
Thu Aug 05 16:01:27 1993

Search Criteria:
    within 500 miles of (78.756352,35.730944) (12 found)

Points found:

  BEULAH SANITARY LANDFILL
  CID LANDFILL
  COUNTYWIDE LANDFILL
  GREENTREE LANDFILL
  LAKE COUNTY LANDFILL
  MODERN LANDFILL
  MOUNTAIN VIEW RECLAMATION
  ROBERTS ROAD LANDFILL
  RUMPKE LANDFILL
  SUBURBAN SOUTH LANDFILL
  SYCAMORE LANDFILL, INC.
  UNITED WASTE LIMITED
```

There are more complex searches and sorts that can be conducted with the PCS database system. The ones presented above will be, for all practical purposes the ones typically run during most spill response situations.

APPLICATIONS OF THE PCS DATABASE SYSTEM

The most obvious use of the database system is the management of multiple petroleum production, storage, distribution and/or marketing facilities (on the order of hundreds or thousands) with wide geographical distribution. The facility manager has at his disposal a tool to quickly identify the best facility and select this facility on issues outside of just location. The facility manager may for example select a facility 50 miles farther from the spill site than the closest facility because the farther facility recycles treated soils in bricks rather than landfill cover. This type of information was previously only available through extensive telephone interviews with treatment facility operators.

The sector of the oil & gas industry which would most likely find this capability most useful is the petroleum truck and pipeline transportation sector. Due to the nature of the industry, pipelines and trucking companies will almost always be faced with the disposal/treatment of quantities of PCS in remote locations where disposal facilities have not previously been identified. Often the remediation work must be conducted on an emergency response basis resulting in extremely high transportation and disposal cost. Since the response manager has no choice but to go to a distant facility for PCS disposal, such issues as cost, long-term liability, short-term transportation liability and past experiences with the facility are often overlooked. With the use of the PCS database, the response manager has maximized the alternatives available to him for immediate PCS treatment/disposal. This will not only save money and limit liability but will free the response manager up to address the protection of human health and the environment during the emergency.

RELATED & FUTURE APPLICATIONS OF GEOGRAPHICAL INFORMATION SYSTEMS FOR SPILL RESPONSE/REMEDIATION

An unrelated client of ESE must address emergency spill response of fuel oil on a national basis. ESE was asked to develop a spill response network of contractors to address any spill within the continental US within a minimum timeframe. ESE conducted a contractor identification survey in much the same matter as the Phase I identification study for the PCS database. Crucial contractor identification information including emergency response contact procedures where identified and entered into a Dbase III+™ format for 270 contractors nationwide. This database was integrated with MapInfo™ as was the PCS database system. This system therefore became a part of ESE's 24 hour emergency response process to manage the client's spill response issues on a national scale. Through the use of the Spill Response database, the PCS database and ESE internal response network, clients dealing with emergency response scenarios can now address the entire response through one ESE 24 hour contact.

Project Managers now have a large selection of data acquisition and data management tools available for comprehensive site characterization and decision support. Remote data collection techniques such as ground penetrating radar, vertical induction profiling (electromagnetic induction), airborne and spaceborne multispectral and radar scanners present non-invasive methods of acquiring a wealth of information about a site or event. These digital data sources manipulated with powerful and increasingly affordable technologies such as geographic information systems (GIS), 3-Dimensional modeling and visualization, and digital image processing allow project managers and site operators to accurately characterize a site. Beyond characterizing existing conditions at a site, the power of new computer technologies allow project team members to construct intricate, multiparameter predictive models for complex phenomenon like trajectory and fate of a contaminant. Lastly, the powerful visualization tools within GIS, image processing and 3-D modeling allow project managers and site operators to communicate effectively to regulatory agencies and public alike the condition of a site and status of remediation efforts.

In closing, with the increased use of GIS related software such as the PCS database system, the petroleum release remediation manager can now reduce decision making time, limit client liability exposure, ensure the most cost effective solutions are being utilized and address these issues within an emergency response framework. The growth of GIS in the environmental industry is a logical progression as remediation processes are identified, evaluated, streamlined and finally automated. The end result at a minimum will be a more efficient means of addressing industry's environmental goals.

CHAPTER 19

Bioremediation of Petroleum Contaminated Soil From a Crank Case Oil Refining Site

Margaret Findlay and Samuel Fogel, Bioremediation Consulting, Inc., Newton, Massachusetts, and **John Borovsky,** Barr Engineering Co., Minneapolis, Minnesota

INTRODUCTION

Waste oils were reclaimed at a Superfund site from 1945 to 1977, by a process which involved treatment with concentrated sulfuric acid producing an acid hydrocarbon waste sludge, followed by a clay filtration step which produced a clay/hydrocarbon sludge. Site soils, 30,000 cu yd, were contaminated with these wastes at an average concentration of 5% hydrocarbons.

The 1986 record of decision (ROD) for the site required incineration of the contaminated soil. This decision may have been due to the observation that the hydrocarbons in the surface soil had apparently not biodegraded, and the belief that the heavy hydrocarbons present were not biodegradable. However, in 1992, the principle responsible parties initiated an investigation of biotreatment as a possible alternative. The data presented demonstrated that the heavy hydrocarbons at this site are biodegradable, and indicate that the reason for non-biodegradation under site conditions is low pH and the lack of available phosphate in the site soil.

METHODS

Petroleum Hydrocarbons by Infra Red Analysis (TPH-IR). TPH-IR was determined by EPA method 418.1, modified as follows: Soil and compost samples were extracted twice with a total volume of freon equal to 10 ml per gram. The extractions were carried out in sealed containers by shaking 20 minutes in a reciprocal shaker. Silica gel clean-up was employed until a clear extract was obtained. Infra red absorption was determined using the method 418.1 standard solution for calibration. Freon extracts were stored at -20° for later fingerprint analysis.

Petroleum hydrocarbon gas chromatographic fingerprints. Hydrocarbon fingerprints were prepared by analyzing the freon extracts by gas chromatography according to EPA method # 8100. While freon is not always as efficient as methylene chloride in extracting petroleum hydrocarbons, the procedure is reproducible and gives a representation of changes in the amount of bulk contaminant during a treatment simulation. GC fingerprints presented in this report contain one full-scale peak at 23 minutes which is orthoterphenyl, the internal standard added for quantitation. TPH-GC was determined by summing two quantities, the GC instrument integration of the "peaks", and the manually integrated area of the broad band of hydrocarbons, based on the area of the internal standard.

Available Nitrogen and Phosphate. Compost samples were extracted with five volumes of deionized water by shaking for 20 minutes. The extract was separated from the compost by centrifugation and further clarified by passing through a 0.45 micron filter, then analyzed for pH and for NH3, NO3 and PO4 according to modifications of Standard Methods (17th ed) # 4500 NH3 C, NO3 E, and P D. The concentrations of these substances in the test compost were obtained by multiplying these values by 5.

Enumeration of Bacteria. Total bacteria were enumerated by standard plate counting technique, using nutrient agar, incubated at room temperature, and counted after seven days of growth. Bacteria capable of growing on volatile sludge hydrocarbons as their sole carbon source were enumerated by a modification of Standard method 9215C (17th ed.). Colonies were grown on nobel agar mineral media plates incubated in an atmosphere of volatile hydrocarbons, and counted after ten days of growth.

Laboratories. The analytical procedures described above were carried out at ABB Environmental Services Treatability Laboratory in Wakefield MA. PAH analysis according to EPA method # 8270, and analysis for volatile hydrocarbons according to EPA method # 8240 were carried out at ENSECO in Arvada, CO.

SOIL AND CONTAMINANT CHARACTERIZATION

Soil samples were obtained with a backhoe from three site locations, and the loads mixed at the site. A five gallon portion of the site mixture was sent to the treatability laboratory where it was passed through a 1 cm sieve and composited. Of the sieved soil, 45% was greater than 1 mm and 38% was between 0.25 and 1 mm.

The fingerprint of the soil hydrocarbons is presented as the top tracing in Figure 19.1. Eluting prior to the standard is a regularly spaced series of compounds having the same retention times as the linear alkanes, up to C19. Immediately to the right of the standard is a large "hump" of undifferentiated compounds, with an indication of the remaining linear alkanes extending above the hump. Compounds lighter than decane made up 0.2 percent of the total. Most of the soil hydrocarbon content is in the molecular weight range of 20 to 43 carbons. TPH-GC, quantitated based on the internal standard, was 2,300 ppm (dry weight basis). TPH-IR, quantited using the EPA standard solution, was 50,000 ppm.

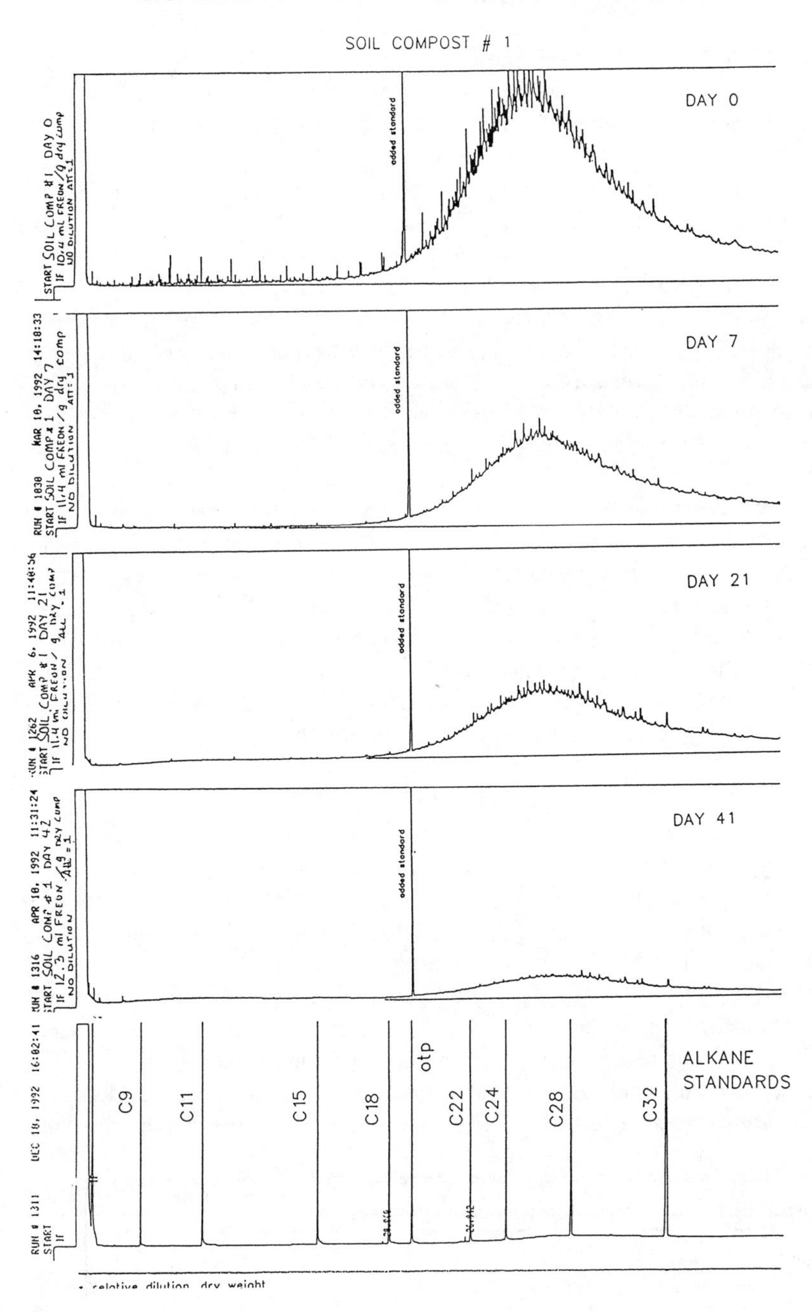
SOIL COMPOST # 1
DAY 0
added standard
DAY 7
DAY 21
DAY 41
ALKANE STANDARDS
C9
C11
C15
C18
otp
C22
C24
C28
C32
* relative dilution dry weight

Figure 19.1.

PRELIMINARY TREATABILITY TEST

A preliminary soil test was carried out to determine the soil modifications necessary to produce growth of hydrocarbon-degrading bacteria. A sample of soil was amended with a complete mineral fertilizer containing nine elements in the proportions required by bacteria. The soil pH of 5.0 was raised to 7.0 with KOH, and 1% organic matter (manure) was added to improve soil moisture-holding ability. Aeration was provided by mixing daily.

The soil had a high acidity, requiring 185 meq of alkali to stabilize the pH at 7.0. Repeated additions of phosphate fertilizer were not recoverable as readily available phosphate. Over a 14 day period, nearly 3,800 ppm PO4 was required in order to maintain available phosphate above 10 ppm. This soil contained approximately 4% iron, which may have reacted with the phosphate. During the first seven days of this preliminary test the hydrocarbon-degrading bacteria increased from less than 0.1 million per gram to 200 million per gram.

The rapid reproduction of the hydrocarbon-degrading bacteria during the preliminary treatability test indicated that hydrocarbons could be biodegraded in this soil if conditions were optimized by adjusting pH, and providing mineral nutrients, moisture, and oxygen. It was observed that a slight excess of water caused the soil to become compacted and lose porosity. Therefore the addition of a bulking agent would be necessary to produce a texture that could be aerated by mixing. Thus, the process would be termed soil composting.

SOIL COMPOST TREATMENT SIMULATIONS

Approach The simulation of soil treatment by composting was carried out in two separate experiments, designed to demonstrate the reproducibility of the process. Soil treatment mixtures of 0.6 and 3 Kg were prepared, and subsamples were removed at intervals for process monitoring.

Method of Determining Compost Bulking Agent Ratios. The bulking agent, shredded branches, and the moisture-holding agent, manure, were added gradually with water to site soil until a mixture was obtained which had high moisture content but would not compact under pressure, and had high porosity and good drainage characteristics. The ratios determined are given in Table 19.1.

Table 19.1. Soil Compost Amendment Weight Ratios

soil (25 % water)	100
Shredded tree waste (dry)	13
Manure (dry)	2
Bulk per dry soil	0.2
Dry soil/tot dry compost	0.83

Process Initiation, Moisture and Aeration.

The mixture of soil and bulking agents had a moisture content of about 38%. Compost samples were analyzed every seven to ten days to determine the moisture content, and water was added as necessary to maintain 38% moisture. The composts were aerated daily by mixing for the first week, then three times per week. Biodegradation was initiated by the addition of the nine element fertilizer to give a concentration of 200 ppm nitrogen (wet weight) in the compost. Extra buffered phosphate solution, over 600 ppm, was also added initially, in an attempt to correct the soil phosphate binding problem.

Process Monitoring and Process Adjustment.

Treatment of Acidity. Compost samples were analyzed for pH approximately at weekly intervals, and adjusted immediately. Soil compost #1 was maintained at pH=7 and required 6.3 grams of hydrated lime per Kg wet compost added over four days to stabilize the pH at the desired level. Compost #2 was maintained at pH = 6.4 , and therefore required only 2.3 g lime per Kg compost, and only one day to adjust the pH.

Available N and PO_4. At approximately weekly intervals, samples were removed for analysis of available nitrogen and phosphate, and additional complete fertilizer and extra phosphate were added to maintain an average concentration of available N and PO_4 of about 100 ppm each. The averages were estimated based on the amounts present at analysis and the amounts added immediately after analysis. These data are shown in Figure 19.2. The total amount of N and PO_4 required in 40 days of composting was about 900 ppm and 3,200 ppm respectively, wet weight compost.

Phosphate binding. Bacteria incorporate about 4 grams phosphate for 10 grams nitrogen. Therefore, 360 ppm PO_4 would be needed for 900 ppm N. Thus the phosphate that reacted with the soil and became unavailable for bacteria amounted to about 2,800 ppm wet weight compost (5,600 ppm dry soil).

Bacterial Growth, Soil Composts # 1 & # 2.

Samples of Soil Compost # 1 were analyzed at five time points for bacterial numbers. Total plate count bacteria increased rapidly from two million per gram wet compost to 300 million in 18 days, and remained high during the active treatment period of 41 days. These data are presented in Figure 19.3.

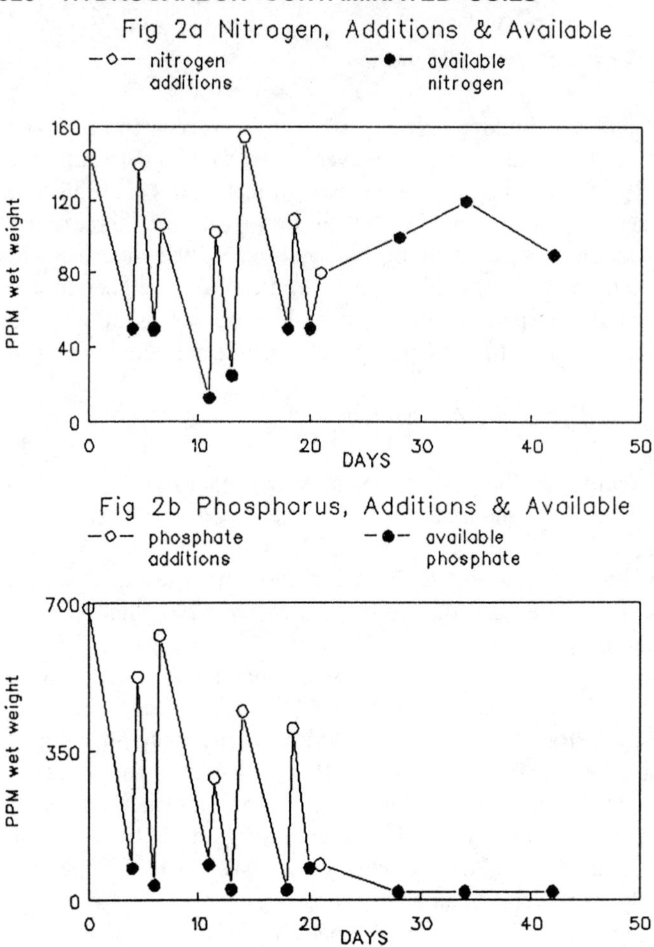

Figure 19.2

TPH-IR Hydrocarbon Reduction, Soil Composts # 1 and # 2.

Rate and Treatment Time. Samples were removed from the soil composts at intervals and analyzed for bulk hydrocarbon content by TPH-IR. The data for both compost experiments is presented in Table 19.2, and plotted in Figure 19.4. The data indicate that the bulk contaminant is about 50% degraded in about seven days, and 70% degraded by day 20. After one month the rate of decrease was very slow, and it therefore appears that the active treatment period at 68°F is one month. The final percent TPH-IR reductions were 89 and 83% respectively.

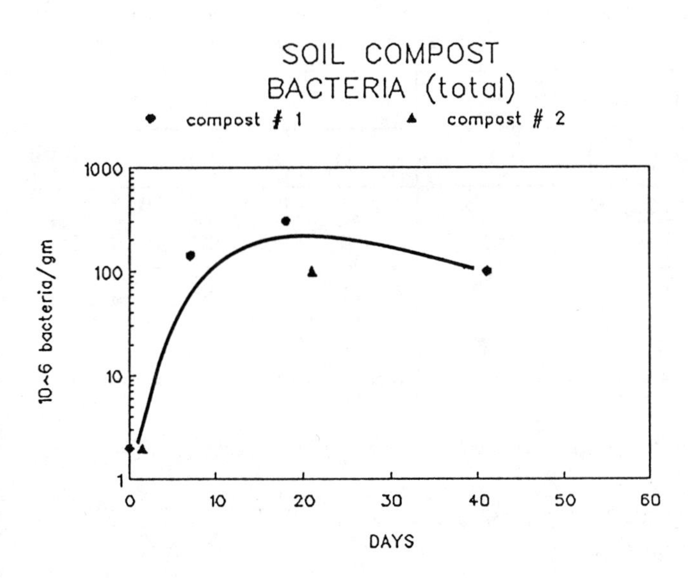

Figure 19.3

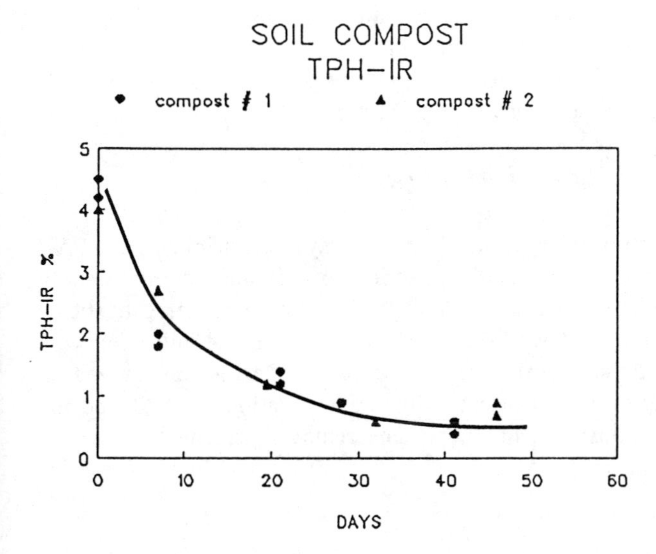

Figure 19.4

In addition to the duplicate TPH-IR analyses shown in Table 19.2, a spike recovery experiment was carried out on Day 53 of experiment # 2, in which an

8000 ppm (dry weight) spike of EPA method 418.1 TPH calibration standard was spiked into the finished compost, with 98% recovery.

Table 19.2 TPH-IR reduction during soil compost treatment percent, EPA Method 418.1, dry weight basis

SOIL COMPOST # 1			SOIL COMPOST # 2		
DAY	TPH	DUP	DAY	TPH	DUP
0	4.2	4.5	0	4.0	
7	1.8	2.0	7	2.7	
21	1.3	1.3	20	1.2	
28	0.9		32	0.6	
41	0.5	0.5	46	0.8	0.8
			74	0.7	

Reduction of Gas Chromatographable (Fingerprint) Hydrocarbons

The GC fingerprints for the freon extracts of day 0, 7, 21, and 41 for Soil Compost #1 are presented in Figure 19.1. These illustrate that the more volatile compounds (less than about 16 carbons, to the left of the added standard in Figure 19.1) are degraded in the first week, and that thereafter the heavier compounds are degraded, resulting in a dramatic reduction in the fingerprint height. The concentration of chromatographable hydrocarbons (TPH-GC) were quantitated by integration and are noted on Figure 19.1. The reductions in TPH-GC were 91% and 77% for soil composts #1 and #2 respectively.

Polynuclear Aromatic Hydrocarbons (PAH)

A separate soil composite from the site was analyzed in triplicate for PAH according to EPA method 8270. The data indicated that the concentration of PAH is low in this soil. Only four PAH were detected in all three triplicate samples. The finished compost was also analyzed for PAH, but only four were detected, and three of these in only one sample. This data is summarized in Table 19.3. The results are consistent with biodegradation of PAH during treatment, but the data is insufficient to calculate removal percents.

Table 19.3. VOC & PAH in starting soil and finished compost
PPM dry weight triplicates ND - not detected
Compounds not listed were not detected

	STARTING SOIL			FINISHED COMPOST		
naphthylene	1.7	2.1	2.2	ND	.06	ND
1 methylnaphthylene	1.3	.15	1.7	ND	ND	ND
phenanthrene	0.8	1.0	1.2	ND	.07	ND
fluoranthene	0.5	0.4	0.6	ND	.10	ND
chrysene	ND	ND	1.2	.31	.35	ND
benzo(b)fluoranthene	.43	ND	.43	ND	ND	ND

Volatile Organic Compounds

Toluene, ethylbenzene and xylene were present in the starting soil at concentrations of 1 to 12 ppm. Benzene could not be detected below 3.8 ppm. For the finished compost, detection limits were much lower, since there had been extensive removal of hydrocarbons. Toluene in the treated material was detected at 0.003 ppm, while benzene, ethylbenzene and xylenes were not detected at detection limits of 0.015 ppm. These data are presented in Table 19.4. While three of these compounds are greatly reduced in the treated material, it is not known what fraction biodegraded and what fraction volatilized.

Table 19.4 VOC in Starting Soil & Finished Compost
PPM dry weight Ave of triplicates

	STARTING SOIL	FINISHED COMPOST
benzene	< 3.8	ND < .015
toluene	1.2	.003
ethylbenzene	1.8	ND < .015
xylenes	12.0	ND < .015

SOIL COMPOST EXPERIMENT WITH INHIBITED CONTROL

Purpose. The purpose of this experiment was to demonstrate that biotic processes were responsible for TPH-IR reduction in the site soil, rather than abiotic processes. The experiment was designed with 5 gram portions of compost in sealed containers, to measure oxygen use, CO_2 production, and TPH reduction on the same sample, and to compare the results with those from three control conditions.

Procedure. A new batch of soil compost was prepared having the same bulking agent and fertilizer as described above, and passed through 4 mm sieve.

Duplicate 5 gram portions were sealed in 160 ml serum bottles. Three controls were set up in duplicate as follows. Heat-treated starting compost, live finished compost, and live unamended soil (no bulk, no fertilizer). At six days, 0.2 ml samples of headspace were withdrawn by syringe and analyzed by gas chromatography with thermal conductivity detection (GC/TDC) for O2 and CO2. The values were recorded, and bottles having low oxygen content were flushed with air and re-sealed. At 15 days, the test bottles were extracted with freon for TPH-IR analysis. The results are shown in Table 19.5.

Conclusion. The live starting compost biodegraded 50% of the TPH-IR in 15 days, but the heat treated starting compost biodegraded only 13% of the TPH, while using significantly less O_2 and producing significantly less CO_2. This result indicates that the disappearance of TPH is linked to the production of CO_2 and is a biotic process. The live finished compost, which contained bacteria but did not contain readily degradable "food" for the bacteria, did not show a decrease in TPH, and used very little O_2, probably in the slow biodegradation of bulking agent. The unamended soil, which had live bacteria and was well aerated, but had no fertilizer or bulking agent, achieved only 12% TPH degradation, indicating that these compost amendments provide a significant stimulus to biodegradation.

Table 19.5. CO_2 Production, O_2 Use, and TPH reduction
Treatment vs. Control Conditions
Av of dup analyses TPH, dry wt CO_2 & O_2 as vol %

	LIVE STARTING COMPOST	HEATED STARTING COMPOST	LIVE FINISHED COMPOST	SOIL, NO BULK NO FERT
TPH START	5.4%	5.4%	0.7%	6.0%
TPH 15 DAYS	2.7%	4.3%	0.7%	5.3%
O2 USE	10.4	1.1	0.9	2.4
CO2 PRODUCED	7.4	0.9	0.9	1.6

SUMMARY

Soil at this site was contaminated by 50,000 ppm heavy hydrocarbons produced by waste oil reprocessing. This study was undertaken to demonstrate that biological remediation could be achieved with this soil, as an alternative to incineration required by an EPA record of decision. Preliminary treatability tests demonstrated that the soil contained acclimated hydrocarbon-degrading bacteria which could be stimulated to grow by correcting the acid pH and by adding excess phosphate to overcome the soil phosphate binding. The addition of a bulking agent (soil composting) was necessary to insure correct soil texture and drainage and allow aeration by mixing. The laboratory treatment simulation demonstrated that petroleum hydrocarbons could be reduced 50% in 7 days and about 85% in one month. The study also identified the process requirements in terms of the amounts of fertilizer, bulking agent, and lime needed. These parameters were employed in design and cost estimation of the full scale remediation.

CONCLUSION

Treatability tests demonstrated that the soil contained acclimated hydrocarbon-degrading bacteria which could be stimulated to grow by correcting the acid pH and by adding excess phosphate to overcome the soil phosphate binding. The addition of a bulking agent (soil composting) was necessary to insure correct soil texture and drainage and allow aeration by mixing. The laboratory treatment simulation demonstrated that petroleum hydrocarbons could be reduced 50% in 7 days and about 85% in one month. The final material was odor free, and easily worked. Thus, it can be concluded that the treatment is satisfactory and that the treated soil is suitable for replacement on site.

CHAPTER 20

Site Closure Using *In-situ* Hot Air/Steam Stripping (HASS) of Hydrocarbons in Soils

Phillip N. La Mori, NOVATERRA, Inc., Los Angeles, California

INTRODUCTION

The remediation of soils containing volatile (VOC) and semivolatile (SVOC) hydrocarbons is most desirably acomplished *in-situ,* i.e., without removal of the contaminated soils from the ground. This approach mitigates the environmental problem, i.e., does not transport it to another location, and when properly applied, does not impact on the local environment during remediation. NOVATERRA has demonstrated commercially an *in-situ*, hot air/steam stripping (HASS) technology to remove VOC and SVOC from soils both in the vadose and saturated zones. The technology consists of a drill tower which injects and mixes steam and hot air continuously into the soil below ground and a method to immediately capture all vapors escaping to the surface and remove the vaporized VOC/SVOC using condensation and carbon beds. The air can be recompressed and recycled. The condensed liquid containing hydrocarbons is purified by distillation. The recovered hydrocarbons can be destroyed or recycled.

The technology has successfully removed various chlorinated aliphatics and aromatics, glycol ethers, phthalates, polyaromatic compounds, ketones, petroleum hydrocarbons and many other compound types from sand to clay soils to risk based standards; e.g. 1 increased cancer risk in 1,000,000, using currently acceptable risk assessment standards. This chapter presents an introduction to the technology of NOVATERRA's hot air/steam stripping (HASS) process. This will include an introduction to the physical and chemical properties of *in-situ* hot air/steam stripping, as well as the examination of the equipment that performs the HASS remediation. Finally, typical achievable results are presented in the case study of a successful remediation project that was completed in the end of 1992 and which achieved site closure for the soils remediation in 1993.

Advantages of the HASS System

The main advantages of the NOVATERRA HASS System are:

(1) It completely treats all soil *in-situ* by mixing and application of treatment agents. Thus treatment is performed in place without incurring the future liability of off-site disposal.

(2) The treatment is not affected by varying strata, permeability, preferred off-gas pathways, or the water table.
(3) It is effective in both the vadose and saturated zones.
(4) It remediates sites quickly and economically.
(5) It can attain 95 to 99 plus percent removal of VOC and SVOC.
(6) The technology has been commercially demonstrated.
(7) It has regulatory approval.
(8) Soil is not a hazardous waste under the Resource Conservation and Recovery Act (RCRA) because of the *in-situ* treatment method. The only hazardous waste is the condensed off-gas which is fully contained and captured.
(9) It can serve as both the first and second steps in a treatment train for mixed waste types.

THE DETOXIFIER

Drilling Equipment

The NOVATERRA "Detoxifier" can easily provide *in-situ* treatment of soils contaminated with volatiles (VOC), semi-volatiles (SVOC), petroleum hydrocarbons (TPH), metals, as well as polychlorinated biphenyls (PCB's), pesticides, and other contaminant materials. The basic process provides the *in-situ* soil mixing with simultaneous injection of the appropriate reagents or physical treatment systems.

The typical *in-situ* soils treatment rig, shown schematically in Figure 20.1, consists of a drill tower with two kellys and two drills as an integral unit and they are mounted on a sturdy metal box called the shroud. The tower holds the two counter rotating kellys to which five foot diameter drills are attached. The counter-rotation provides for balanced forces and excellent stability of the tower. The fixed tower design currently has depth capabilities of 34 feet.

The shroud's bottom is a knife edge that sits firmly on flat ground so that it automatically creates an excellent seal. Thus, the shroud maintains a physical environmental barrier, excluding what is occurring as part of the treatment from the surrounding area. The shroud traps the dust from drilling, it contains the expansion of the soil caused by injection (up to 25%) and captures the gases coming to the surface as a result of the treatment and channels them to the process. The shroud operates under vacuum of 2-28 inches of water to prevent contaminant gas from escaping into the atmosphere. During actual operation, the shroud seals are routinely measured for VOC gases to document their effective-

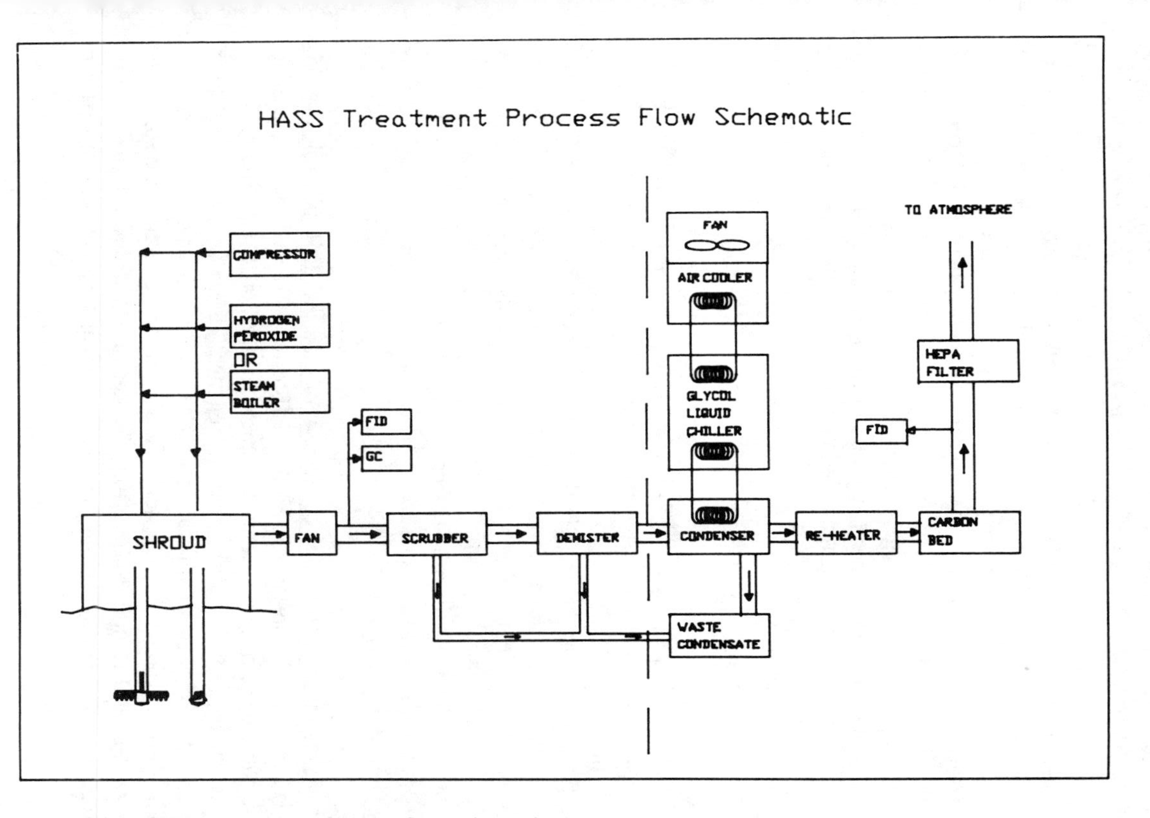

Figure 20.1. HASS treatment process flow schematic.

ness. The operational protocols contain specific instructions if shroud leaks are found. This includes stopping operations.

The drills at the bottom of the kellys are designed for slicing through the soil and have high mixing shear close to the top surface. Each drill blade is equipped with two manifolds for injection of liquids, gases or slurries. These can be injected simultaneously (as in HASS) or sequentially as in stabilization, solidification or neutralization. The kellys have specially designed concentric tubes and swivels to accommodate the dual injection system. The kelly design is such that it's rotation creates an annulus which is the pathway for vapors to escape to the surface and be captured in the shroud.

Treatment using the Detoxifier process proceeds in a batch wise manner. Figure 20.2 shows how this is accomplished for a typical dual five foot diameter drill configuration. The site can be laid out as treatment areas of close packed overlapping circles. The "effective treatment area" can then be described by rectangles contained within the two circles of the blades. The area of each rectangle is 29 ft^2. This arrangement provides sufficient overlap to insure no untreated zones as long as surface control of tower placement and verticality is maintained. Tower placements are surveyed in with a transit. This approach also permits unique identification of each treatment block (as they are called) from a known survey point. Before treatment commences, the site is laid out by rows and columns so that when remediation commences the operational plan is complete.

Hot Air/Steam Stripping (HASS)

Hot Air/Steam Stripping (HASS) is the *in-situ* removal of VOC and SVOC by the simultaneous injection of steam and heated air into soil during mixing by the equipment described above.

The function of the heated air is to vaporize VOC and SVOC and then provide the mechanism to carry them to the surface, thus, reducing their soil concentration. Steam augmentation is used to increase the removal rate because:

1. it permits the soil to be heated more quickly,
2. steam forms azeotropes with many of the SVOC and VOC, thus, improving removal efficiency.

Air is sent through the outer concentric tube to the drill manifolds at 250 p.s.i. and 125°C at a constant 700SCFM. Steam is sent through the inner concentric tube to the drill manifolds at approximately 200°C and 400 p.s.i. The steam flow varies from full at the start of treatment (3000 lbs/hr., i.e. 3.0 (10^6) BTU/hr) until the operating temperature of 75°C-88°C is reached. At that point, the steam flow is reduced to a level sufficient to maintain the operating temperature, i.e. 300 to 600 lbs/hr. Both the steam and air are injected into the soil through appropriately sized nozzles which not only reflect the properties of the fluids, but also the increasing area of the outside diameter. After expansion, the steam is slightly superheated.

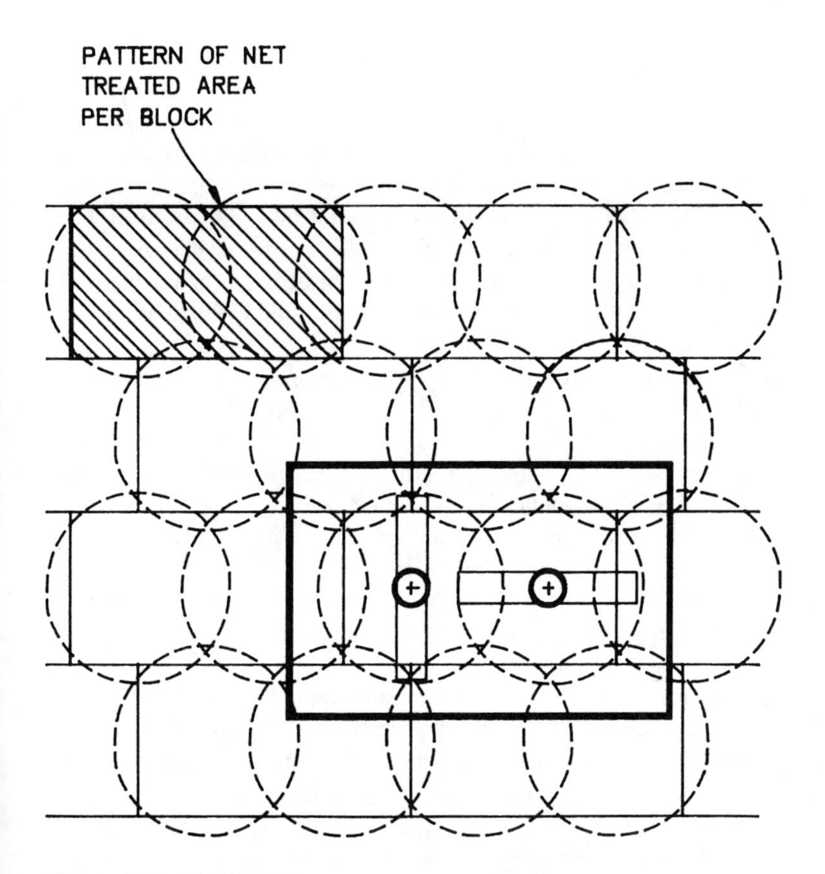

Figure 20.2. DETOXIFIER treatment block pattern.

Thus, while there is a net gain of water in the treatment volume until the operating temperature is reached, after that there is loss of water. The top sides of the blades are equipped with shear inducing surfaces which provide good horizontal mixing of four to six inches thickness. The steam and air are directed into the shear zone and provide kinetic as well as thermal energy to remove material from the soil. The air, steam and contaminant gases flow to the center of the drill and are transferred to the surface along the kelly via a special annulus maker that also serves as the kelly drive bar.

The size of the process equipment is designed to continuously handle the maximum flow expected. To define it simply is to say that the process equipment will handle 700 SCFM of air that is saturated with steam at 85°C and 1 atmosphere. The ambient air temperature is 20°C.

Because the drills are 60 inches in diameter and the annulus is 16 inches in diameter, the air has only 22 inches to flow before it can escape to the surface. This short distance and high shear above the blade helps insure that all the air is channeled to the surface and not to the surrounding soil. The specially designed annulus maker then assures easy passage to the surface shroud operating under negative pressure.

The contaminated off-gas is then water scrubbed to remove dust particles and then sent to a cyclone demister to separate the entrained water. At this point the off gas can be treated in one of two ways. The first option, uses refrigeration to separate the liquid from the air (Figure 20.1 to the right of the dashed line). The air is further treated with carbon beds and then recycled through the compressor or exhausted to the atmosphere. The carbon beds can be regenerated when there are high levels of soils contamination. The liquid stream is further treated to separate the hydrocarbons from the water by gravity separation and distillation, filtered through a wet carbon bed, or dealt with as a hazardous waste. This approach is commercially proven. The second option, is thermal or catalytic oxidization which is simpler than the closed loop refrigeration. Here a commercially proven catalytic oxidization system is used to remove almost all hydrocarbons to acceptable air quality levels. The main advantage of catalytic oxidization is that most of the waste is treated and destroyed on site.

The key to successful operation of the HASS system is the real time process control developed by NOVATERRA. The process control instrumentation relates surface off-gas chemistry to below ground soil chemistry; it is also used to direct and manage the process of remediation. There are two primary instrument types used for process control, a continuous reading THA (Total Hydrocarbon Analyzer) sometimes called FID, and two GC's (Gas Chromatographs). The THA profiles the hole chemistry with depth, i.e. it acts to characterize the contamination (Figure 20.3). It directs the remediation to those depths of high contamination and also acts as an indicator of the progress of the remediation. Even in cases where there are several contaminants of concern, the absolute THA level can be used as the determinate of when remediation is complete, Figure 20.4. Once the THA is below the control point, the block is clean in 98% of the cases.

The THA is generally adequate for process control, even for multicomponent contamination. However, for cases where a key contaminant must be remediated to a specific level, when contamination species is variable over the site and when one needs to document the presence or absence of a critical compound, e.g. benzene, vinyl chloride, etc., the on board GC is used to control the remediation process.

Typical THA or Total VOC Readings as a Function of Depth

DEPTH (ft)	TOTAL (ppm)
0	NA
5	28,980
10	3,056
15	3,317
20	14,000
25	2,617
30	2,900

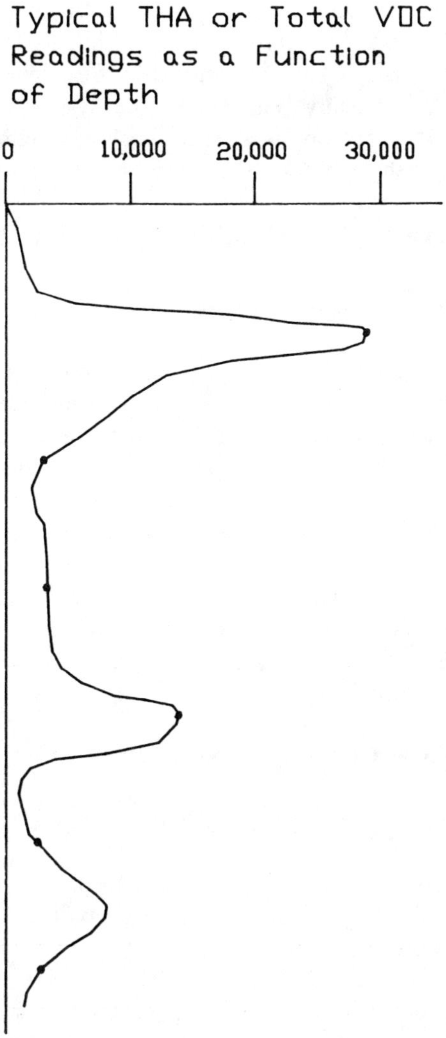

0 10,000 20,000 30,000

Figure 20.3. Typical THA vs. Depth Profile.

Instrumentation

In addition to the remediation control instrumentation, the process is also instrumented to measure key flows, pressures, temperatures, operational status, levels, etc. of all the process equipment. The operator also has depth, rotation rate, downhole temperature, steam flow and air flow available as a separate control group. Hard copy in the form of a strip chart record is maintained for depth, downhole temperature, process THA, and THA after the carbon beds. This last information assures meeting air quality standards. All this information plus the GC data is computer stored by treatment block as a permanent record as part of a proprietary Data Acquisition System. This is important because the record serves as proof that each block was remediated to the agreed upon standards for those blocks where there are no post-treatment chemistry samples.

THE PHYSICAL AND CHEMICAL PROPERTIES OF HASS

HASS Removal Mechanisms

The HASS System is based on the use of continuous steam injection to provide the heat to volatilize and perhaps react with soil hydrocarbons. Continuously injected hot air is the transfer medium for removal of contaminates out of the soil. The process takes place at a fairly low bulk soil temperature (85°C) but at a reasonably moderate application temperature, 200°C. Thus, it is most effective on VOC and generally becomes less effective as the VOC boiling temperature increases, i.e. with decreasing vapor pressure. The compounds of concern for this technology are almost always liquid at normal temperature (20°C). Gaseous contaminates would have dissipated and solid contamination is usually surfacial. Solid contaminants are usually dealt with by surface collection schemes.

The liquid contamination in soil can be classified as:

Vadose Zone	Saturated Zone
Vapor in pore spaces	Liquid floating on water (density < 1)
Liquid in pore spaces	Liquid (undissolved) in pore spaces (density > 1)
Liquid dissolved in water	Liquid dissolved in water
Liquid absorpted on soil	Liquid absorpted on soil

When using the HASS *in-situ* mixing technology there are four main types of removal mechanisms to consider in the above classification.

(1) Removal of vapor.
(2) Volatilization of the liquid in water or removal of pure liquid.
(3) Thermal desorption of the contamination from the soil-followed by removal by (1) or (2).
(4) Possible chemical reactions.

The difficulty of removal increases from (1), (2), and (3) above and removal by chemical reaction is determined by other factors. Note that using these concepts treatment of NAPL and DNAPL does not take any special significance. Their removal is relatively easy!

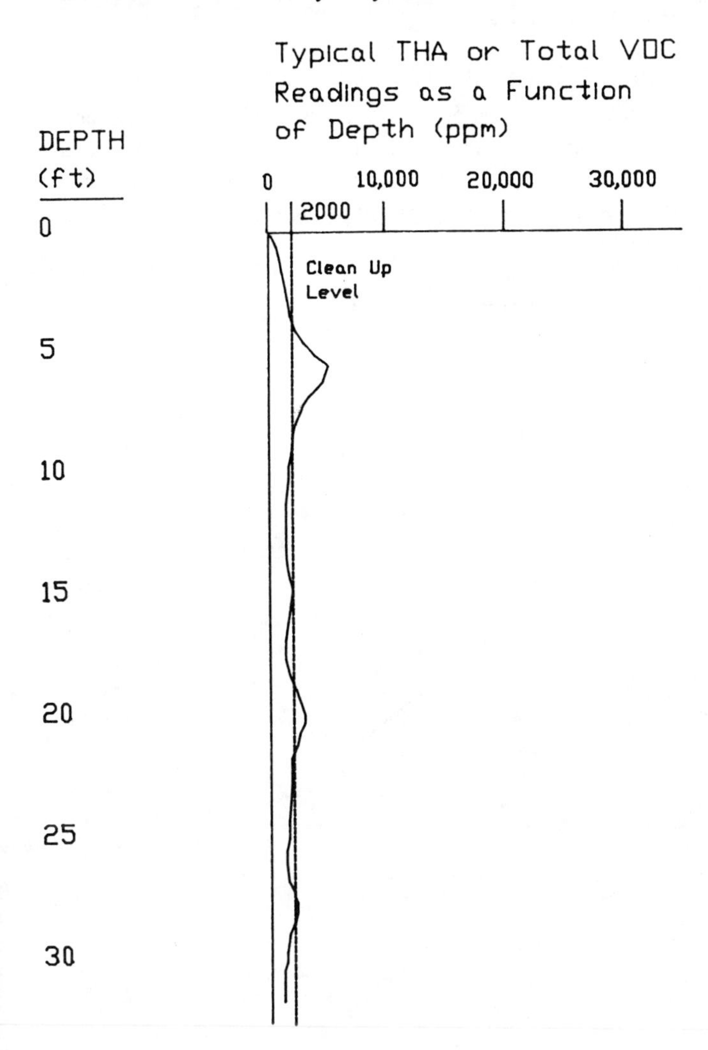

Figure 20.4. Typical THA vs. Depth Profile.

Generally at the start of remediation the assumption is that the relative amounts of vapor, liquid, and absorpted material in the soil are in quasi-equilibrium. Since volatilization is the major mechanism of removal using HASS, the removal efficiency of compounds is generally determined by the vapor pressure. However, because the physical process being applied here is really distillation of organic compounds using direct contact with steam (water), their removal from soil occurs by azetropic distillation. A simple way to do this is to review the vapor phase/liquid phase relationships of steam and a single organic compound. Having done that it is possible to generalize the result to steam and multicomponent organic compounds.

Liquid/Liquid Systems

Most of the organic compounds of concern are considered slightly soluble to insoluble in water/steam. Some compounds such as alcohols, organic acids, some ketones, phenol, etc. are completely or highly soluble in water/steam. Figure 20.5 shows the vapor pressure curve for two components which are completely soluble and "ideal" at the boiling point temperature. These liquids are said to obey Raoult's Law, i.e.

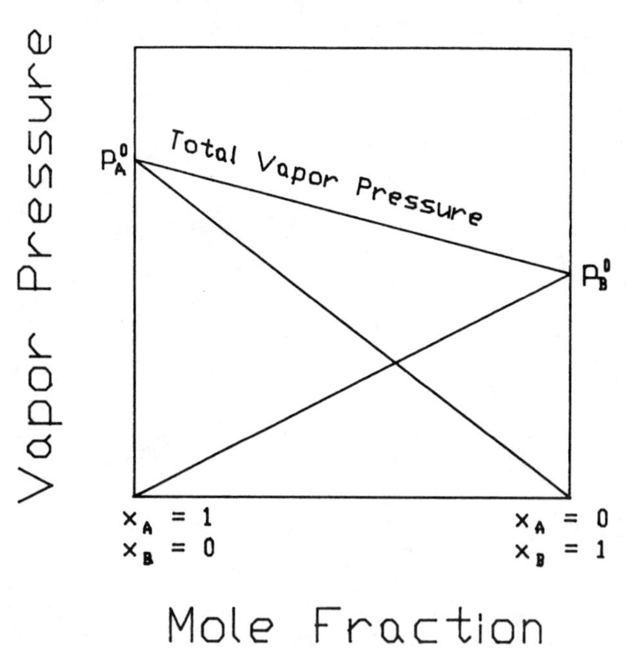

Figure 20.5. System obeying Raoult's Law

$$P_A = X_A P^O_A \qquad (1)$$

Where

P_A = partial pressure of component A

X_A = mole fraction of component A

P^O_A = vapor pressure of pure component A at temperature

Very few liquids which are completely soluble are "ideal". Most have been found to show positive deviations from Raoult's Law, i.e. their vapor pressure is greater than "ideal" (Figure 20.6).

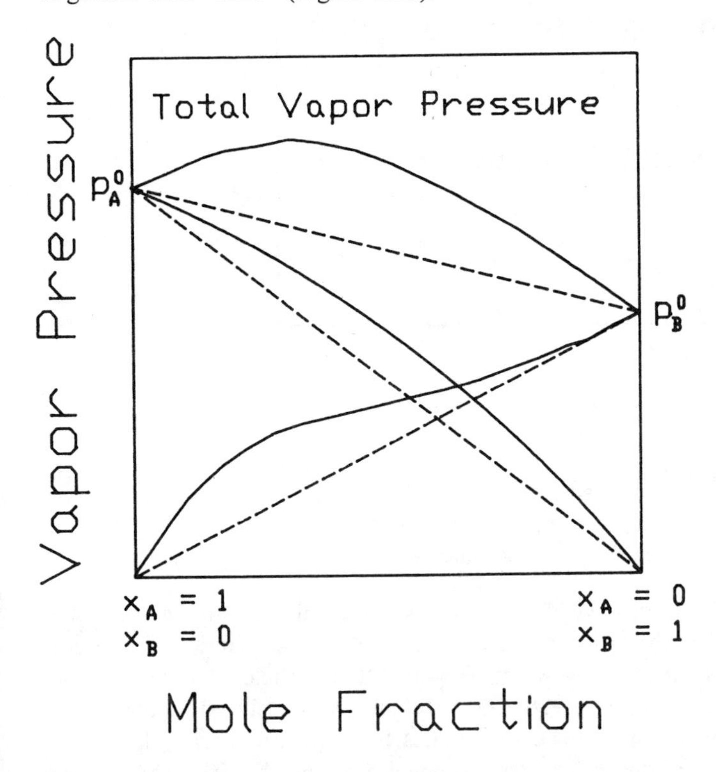

Figure 20.6. Positive deviations from Raoult's Law.

Compounds which are completely immiscible have a radically different behavior. This is shown in Figure 20.7. Here, the vapor pressure is a constant at all amounts of components A and B, as long as both liquids are present. One can see that this must be so by consideration of the phase rule

$$P + F = C + 2 \qquad (2)$$

where P is the number of phases present, F is the degrees of freedom and C is the number of components. Here P = 3, two liquid phases and one vapor phase, C = 2 components. This means F = 2 + 2 - 3 = 1, but since the temperature is determined the total vapor pressure must remain constant over all amounts of A and B, as shown in Figure 20.7.

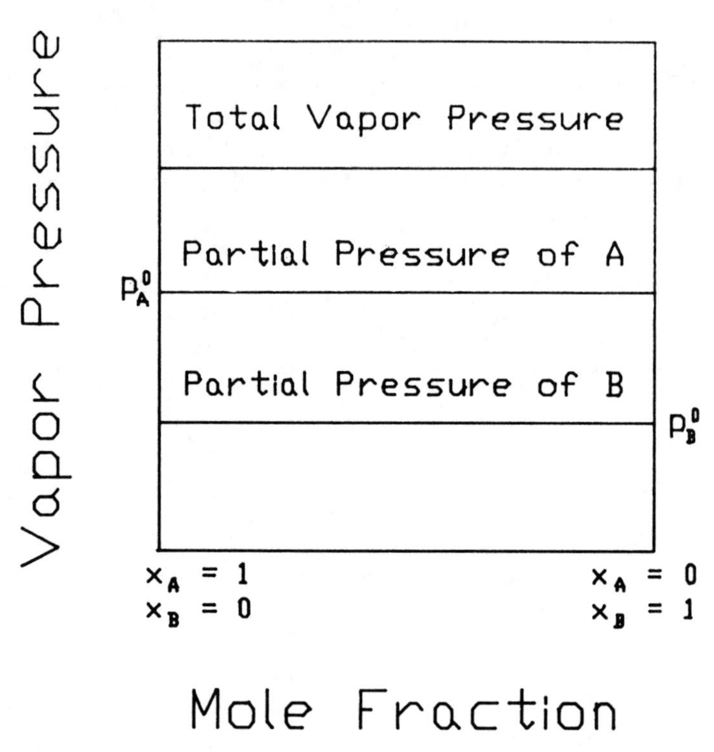

Figure 20.7. Vapor pressure for immiscible liquids.

It is interesting to observe that in the case of immiscible liquids the total vapor pressure can reach 1 atmosphere at a temperature well below 100 degrees C, if one of the components is water, (Figure 20.7). Thus, even though the boiling point of neither liquid is reached, distillation will occur. This obviously is an important removal mechanism of organics from soil when using the HASS technology. It is called steam distillation in the organic process industry. To see how this can be used, let us take the case of chlorobenzene and water and calculate how much can be removed assuming equilibrium and a perfect gas.

The total vapor pressure P is the sum of the vapor pressures of the two immiscible components

$$P = P^O{}_A + P^O{}_B \tag{3}$$

Now

$$\frac{P_A^o}{n_A} = \frac{P_B^o}{n_B} \qquad (4)$$

Where n = number of moles

To express the weight (w) of each component in the gas we must use the expression W = (M) (n) where M is the molecular weight. Thus,

$$\frac{W_A}{W_B} = \frac{M_A n_A}{M_B n_B} = \frac{P_A^o M_A}{P_B^o M_B} \qquad (5)$$

The boiling point is defined as the temperature when the total vapor pressure equals 760 mm Hg. This occurs for water and chlorobenzene at 90.3°C. At this temperature the sum of vapor pressure of the individual components equals 740.2 mm Hg; water = 530.1 mm Hg and chlorobenzene = 210.1 mm Hg. This is very close to 760 mm Hg, showing that the boiling mixture has a slight positive deviation from Raoult's Law. The ratio of the

$$\frac{W_A(ClBz)}{W_B(H_2O)} = \frac{M_A P_A^o}{M_B P_B^o} = \frac{(112.6)\,(210.1)}{(18)\,(530.1)} = 2.48 \qquad (6)$$

that is, the distillate should contain 71.2% chlorobenzene by weight. The measured value is 71.4%: a good agreement considering the assumption of a perfect gas. It does prove the point of the importance of steam distillation to the HASS process. Chlorobenzene, which has a boiling point of 132°C is readily distilled at the higher operating temperatures of the HASS System. Operating at temperatures of 85°C reduces the effect somewhat; however, addition of a third and more components will continue to lower the distillation temperature. Thus, multicomponent systems will remove significant quantities of hydrocarbons by steam distillation at 60° - 80°C.

Aniline (b.p 184.1°C) is another example of a chemical that is steam distilled in industrial practice. The aniline - water mixture should boil at 98.5°C when the aniline and water vapor pressures are 43 mm Hg and 717 mm Hg respectively. With molecular weights of 98 and 18 grams per mole, the distillate should contain 23% aniline by weight. Because aniline is soluble in water this is reduced somewhat.

This analysis also explains why polyaromatic hydrocarbons (PAH) are removed from the soil by steam distillation using the HASS process. We have found measurable quantities of PAH in the process after treatment - even when PAH was not detected in the soil chemical analysis. This also explains why good removal for other semivolatiles as well as pesticides is also observed.

The case of two immiscible liquids is really the limiting case for compounds with a positive deviation from Raoult's Law. Consideration of Figures 20.6 and 20.7 should easily convince one of that. As stated above, these positive deviations from Raoult's Law occur from dissimilar compounds. On the other hand, negative deviations from Raoult's Law occur in, and are caused by, compounds that have a strong attraction to each other. While negative deviations generally do not occur between water and organics, they can occur between water and inorganic salts, water and strong acids and organic/organic compounds, e.g. phenols/alcohols, phenols/amines etc.

Referring back to Figure 20.6, we see that positive deviations from Raoult's Law raise the vapor pressure, i.e. they lower the boiling temperature. (Conversely negative deviations raise the boiling temperature.) These positive and negative deviations can create what is called an azeotrope, i.e. a minimum or maximum boiling point temperature. Figure 20.8 shows the two component azeotrope boiling point for a system with positive deviation from Raoult's Law. (Note this results in a decrease in boiling temperature).

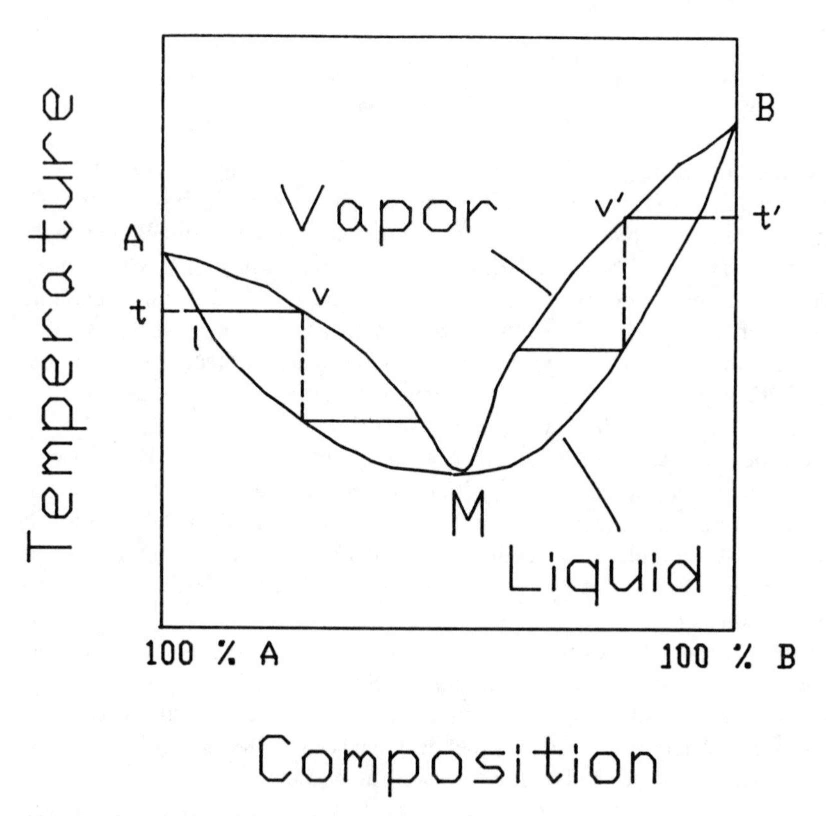

Figure 20.8. System with minimum boiling point.

As stated earlier, the great majority (90%) of liquid systems show a positive deviation from Raoult's Law. This is true for water-organic and organic-organic systems. Many of these positive deviations are large enough to form an azeotrope. As in the case of steam distillation, additional components will lower the azeotrope temperature. Thus, the presence of an azeotrope is an important mechanism for the removal of organic compounds from soil by the HASS System. This is especially true when water is the lower boiling point component because there exists a constant boiling point mixture which boils at less than 100°C, i.e. at or near the temperature of HASS operations (80° - 90°C). As the boiling point of the organic increases, the composition of the azeotrope becomes more concentrated with water and the boiling temperature of the azeotrope moves closer to 100°C. Examples for several two component azeotropic systems of water/hydrocarbon are given in Table 20.1 and Figure 20.9.

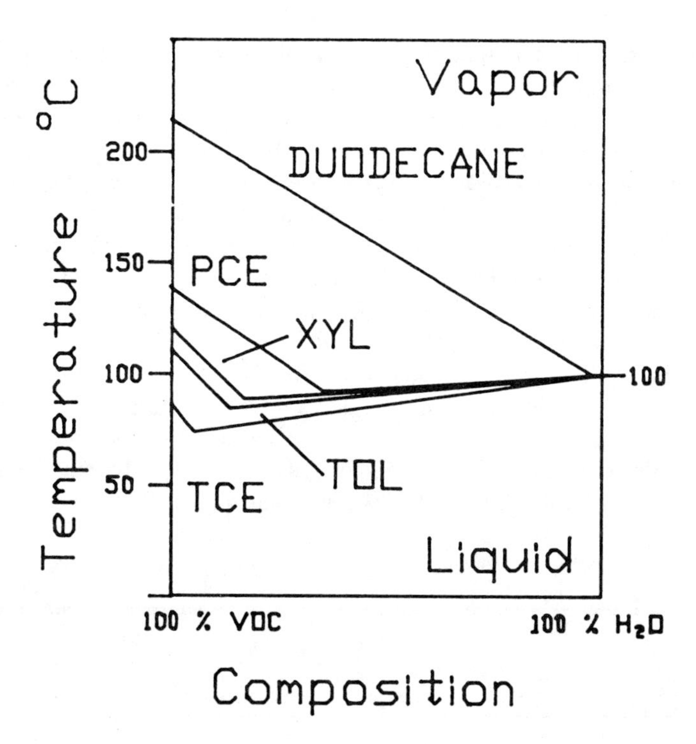

Refer to Table 1

Figure 20.9. Schematic of azeotropic boiling points.

Table 20.1. Water/hydrocarbon azeotropes boiling points and weight percent

Water	Hydrocarbon, b.c.	Azeotrope Temperature	wt. % Water	wt. % VOC
100°C	Trichloroethylene 86.2° - 86.6°C	73.6°C	5.4	94.6
100°C	Toluene 110.7°C	84.1°C	13.5	86.5
100°C	m-Xylene 139°C	92.0°C	35.8	64.2
100°C	Tetrachlorethylene 121°C	85.5°C	17.2	87.8
100°C	Duodecane $C_{12}H_{26}$ 214.5°C	99.45°C	98.0	2.0

The above discussion indicates that in addition to volatilization, liquid phase equilibria is an important mechanism for the HASS remediation of hydrocarbons from the soil. This occurs because in the HASS system steam is continuously supplied. NOVATERRA has extensive laboratory and field data which demonstrate these facts. Tables 20.2 and 20.3 show an example of a field remediation of a clay/silty sand for USEPA Method 8240 (VOC) and USEPA Method 8270 (SVOC). These data are the average of nine soil samples pre-treatment and eight soil samples post-treatment. This particular site has over 49 chemicals of concern and thus provides an excellent example of the range of capabilities of the HASS system for both VOC and SVOC. (This site is examined in depth in the case study below.)

As might be deduced from the above theoretical discussion, multicomponent systems should remediate faster than systems with only a few chemicals. The extensive work done at this site shows that soils with the multicomponent contamination of Tables 20.2 and 20.3 remediate quickly.

Table 20.2. San Pedro site results (VOC)

Treatment Block A-10-g Average Concentration (ppm)		
Volatiles	Pre-Treatment	Post-Treatment
acetone	2.10	--
1,1-dichloroethane	2.18	--
tetrahydrofuran	7.97	--
2-butanone	3.33	--
1,1,1-trichloroethane	95.33	--

Table 20.2 (cont.)

Treatment Block A-10-g Average Concentration (ppm)		
Volatiles	Pre-Treatment	Post-Treatment
trichloroethene	250.04	0.33
chlorobenzene	451.26	10.00
C9-C10 aliphatic hydrocarbons	100.00	--
C7-C11 aliphatic/alicyclic hydrocarbons	433.33	--
C9-C10 aromatic hydrocarbons	15.00	--
dimethoxymethane	5.00	--
2-butanol	0.03	--
pentane	1.17	--
unidentified compounds	1.33	--
trichlorofluoromethane	--	0.33
Total Volatiles:	1,368.07	10.67

Table 20.3. San Petro site results (SVOC)

Treatment Block A-10-g Average Concentration (ppm)		
Semi-Volatiles	Pre-Treatment	Post-treatment
acenaphthene	1.33	--
anthracene	1.00	--
benzo(A)anthracene	0.83	--
benzo(B&K)fluoroanthenes	0.50	380.00
bis(2-ethylhexyl)phthalate	1,043.33	--
chyrsene	1.33	--
dibenzofuran	1.00	--
fluoranthene	3.00	--
fluorene	1.33	--
isophorone	4.33	--

Table 20.3 (cont.)

Treatment Block A-10-g Average Concentration (ppm)		
Semi-Volatiles	Pre-Treatment	Post-treatment
2-methylnaphthalene	1.00	--
naphthalene	6.00	--
phenol	0.83	--
pyrene	2.67	--
butyl cellosolve	90.00	--
hexanoic acid	1.67	3.33
diethyl carbitol	106.67	--
2-ethyl-l-hexanol	3.33	--
octanoic acid	1.67	--
cutyl carbitol	91.67	46.67
2-ethylhexanoic acid	3.33	--
2-phenoxyethanol	70.00	9.00
C8-C12 hydrocarbon matrix	166.67	--
C8-C14 hydrocarbon matrix	333.33	--
1-(2-(2-methoxy-1-methylethoxy)-1-methylethoxy)-2-propanol	18.00	5.00
bis(2-ethylhexyl) adipate	16.67	--
Phthalate matrix	5,333.33	60.00
Glycol ethers	18.17	56.67
Unidentified compound	126.67	3.33
1-(2-methoxypropoxy)-2-propanol	--	2.00
1-(2-methoxy-1-methylethoxy)-2-propanol	--	9.67
2-(2-methoxyethoxy)ethanol	--	16.67
Total Semi Volatiles	7,453.16	592.35

Thermal Desorption

The above discussion indicates that HASS removal of the vapor and liquid phases of contamination in soil will be effective and rapid. The field data of THA versus time indicates their rapid early removal, i.e. removal of the majority of material.

The thermal desorption of organics from soil is a different process and much slower. At the 80° - 90°C HASS bulk soil operating temperature, the rates of desorption are low. The process operates at about 200°C at the steam injection nozzles and this clearly improves the desorption mass transfer. This means that for 200°C to be applied to all the soil the drill must by moved continuously over the contaminated depths. Field THA versus time readings document this effect by showing much slower removal rates during the desorption part of the remediation.

Both soil types and the organic compound types influence the rate of thermal desorption. As expected and found by others, thermal desorption in clay is more difficult than in sand or silt. The data in Tables 20.2 and 20.3 were in soils with about 40% clay and 60 % silt/sand and show that cleanup is occurring. We have found that perchloroethylene particularly, and chlorobenzene to a lesser degree, is slower to remove from heavy clay soils.

Qualitatively we find that in heavy clay, the first 90% of the material is removed as liquid, vapor, or is easily thermally desorpted. Treatment to 95% and 99% becomes progressively more difficult and will increase treatment time. On the other hand, treatment efficiency in sands and sandy silts quickly reaches 98 to 99% removal. Removals of 99.5-99.9% have been achieved in non clay soils.

Chemical Reactions

The possibility of chemical reactions contributing to hydrocarbon removal in the HASS System is not large. Clay catalyzed cleavage is possible in some cases as is oxidation. The addition of hydrogen peroxide, or other oxidants, would enhance the oxidation potential. In both the field and the laboratory NOVATERRA has observed the disappearance of large amounts of phthalate ester compounds and the appearance of olefins in the recovered material when no olefins were present in the pre-treated soils. In addition, NOVATERRA has been unable to find as many phthalate esters in the recovered material or in the treated soils as indicated by pre-treatment analysis.

NOVATERRA postulates that the phthalate radical has reacted with some ion in the clay (possibly sodium) and, thus, is structurally immobilized at temperatures below thermal destruction. An olefin would result from this reaction. Thus, where it is important to track the fate of each species of contaminant, chemical reactions must be considered.

CASE STUDY: RESULTS OF A SITE REMEDIATION

The largest and most successful site that NOVATERRA has provided the *in-situ* treatment of contaminated soils was at a Bulk Chemical Storage and Transfer Facility, located in San Pedro, California, this site was decommissioned in 1983. The largest source of contamination occurred in 1971 when a fire destroyed some of the tanks. Operational spillage caused additional contamination. Subsequent soil sampling revealed that extensive chlorinated volatile and semi-volatile soil contamination had occurred over 2.5 acres of the 5.0 acre site, see Table 20.4. Additional minor amounts of TPH were found. The site was listed on the California State Superfund list and NOVATERRA was contracted by the Responsible Party (RP) to remediate the site using the HASS system.

The California Department of Toxic Substance Control (DTSC) mandated cleanup levels for each of 21 volatile chemicals and 28 semi volatile chemicals. These same levels were to be met for both the three foot and eight foot soil samples (treatment was performed to a depth of ten feet where the water table was at an average depth of six feet). While each of the 49 chemicals was given a different cleanup level (volatiles generally in the 2-10 ppm range and semi volatiles in the 10-100 ppm range) the cleanup level was risk based in that it

Table 20.4. Summary of average pre and post treatment soil contamination levels San Pedro site

Major Volatiles			
	Clean Up Level (ppm)	Pre Treatment Levels (ppm)	Post Treatment Levels (ppm)
1,1-dichloroethane	2.33	11.50	0.81
1,2-dichloroethane	3.24	19.89	0.47
1,1-dichloroethylene	2.00	1.70	0.22
cis-1,2-dichloroethylene	3.18	16.91	2.25
trans-1,2-dichloroethylene	2.05	0.80	0.23
methylene chloride	16.05	23.47	1.07
tetrachloroethylene	19.50	534.11	14.60
1,1,2-trichloroethane	1.94	2.30	0.22
C5-C11 aliphatic & ahevelic	90.00	985.74	10.62

Table 20.4 (cont.)

C9-C10 aromatic	123.30	84.00	17.53
Major Semi-Volatiles			
	Clean Up Level (ppm)	Pre Treatment Levels (ppm)	Post Treatment Levels (ppm)
bis(2-ethyl-hexyl)phtha	680.70	988.43	52.09
phenanthrene	4.89	0.90	0.60
butyl cellosolve	60.60	1086.04	2.81
butyl carbitol	82.80	589.49	4.15
2-phenoxyethanol	59.10	132.07	4.84
triethylene glycol	60.00	433.70	2.32
phthalate ester matrix	510.30	6268.20	217.00
unidentified glycol ethers	63.30	1866.33	4.88
2-(2-methoxyethoxy)-ethanol	124.80	140.40	4.27

mandated a site average for each chemical such that the total increased cancer risk from all chemicals remaining at the site would be 1 in 1,000,000 for a construction worker scenario. Additionally, the chemical levels in any grid (a well defined sub-area of the site of 36 treated blocks, approximately 1054 square feet in size) could not be greater than ten times the mandated site average cleanup value for any of the 49 chemicals and the average of any chemical in any three contiguous grids could not exceed five times the site cleanup level. Levels in excess of the averages had to be offset by over treatment in other areas. A summary of the cleanup values for the most important chemicals, identified as "Major Chemicals" is given in Table 20.4.

NOVATERRA treated over 3,000 blocks (a block is the 29 square feet effective treatment area by a 10'0" foot depth) at the San Pedro Site. A record of the treatment including a strip chart of the FID, steam flow, depth of treatment, and block temperature, as well as any GC's taken, was generated during the treatment process and archived for future reference and independent QA/QC.

Baseline testing and sampling, as well as an internal program of QA/QC soil sampling of approximately 10% of the completed blocks, insured that target levels were being met and that differences in soil or chemical distribution were accounted for by adjusting the operational criteria.

For example, during the treatment of the final 200 blocks of the San Pedro Site levels of cis-1,2-dichloroethylene (cis-1,2-DCE) were found to be 10 to 100 times greater than elsewhere on the site. While cis-1,2-DCE was a major chemical of concern it had always been present in levels low enough that when other chemicals, such as tetrachloroethylene, were removed to the cleanup levels required (as indicated by the FID and GC) cis-1,2-DCE would also achieve the cleanup level. This was no longer the case during the final 200 blocks of treatment. Cis-1,2-DCE became the driving chemical, e.g. once cis-1,2-DCE was removed to below the required cleanup level all other chemicals were also below their respective cleanup levels.

Operational criteria are also adjusted for soil type. For example, the level to which tetrachloroethylene had to be treated, as indicated by the FID and GC, was not the same in silty soil as in soils with a greater clay content. NOVATERRA's internal program of QA/QC sampling quantified the results of treatment subject to these types of changes in soil and chemical distribution. The operational criteria for the treatment of blocks, such as treatment time or temperature, could then be adjusted to account for these types of changes and provide proper remediation. The QA/QC sampling also provided the information on whether a selected area required retreatment or a small area of higher than average results could be absorbed in the site and grid averages.

After treatment the California DTSC took a random sample(s) in each grid for treatment verification. At the end of soil treatment all DTSC mandated levels were meet. Table 20.4 summarizes the results for major chemicals of concern. In early 1993, the agency sent a letter to the client saying that the soil cleanup met the mandated levels and closure would occur.

CONCLUSION

The preferred method for the remediation of contaminated soils is to treat the soil *in-situ.* This approach mitigates the environmental problems, i.e., does not transport it to another location, limits future liability, and when properly applied, does not impact on the local environment during remediation. NOVATERRA has demonstrated commercially an *in-situ*, hot air/steam stripping (HASS) technology to remove VOC and SVOC from soils both in the vadose and saturated zones to stringent mandated cleanup levels.

Although the technology operates at a low temperature of 80-90° C, it is effective in removing liquid VOC and SVOC, including higher boiling point chemicals. The lower boiling point chemicals are volatilized by heat and carried to the surface by the injected air. The higher boiling point chemicals are removed by steam distillation and azeotropic boiling. These last two mechanisms occur because steam is continuously applied to the treatment. The continuous application of steam is different from other low temperature thermal desorption methods which dry the soil. The presence of steam offers a very effective mechanism for removal of hydrocarbons from soil once the thermal desorption process occurs.

This chapter presented the results of treating *in-situ* 30,000 yd^3 of soil using this technology. The results showed that the remediation met the risk based criteria of the regulators for the 49 chemicals of concern. The operational record demonstrates that the process as applied met the clean up standards over 98% of the time after the initial treatment. An additional treatment of short duration was all that was required to complete the work. The site obtained closure for the soil remediation in early 1993.

CHAPTER 21

Generic Biocell and Biopile Designs for Small-Scale Petroleum Contaminated Soil Projects

Susan M. Lasdin, P.E. and Christopher M. O'Neill, P.E., New York State, Department of Environmental Conservation, Division of Spills Management, Albany, New York

INTRODUCTION

The New York State Department of Environmental Conservation's Division of Spills Management (DSM) has been regulating petroleum spills and releases to the environment since the 1970's. With the advent of New York State's underground storage tank regulations, the number of reported spills has increased steadily, and is reflected by an increase in groundwater cleanup projects being managed by DSM. As the number of petroleum-contaminated sites requiring cleanup in New York State increases, so does the desire for better, faster and more cost-effective ways to investigate and remediate these sites. In the past, nearly all petroleum-contaminated soil in New York State was landfilled. The option of landfilling petroleum-contaminated soils has been decreasing due to the closing of more and more landfills to this type of waste. Landfilling has become cost prohibitive for the few which remain in operation and it is the Department's least preferred environmental solution. The New York State Department of Environmental Conservation (NYS DEC) has been investigating alternatives to landfilling which meet environmentally-protective limits for contaminants in air, water and soil. DEC is also seeking alternatives which lend themselves to the development of a generic design standard for small-scale projects. Development of generic design standards is desirable as it will reduce the time lag and the overall costs of a spill cleanup of small-scale projects, by providing the preliminary design work for a responsible party (RP) or contractor to adapt to similar projects and eliminating the engineering design phase. Generic design standards will also educate many RPs and contractors who do not have knowledge and experience in these innovative remedial technologies.

BACKGROUND

Until 1985, the New York State Department of Environmental Conservation (DEC) and the New York State Department of Transportation shared response and remediation responsibilities for petroleum spills. In 1985, DEC assumed full responsibility for regulating petroleum releases and registration of petroleum storage facilities. The Bureau of Spill Prevention and Response was formed to regulate the storage of petroleum to respond to petroleum emergencies, and to remediate petroleum spills. The Bureau of Spill Prevention and Response has evolved into the Division of Spills Management, and is commonly referred to as the Spill Program. DSM has grappled with an ever-increasing workload since 1985. The total number of spills reported in Fiscal Year 1985 was 8,132. The total number for Fiscal Year 1992 was approximately 15,000, amounting to over $14 million in state and federal funds plus many millions spent by responsible parties, for investigative and cleanup costs. The reported spills can vary from pints to millions of gallons, so the increase does not necessarily reflect a large increase in major incidents. Much of the increase in reported spills may be attributed to a greater public awareness of the Spill Program and its regulations. Nonetheless, the number of spills related to underground storage tanks increased dramatically in 1987, coinciding with the first tank testing deadline under DEC's bulk storage regulations. The number of spills from underground storage tanks has leveled off at about 2,000 spills per year since then, reflecting routine tank testing, inventory monitoring, overfilling, accidents and piping leaks.

Many of the underground tank spill reports result in groundwater investigations and cleanups. There has been a steady increase in the number of active groundwater projects for the Spill Program to fund, supervise and manage, amounting to approximately 800 new projects annually. This increased number of petroleum-contaminated sites in New York has driven DSM and responsible parties (RPs) to look for ways to investigate and remediate spill sites in a more timely and cost effective manner. The option of landfilling petroleum-contaminated soils is decreasing due to the closure of more and more landfills, and may be cost prohibitive for the few which remain in operation. DSM is concerned that the RPs get their money's worth so they will continue to be responsible and cooperative in remediating petroleum releases to the environment. In addition, DSM wants to control expenditures from the New York State Spill Fund, which is a revolving fund of State and federal money used to investigate and remediate spills when an RP is unidentifiable, or is unwilling or unable to perform the work deemed necessary by DSM. By developing generic design standards for small-scale projects, the time lag and the overall costs of cleaning up small spills can be reduced. By providing preliminary generic design work for an RP or contractor to adapt to similar projects, the time and cost of the engineering design phase is eliminated. In addition, such design standards will also provide education for many RPs and contractors who do not have knowledge of experience in innovative remedial technologies.

The limited availability of landfill space and the long-term liability of landfilling petroleum-contaminated soil have made it necessary to develop alternatives to soil disposal. It has also fostered the beneficial re-use and on-site treatment of soils. Reuse options for treated soils include reuse as a construction material, returning soil to the original excavation, placing the soil elsewhere on site, and reuse off-site at a pre-approved location. On-site treatment options which are being used in New York State by DEC include thermal treatment, soil venting, hot and cold-mix asphalt manufacturing, and bioremediation. Several limitations on each of these technologies, including site size, soil type, contaminant type, and equipment needs, may prevent these technologies from being used on small-scale projects. Soil washing and thermal treatment are not cost-effective for small-scale projects. Venting is not effective for fuel oils. Hot-mix asphalt manufacturing is conducted off site. Cold-mix asphalt manufacturing specifications vary by manufacturer for contaminant concentration and particle size distribution of the soil. Bioremediation technology can be scaled down to be cost-effective for small-scale projects and can be adjusted to provide effective treatment for a wide range of soil contamination conditions.

Bioremediation stimulates microorganisms, by creating and maintaining a favorable environment, to use contaminants in soil as a food source. Under proper conditions, microorganisms, either indigenous or non-indigenous, i.e., naturally existing or genetically engineered, can break down the contaminants into non-hazardous inorganic substances. Small-scale bioremediation lends itself to a generic design standard because the design criteria, which include moisture content, temperature and pH of the soil, can be measured simply and adjusted to optimum conditions for the process. The additional design criteria, nutrient and oxygen requirements, can be estimated based on contaminant concentrations in the soil. It is understood that generic parameters established by a standardized method may not provide the same remedial efficiencies as those based on a site-specific feasibility study; however, it is anticipated that the results will be adequate for small-scale projects.

Some of the advantages of bioremediation, include the following: it can be conducted on site, the waste is permanently eliminated, capital costs for these small-scale applications are cheaper than other processes, there is positive public acceptance because it provides for recycling, the long-term liability risks associated with leaving contamination on site are eliminated, there is minimum site disruption, transportation costs and liability are eliminated, and it can be coupled with other treatment techniques. Some of the general disadvantages include: there is a potential for the production of unknown byproducts, the design criteria is site-specific, and extensive monitoring is necessary.

The design standard which DEC is developing will consist of using indigenous microorganisms. It will apply to petroleum-contaminated soils of approximately 30 - 100 yd^3, typical of the removal of an underground storage tank. This volume of soil was chosen recognizing that a standard approach to cleaning up this amount of soil would reduce costs for many responsible parties. The cost to hire professionals with experience in bioremediation is prohibitive for such small quantities and this would be a manageable quantity of soil for application of a generic design standard.

This chapter describes the engineering conditions of bioremediation and establishes design standards for a small-scale cell and pile, both *ex-situ* designs. The design standards and engineering conditions are summarized in Appendix A: Small-Scale Bioremediation Design Specifications and Operating Conditions.

BIOREMEDIATION

Bioremediation consists of creating and maintaining a favorable environment for microorganisms, either indigenous or non-indigenous, to use contaminants in soil as a food source. The basic requirements for a compatible environment include proper pH, temperature and moisture. Nutrient requirements, other than the contaminants in the soil, which provide a carbon source, include hydrogen, oxygen, nitrogen, and phosphorous. Other elements, such as potassium, calcium, iron, manganese, cobalt, copper, and zinc, are generally present in adequate concentrations in most soil and aquifer systems, and usually need no further attention in the design of a bioremediation process.

Two commonly used designs for *ex-situ* bioremediation are the biocell and the biopile. These are described in the Bioremediation Technologies section of this chapter.

pH

Petroleum-consuming microorganisms grow best at pH near 7. Where high concentrations of aromatic compounds are present and where soils have low alkalinity, liming may be necessary. Adding enough lime to attain a pH of 7.2 to 7.5 should be sufficient to maintain appropriate pH throughout the life of the project without having to monitor the pH. The lime added should be in the form of ground agricultural limestone ($CaCO_3$). Ground limestone is recommended because it is less expensive than other forms and because it is harmless to add too much. Soil samples can be collected and taken to a local garden store for pH measurement and liming requirements to achieve pH near 7.

Temperature

The microorganisms will operate at ambient temperatures above 40° F. The heat generated by covering the soil, and from the biodegradation reactions should allow operation of a bioremediation process in most of New York State for approximately nine months per year. Additionally, petroleum hydrocarbon degradation does not generate enough heat to be concerned with temperature highs.

Moisture

Moisture content should be maintained at 50-60% field moisture capacity, which means that the soil should be wet but not puddly. (Values of field moisture capacity for various soil textures are tabulated in Appendix C: Small-Scale Bioremediation Nutrient Requirements.) Moisture can be measured once per week using a lysimeter. Initially, water can be applied and measured until the proper moisture is obtained. Moisture can be monitored visually. Moisture can be added to a cell using a spray applicator and distributed by the weekly tilling process. If spraying is not expected to provide enough moisture throughout a pile, then moisture should be added through a system of slotted pipes woven through the pile, to ensure even distribution.

Dechlorinated water must be used. Otherwise, chlorine will kill the microorganisms. Potable quality water must be used to avoid propagation of pathogens.

Nutrient Requirements

Nutrient requirements to be determined include nitrogen, phosphorous and oxygen. These requirements are calculated based on the composition of contaminants in the soil and the amount of soil to be treated. These compositions are measured or are assumed to be the average for the type of petroleum product which was spilled.

Hydrocarbons are degraded by microorganisms through chemical reactions (reduction-oxidation (redox) reactions) between the microbial enzymes and the hydrocarbons. The total reaction includes the organic specie being oxidized (hydrocarbons), the electron donor being reduced (oxygen), and the major nutrients for cell growth, which are nitrogen and phosphorous. The amount of nutrients required can be calculated by solving the chemical reaction equations. The overall redox stoichiometric equation is a result of the summation of half reactions as performed for nitrite oxidation, plus a reaction for cell synthesis. The derivation of this equation is included in Appendix C. Nutrient requirements based on these calculations are also found in Appendix C.

Oxygen can be added to a biocell by tilling approximately once per week, and to a pile through a system of slotted pipes to ensure even distribution of oxygen. Oxygen rates need to be kept close to the calculated requirements. An excess oxygen supply is desirable to ensure adequate distribution of oxygen throughout the pile. However, too much air can dry out the soil and volatilize the contaminants. Based on the tabulated oxygen requirements found in Appendix C and the operating capabilities of a 1 hp pump, a 1 hp can be operated at a low flow rate while monitoring moisture content. If the soil is drying out, then the pump flow rate should be decreased or water should be added.

Nitrogen and phosphorous requirements can be satisfied by applying the appropriate fertilizer or a custom fertilizer blend based on the calculated requirements. If in doubt, more phosphorous could be used because it is not very mobile in soil. Therefore, it is assumed for this small-scale design that phosphorous already present in the soil is negligible and that there is no need to calculate the amount to be added based on amount already present in the soil. The amount to be added will be the amount required based on the calculations. Ammonia is the preferred source of nitrogen for hydrocarbons and it should be assumed that there is no nitrogen in the soil before adding the required amount because there are no reliable soil tests for nitrogen.

Nitrogen and phosphorous can be added in the form of "off-the-shelf" fertilizer. If it was assumed that nitrogen and phosphorous initially in the soil is negligible, then a 6:1, Nitrogen: Phosphorous ratio is desirable. Therefore, a lawn fertilizer of 19:3:3 ratios can be used. All the fertilizer can be applied at the start of the project. The bacteria will consume the nutrients as they need them.

Monitoring Requirements

Regular sampling and analysis of contamination levels and microbial counts is necessary to monitor the amount of biodegradation taking place. Low microbial counts and high contamination levels can indicate that the environmental conditions are not ideal for microbial growth. High microbial counts and lower contamination levels probably indicate the process is working well. Low microbial counts and low contamination levels can indicate that biodegradation was successful and that the microbes are dying off due to lack of contamination to consume. Types, numbers and frequencies of monitoring are outlined in Appendix B: Small-Scale Bioremediation Sampling and Analysis Protocol.

BIOREMEDIATION TECHNOLOGIES

The engineering technologies for bioremediation can be characterized as physical controls, pump and treat, excavate and treat (*ex-situ*), and in-place (*in-situ*) technology. Physical controls consist of impermeable barriers designed to prevent contaminant migration and to allow natural biodegradation to occur. Pump and treat, and excavate and treat methods bring contaminated groundwater or soil to the surface where it is treated by biological reactors possibly coupled with physical and chemical processes. *In-situ* technologies process the contaminated groundwater or soil in place in the subsurface. This chapter addresses excavating and treating soil in a pile, also known as a biopile, or in a layer, also known as a biocell.

Biopile

A biopile consists of piling contaminated soil in a pile of four to five feet in height with a flat top. A double-layered 8 mil polyethylene liner is laid under the pile. The soil is completely covered with a nylon-reinforced tarp or placed under a greenhouse cover to protect the soil from rain and to keep it warm. The cover can be anchored using tires or hay bales around the perimeter and ropes run over the top of the cover and tied to the tires or bales. Spacers, such as tires or bales, should also be placed on top of the soil, under the cover to promote ventilation. A two-foot earthen berm is built around the pile to prevent run-on of surface waters and run-off of leachate. If this curb is constructed of soil, it should also be covered with the polyethylene liner to protect the curb from erosion. The entire set-up should be surrounded by a safety fence.

Ventilation is provided by pulling air through a network of slotted PVC piping woven throughout the pile. Slotted PVC pipes should be wrapped in a geotextile cloth to prevent soil from clogging the screens. A barrier should be placed between the pile and the cover to allow better air circulation. The pump should be explosion proof, have a particle filter, a moisture trap and a muffler, and should be enclosed to muffle noise. The piping system includes shut-off valves at each elevation of piping to allow varying air flow rates depending on moisture and contamination levels. The pump and piping should be installed following manufacturer's recommended procedure.

Moisture is provided by spraying the soil with dechlorinated water until it is wet but not puddly, when the soil appears dry. Dehydration can be somewhat controlled by increasing or decreasing flowrate of the vacuum pump. Lime and nutrients are mixed in the pile while it is being constructed.

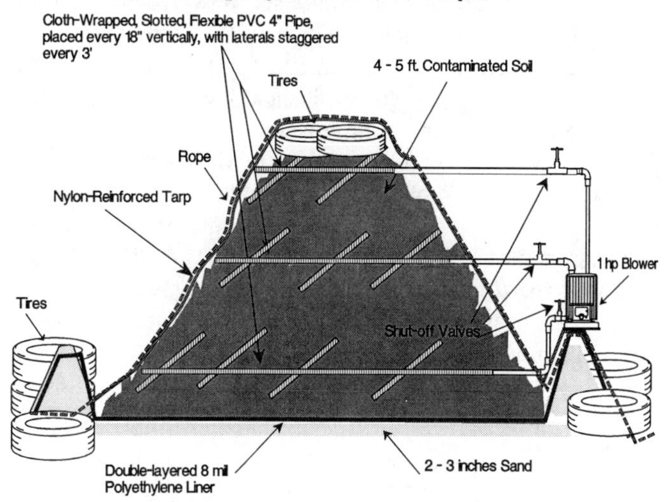

Figure 21.1. Design specifications for a generic biopile.

Biopile Design Specifications and Engineering Conditions

The basic process specifications include proper pH, temperature, moisture, nutrients and aeration

pH: The amount of lime ($CaCO_3$) to be added to obtain pH 7 is based on the existing pH of the soil and the amount of soil to be treated. This can be accomplished by taking a soil sample to a local garden store to be tested for pH and referring to a liming chart. Lime is added and mixed with soil and fertilizer as the soil layer is constructed.

Temperature: Soil temperature should be above 40° F.

Moisture: When the soil appears dry, moisture is added by spraying it with potable, dechlorinated water until soil is wet but not puddly. Dehydration can be somewhat controlled by increasing or decreasing flowrate of the vacuum pump.

Nutrients: The amount of fertilizer to be added is tabulated based on the amount of soil to be treated and the TPH. Fertilizer is added and mixed with the soil and lime as the cell is constructed.

Aeration: Aeration can be provided by a pump system of slotted pipes woven throughout the pile.

Biocell

A biocell consists of spreading the soil into 18 to 24 inch layers on a double-layered 8 mil polyethylene liner laid to collect leachate. The foundation should be sloped towards a sump to collect leachate. The liner is laid on top of a two to three inch layer of sand and covered with a six to twelve-inch layer of sand or gravel to protect it against tilling equipment. A six to twelve-inch earthen berm is built around the pile to prevent run-on of surface waters and run-off of leachate. If this curb is constructed of soil, it should also be covered with the polyethylene liner to protect the curb from erosion.

The biocell should be covered to protect against rainfall and the resulting leachate. A durable peaked or sloped roof cover is desirable to prevent puddling on top of the liner.

Lime and nutrients are mixed in when the cell is constructed. When the soil appears dry, the cell is sprayed with dechlorinated water until wet but not puddly and moisture is distributed. Ventilation is provided by tilling the soil or by forced aeration using a pump and piping system.

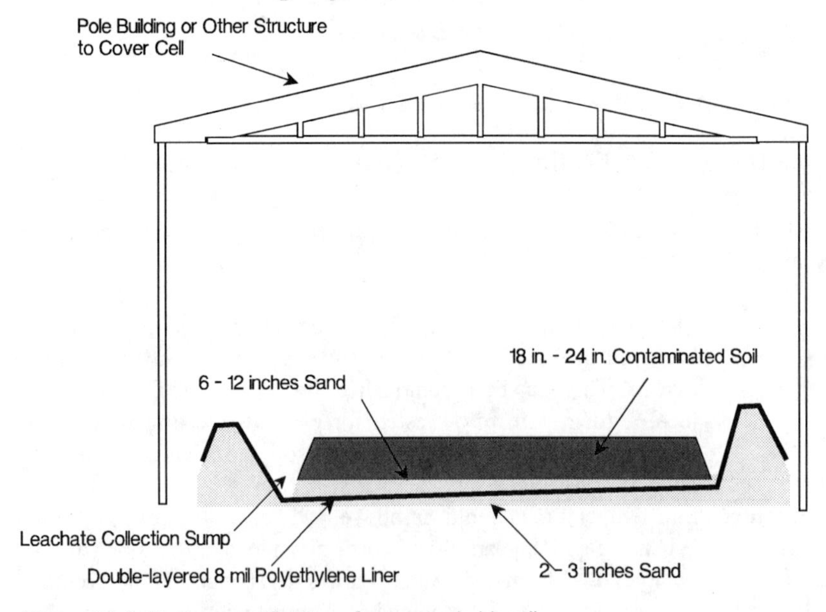

Figure 21.2. Design specifications for a generic biocell.

Biocell Design Specifications and Engineering Conditions

The basic process specifications include proper pH, temperature, moisture, nutrients and aeration

pH: The amount of lime ($CaCO_3$) to be added to obtain pH 7 is based on the existing pH of the soil and the amount of soil to be treated. This can be accomplished by taking a soil sample to a local garden store to be tested for pH and referring to a liming chart. Lime is added and mixed with soil and fertilizer as the soil layer is constructed.

Temperature: Soil temperature should be above 40^0 F.

Moisture: When the soil appears dry, moisture is added by spraying it with potable, dechlorinated water until soil is wet but not puddly, and distributed by the tilling process.

Nutrients: The amount of fertilizer to be added is tabulated based on the amount of soil to be treated and the TPH. Fertilizer is added and mixed with the soil and lime as the cell is constructed.

Aeration: Aeration can be provided by tilling the soil once per week.

ACKNOWLEDGEMENTS

This chapter, which was prepared by the New York State Department of Environmental Conservation Division of Spills Management, presents guidelines and recommended practices for bioremediation of small-scale amounts of petroleum-contaminated soil. A research project substantiating this paper is currently underway and is being funded by the U.S.E.P.A. LUST Trust program.

The Division wishes to extend thanks and appreciation to the following individuals and their companies for both their financial and professional support:

Chad Fowler - Stewart's Ice Cream Shops, Inc.

Bill Black - Lebanon Valley Landscaping, Inc.

George Longworth and Bill Toran - American Spill Abatement, Inc.

Mike Barnhart and Jim Hyzy, Ph.D. - Waste Stream Technology, Inc.

Additional appreciation is extended to the DEC Central Office and Region 5 Divisions of Solid Waste and Regulatory Affairs for their support in expediting construction and operation of this project.

REFERENCES

1. American Spill Abatement, Inc., Galway, New York, Professional Consultation, Summer 1993.
2. General Physics Corporation, GP Environmental Services, Columbia, Maryland, Bioremediation Engineering: Principles, Applications, and Case Studies, 1990.
3. Lebanon Valley Landscaping, Inc., West Lebanon, New York, Professional Consultation, Summer 1993.
4. McCarty, P.L. 1987. Bioengineering issues related to *in-situ* remediation of contaminated soils and groundwater, pp. 143-162, In: Omenn, G.S., Ed. *Environmental Biotechnology*, Plenum Press, New York.
5. New York State Department of Environmental Conservation, Division of Construction Management, Bureau of Spill Prevention and Response, Albany, New York, "STARS Memo #1: Petroleum-Contaminated Soil Guidance Policy," August 1992.
6. New York State Department of Environmental Conservation, Division of Water, Bureau of Spill Prevention and Response, Albany, New York, "Sampling Guidelines & Protocols: Technical Background and Quality Control/Quality Assurance For NYS DEC Spill Response Program," March 1991.
7. Stewart's Ice Cream Shops, Inc., Saratoga Springs, New York, Professional Consultation, Summer 1993.
8. Waste Stream Technology, Inc., Buffalo, New York, Professional Consultation, Summer 1993.

APPENDIX A

Design Specifications and Operating Conditions for a Biopile

Setup

Set up pile according to these design specifications and accompanying sketch.

1. Clear and grade a sloped area for construction.
2. Lay a double-layered 8 mil polyethylene liner on top of a two to three-inch layer of sand with two-foot berms.
3. Pile the soil into a four to five-foot flat-top pile on the tarp.
4. While constructing the pile, install the ventilation system (4", slotted PVC piping, shut-off valves, explosion-proof blower, particle filter, moisture trap, and muffler) according to manufacturers' recommended practices. The piping system includes shut-off valves at each elevation of piping to allow varying air flow depending on moisture and contaminant levels. Slotted PVC pipes should be wrapped in a geotextile cloth to prevent soil from clogging the screens. Also add lime and fertilizer, and spray with dechlorinated water until soil is wet but not puddly.
5. Place tires or hay bales on top of the pile to provide air space between the soil and the cover, to promote aeration.
6. Cover the pile with a nylon-reinforced tarp.
7. Anchor the cover using tires or bales around the perimeter of the cover, and ropes run over the top of the cover and tied to the tires or bales.
8. Surround the entire area with a safety fence.

Operation

The process specifications include proper pH, temperature, moisture, nutrients and aeration:

pH

1. Determine the amount of soil to be treated.
2. Take one composite soil sample to a local garden store to be tested for pH. Refer to a liming chart for amount of lime ($CaCO_3$) to be added to obtain pH 7.
3. Add lime and mix with soil and fertilizer as the pile is constructed.

Temperature

1. Operate at soil temperature above 40° F.
2. When soil temperature is below 40° F, follow end-of-season sampling procedures and secure site.

Moisture

1. When the soil appears dry, remove cover, spray soil with potable, dechlorinated water until it is wet but not puddly. (Dehydration can be somewhat controlled by varying flowrate of vacuum pump. Water can be dechlorinated with tablets purchased at a local aquarium store.)

2. Check soil weekly, if soil appears dry, remoisten. Adjust schedule or pump flowrate based on results.

Nutrients

1. Determine the amount of soil to be treated and the TPH of the soil. TPH analysis should be conducted using EPA Modified Method 418.1. Refer to nutrient addition table in this appendix.

2. Add fertilizer and mix with the soil and lime as the pile is constructed.

Aeration

1. Supply air through a system of slotted pipes to ensure even distribution of oxygen. Oxygen rates need to be kept close to the calculated requirements found in Appendix C: Small-Scale Bioremediation Nutrient Requirements. An excess oxygen supply is desirable to ensure adequate distribution of oxygen throughout the pile. However, too much air can dry out the soil and volatilize the contaminants.

   Based on the tabulated oxygen requirements found in Appendix C and the operating capabilities of a 1 hp pump, a 1 hp pump can be operated at a low flowrate while monitoring moisture content to meet oxygen requirements. If the soil is drying out, then the pump flow rate should be decreased or water should be added.

Monitoring

1. Perform types, numbers, and frequency of sampling as outlined in Appendix B: Small-Scale Bioremediation Sampling and Analysis Protocol.

Project Close-out

1. Conduct process under the guidance of NYS DEC until the soil reaches the guidance values listed in STARS Memo #1 or until determined appropriate by NYS DEC. Perform closure samples as described in STARS #1.

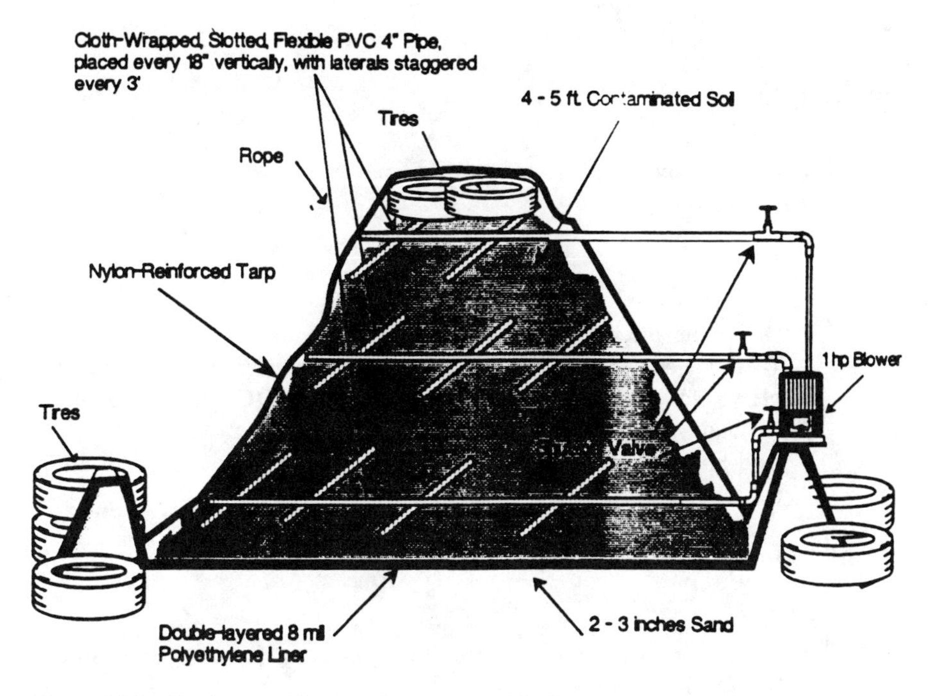

Figure 21.A1. Design specifications for a generic biopile.

Design Specifications and Operating Conditions for a Biocell

Setup

Set up pile according to these design specifications and accompanying sketch.

1. Clear and grade a sloped area for construction. The foundation should be sloped towards a sump to collect leachate.

2. Lay a double-layered 8 mil polyethylene liner on top of a two to three-inch layer of sand with six to twelve-inch berms. Cover the liner with a six to twelve-inch layer of sand or gravel.
3. Spread the soil into a 18 to 24-inch layer on the tarp.
4. While constructing the cell, add lime and fertilizer, and spray with dechlorinated water until soil is wet but not puddly.
5. Cover the cell with a durable peaked or sloped-roof cover to prevent puddling on top of the liner and to protect against rainfall and the resulting leachate.
6. Surround the entire area with a safety fence.

Operation

The process specifications include proper pH, temperature, moisture, nutrients and aeration:

pH

1. Determine the amount of soil to be treated.
2. Take one composite soil sample to a local garden store to be tested for pH. Refer to a liming chart for amount of lime ($CaCO_3$) to be added to obtain pH 7.
3. Add lime and mix with soil and fertilizer as the soil layer is constructed.

Temperature

1. Operate at soil temperature above 40° F.
2. When soil temperature is below 40° F, follow end-of-season sampling procedures and secure site.

Moisture

1. When the soil appears dry, spray soil with potable, dechlorinated water until it is wet but not puddly. Water can be dechlorinated with tablets purchased at a local aquarium store. Distribute by tilling once per week.
2. Check soil weekly, if soil appears dry, remoisten. Adjust schedule based on results.

Nutrients

1. Determine the amount of soil to be treated and the TPH of the soil. TPH analysis should be conducted using EPA Modified Method 418.1. Refer to nutrient addition table in this appendix.

2. Add fertilizer and mix with the soil and lime as the cell is constructed.

Aeration

1. Till once per week or supply air through a system of slotted pipes (see biopile design specifications).

Monitoring

1. Perform types, numbers, and frequency of sampling as outlined in Appendix B: Small-Scale Bioremediation Sampling and Analysis Protocol.

Project Close-out

1. Conduct process under the guidance of NYS DEC until the soil reaches the guidance values listed in STARS Memo #1 or until determined appropriate by NYS DEC. Perform closure samples as described in STARS #1.

Fertilizer Requirements

Table 21.A1 lists the amount of fertilizer required to treat gasoline-contaminated soil for varying levels of contamination and varying amounts of soil to be treated. The nitrogen:phosphorous ratio in the fertilizer should be 6:1, such as 19:3:3 lawn feed which can be found in garden stores.

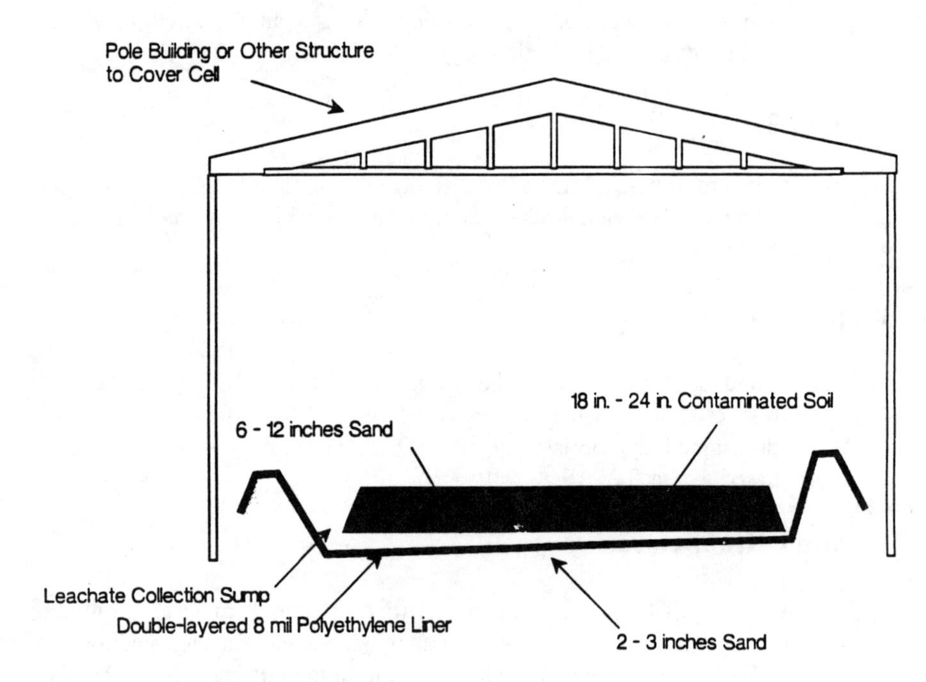

Figure 21.A2. Design specifications for a generic biocell

Table 21.A1: Amount of Fertilizer Required to Treat Gasoline-Contaminated Soil (lbs.) (N:P = 6:1)

		Volume of Soil (yd.^{3})							
		30	40	50	60	70	80	90	100
Total Petroleum Hydrocarbons (TPH) (ppm)	1000	59	79	99	118	138	158	177	197
	2000	118	158	197	236	276	315	355	394
	3000	177	236	296	355	414	473	532	591
	4000	236	315	394	473	552	631	709	788
	5000	296	394	493	591	690	788	887	985
	6000	355	473	591	709	828	946	1064	1182
	7000	414	552	690	828	966	1104	1242	1379
	8000	473	631	788	946	1104	1261	1419	1577
	9000	532	709	887	1064	1242	1419	1596	177
	10000	591	788	985	1182	1379	1577	1774	1971
	12500	739	985	1232	1478	1724	1971	2217	2463
	15000	887	1182	1478	1774	2069	2365	2660	2956
	17500	1035	1379	1724	2069	2414	2759	3104	3449
	20000	1182	1577	1971	2365	2759	3153	3547	3941

Table 21.A2 lists the amount of fertilizer required to treat fuel oil-contaminated soil for varying levels of contamination and varying amounts of soil to be treated. The nitrogen:phosphorous ratio in the fertilizer should be 6:1, such as 19:3:3 lawn feed which can be found in garden stores.

Table 21.A2: Amount of Fertilizer Required to Treat Fuel Oil-Contaminated Soil (lbs.) (N:P = 6:1)

		Volume of Soil (yd.^{3})							
		30	40	50	60	70	80	90	100
Total Petroleum Hydrocarbons (TPH) (ppm)	1000	56	75	93	112	131	149	168	187
	2000	112	149	187	224	261	298	336	373
	3000	168	224	280	336	392	448	504	560
	4000	224	298	373	448	522	597	671	746
	5000	280	373	466	560	653	746	839	933
	6000	336	448	560	671	783	895	1007	1119
	7000	392	522	653	783	914	1044	1175	1306
	8000	448	597	746	895	1044	1194	1343	1492
	9000	504	671	839	1007	1175	1343	1511	1679
	10000	560	746	933	1119	1306	1492	1679	1865
	12500	699	933	1166	1399	1632	1865	2098	2331
	15000	839	1119	1399	1679	1958	2238	2518	2798
	17500	979	1306	1632	1958	2285	2611	2938	3264
	20000	1119	1492	1865	2238	2611	2984	3357	3730

APPENDIX B

Small-Scale Bioremediation Sampling and Analysis Protocol

Sampling and analysis will be conducted in accordance with the DEC Division of Spill Management's *Sampling Guidelines and Protocols* and *STARS Memo #1: Petroleum-Contaminated Soil Guidance Policy.*

The following sampling plan contains minimum guidelines for appropriate sampling and analysis of a small-scale bioremediation project. Small-scale projects, including the sampling and analysis procedures, should be conducted under the guidance of a DEC Regional Spill Responder.

Small-Scale Bioremediation Sampling Plan

Pretreatment Sampling:	TPH, total soil concentration*, TCLP*, microbes, and soil sieve analysis (grain size distribution)***
Sampling During Treatment:	
every 4 - 6 weeks:	TPH and microbes
every 8 - 12 weeks:	TPH, indicator compounds**, and microbes
End of Season:	TPH, total soil concentration*, and microbes
Next Season Start-up:	TPH, total soil concentration*, TCLP*, microbes, and nutrients
Project Closeout:	TPH, total soil concentration*, TCLP*, and microbes

---

* Total soil concentration analysis and TCLP extract analysis will be performed using EPA Method 8021 plus MTBE for gasoline and EPA Methods 8021 and 8270 for fuel oil, in accordance with STARS Memo #1.

** Indicator compounds to be analyzed for gasoline include BTEX using EPA Method 8020. Indicator compounds to be analyzed for fuel oil will be determined based on the total soil concentration analysis results.

*** Soil sieve analysis (grain size distribution) is conducted to classify soil type and to determine whether or not composting would be recommended to promote better aeration, such as in clays. Composting is beyond the scope of this issue of this guidance paper.

APPENDIX C

Small-Scale Bioremediation

Nutrient Requirements

This appendix is quite theoretical and is provided for informational purposes only. The nutrient needs calculated from the following equations are tabulated in Tables A1 and A2 of Appendix A and Tables C1 - C8 in this appendix.

Calculating nutrient requirements is based on balancing a stoichiometric equation representing the redox reaction which occurs when are broken down. The total reaction includes the organic specie being oxidized (hydrocarbons) and the electron donor being reduced (oxygen), in the presence of nitrogen and phosphorous, which are the major nutrients for cell growth.

The overall redox stoichiometric equation is a result of the summation of half reactions as performed for nitrite oxidation, plus a reaction for cell synthesis. The overall reaction can be given in general terms by:

$$H_D + f_e H_A + f_S C_S \quad (1)$$

where:

H_D is the half reaction for organic oxidation:

$$1/e\ (C_a H_b O_c N_d) + 2(a\text{-}c)/e\ (H_2O) = a/e\ (CO_2) + (d/e)\ (NH_3) + H^+ + e^- \quad (2)$$

where $e = 4a + b - 2c - 3d$

H_A is the half reaction for the electron acceptor:

$$1/4\ O_2 + H^+ + e^- = 1/2\ H_2O \quad (3)$$

C_S is the reaction that provides nutrient requirements for cell synthesis

$$1/4\ CO_2 + 1/20\ NH_3 + H^+ + e^- = 1/20\ C_5H_7O_2N + 2/5\ H_2O \quad (4)$$

To determine the nutrient requirement, it is necessary to establish that portion of energy for cellular growth. Thus, a factor must be included for the distribution of energy between cell synthesis and other needs. These factors are represented by:

f_e = fraction of organic oxidized for energy

f_s = fraction associated with conversion to microbial cells

$f_e = 1 - f_s$

The nutrient requirement for cell synthesis is balanced and added to the half reactions.

For aerobic systems:

$$f_s = 0.12 - 0.6 \quad (5)$$

The slower the reaction, the lower the value of f_s.

Nutrient Requirements for Gasoline-Contaminated Soil

The calculations for required nutrients for gasoline-contaminated soil are illustrated in this appendix using the following example problem.

Example Problem

Estimate the nutrient needs for bioremediation of 100 yd^3 of silty sand contaminated with gasoline, where TPH results indicate 5000 ppm contamination.

Assumptions:

For hydrocarbons, oxygen is the appropriate electron acceptor and aerobic microbial activity is the appropriate metabolic mode for destruction of the hydrocarbons. Ammonia is the preferred source of nitrogen. Hydrocarbons oxidize relatively quickly; therefore, a value for f_s of .5 is selected, hence f_e = .5. Based on average compositions of gasoline, the overall chemical composition of gasoline can be estimated as C_8H_{10} (xylene). (See Appendix D) Assume soil density is average, i.e., 100 lb/ft^3.

Step 1. Determine the amount of hydrocarbons to be treated.

Answer: Total Mass Hydrocarbons(HC) = Average Concentration Hydrocarbons(HC) X Soil Density X Soil Volume

$$\text{Total} = \frac{5000 \text{ lbs. HC}}{1X10^6 \text{ lbs. Soil}} \times \frac{100 \text{ lbs. Soil}}{ft^3} \text{ X } 100 \text{ yd}^3 \text{ Soil X } \frac{27 \text{ ft}^3 \text{Hydrocarbons}}{yd^3}$$

= 1350 lbs. Hydrocarbons (See Table 1 for amount of hydrocarbons to be treated for varying levels of contamination and soil volume.)

Step 2. Write the appropriate half reactions and the equation for cell growth using the yield fractions, f_e and f_s.

For $C_aH_bO_cN_d$, $e = 4a + b - 2c - 3d$

for C_8H_{10}; $a = 8, b = 10, c = 0, d = 0$

Answer: $e = 4(8) + 10 = 42$

Half Reaction of Electron Donor (H_D):

H_D: $1/e\ (C_aH_bO_cN_d) + 2(a\text{-}c)/e\ (H_2O) = a/e\ (CO_2) + (d/e)\ (NH_3) + H^+ + e^-$

$$H_D\text{: } 1/42\ C_8\ H_{10} + 16/42\ H_2O = 8/42\ CO_2 + H^+ + e^-$$

Half Reaction of Electron Acceptor (H_A) for Aerobic Reaction:

$f_e = .5$ H_A: $1/4\ O_2 + H^+ + e^- = 1/2\ H_2O$

$$f_eH_a\text{: } 1/8\ O_2 + 1/2\ H^+ + 1/2\ e^- = 1/4\ H_2O$$

Cell Synthesis Equation (Cs) for Ammonia as Nitrogen Source:

$f_e = .5$ Cs: $1/4\ CO_2 + 1/20\ NH_3 + H^+ + e^- = 1/20\ C_5H_7O_2N + 2/5\ H_2O$

$$\text{feCs: } 1/8\ CO_2 + 1/40\ NH_3 + 1/2\ H^+ + 1/2e^- = 1/40\ C_5H_7O_2N + 2/10\ H_2O$$

Step 3. Write the overall reaction by summation of half reactions and cell growth equation.

Answer: $1/42\ C_8H_{10} + 1/8\ 0_2 + 1/40\ NH_3 = 1/40\ C_5H_70_2N + 11/168\ CO_2 + 29/420\ H_20$

Simplifying, one obtains the overall stoichiometric redox equation as:

$$20\ C_8H_{10} + 105\ O_2 + 21\ NH_3 = 21\ C_5H_7O_2N + 55\ CO_2 + 58\ H_2O$$

for 1 lb. HC, the overall stoichiometric redox equation for gasoline (represented by C_8H_{10}) is:

$$C_8H_{10} + 5.25\ O_2 + 1.05\ NH_3 = 1.05\ C_5H_7O_2N + 2.75\ CO_2 + 2.9\ H_2O$$

Step 4. Calculate molecular weights to establish stoichiometric mass ratios.

Answer: MW: C_8H_{10} = 106
5.25 0_2 = 168
1.05 NH_3 = 17.85

Step 5. Calculate the number of pounds of oxygen, ammonia, and phosphorus necessary to degrade the hydrocarbons to be treated.

Answer: **Oxygen:** 1350 lbs. hydrocarbons (step 1) X $\frac{\text{168 lbs. } O_2 \text{ required}}{\text{106 lbs. hydrocarbons}}$ (step 4)

= **2140 lbs. oxygen** (See Table 3 for oxygen requirements for varying levels of contamination and soil volume. See Table 2 for air flow rates which will satisfy these oxygen requirements.)

Ammonia: 1350 lbs. hydrocarbons X $\frac{\text{17.85 lbs. } NH_3 \text{ required}}{\text{106 lbs. hydrocarbons}}$

= 227 lbs. (as ammonia)

or 227 lbs. ammonia X (14 lbs. nitrogen/17 lbs. ammonia)

= 187 lbs. (as nitrogen) (See Table 5 for nitrogen requirements for varying levels of contamination and soil volume.)

Phosphorus: $\frac{\text{1 lb. phosphorous required}}{\text{6 lbs. nitrogen required}}$ X 187 lbs. nitrogen required

= 31 lbs. phosphorous (See Table 7 for phosphorous requirements for varying levels of contamination and soil volume.)

A site contaminated with 1350 pounds of hydrocarbons, having an having an average composition of C_8H_{10}, will require 2140 lbs. of oxygen. The nutrient needs are 187 pounds of nitrogen and 31 pounds of phosphorus.

Step 6. Calculate the number of pounds of fertilizer necessary to degrade 1350 pounds of hydrocarbons.

Answer: Based on the requirement for a 6:1 nitrogen:phosphorous ratio, and the prepackaged fertilizers which are available, 19:3:3 fertilizer is chosen.

$$\text{Amount Fertilizer Required (lbs.)} = \text{Amount Nitrogen Required} \times \frac{\text{100 lbs. 19:3:3 fertilizer}}{\text{19 lbs. nitrogen}}$$

$$\text{Amount Fertilizer Required (lbs.)} = \text{187 lbs. Nitrogen Required} \times \frac{\text{100 lbs. 19:3:3 fertilizer}}{\text{19 lbs. nitrogen}}$$

$$= \text{984 lbs. 19:3:3 fertilizer}$$

(See Table 1 in Appendix A for fertilizer requirements for varying levels of contamination and soil volume.)

Nutrient Requirements for Fuel Oil-Contaminated Soil

The calculations for required nutrients for fuel oil-contaminated soil are illustrated in this appendix using the following example problem.

Example Problem

Estimate the nutrient needs for bioremediation of 100 yd.^{3} of silty sand contaminated with fuel oil, where TPH results indicate 5000 ppm contamination.

Assumptions:

For hydrocarbons, oxygen is the appropriate electron acceptor and aerobic microbial activity is the appropriate metabolic mode for destruction of the hydrocarbons. Ammonia is the preferred source of nitrogen. Hydrocarbons oxidize relatively quickly; therefore, a value for f_s of .5 is selected, hence f_e = .5. Based on average compositions of fuel oil, the overall chemical composition of gasoline can be estimated as $C_{10} H_8$ (naphthalene). (See Appendix D) Assume soil density is average, i.e., 100 lb/ft^3.

Step 1. Determine the amount of hydrocarbons to be treated.

Answer: Total Mass Hydrocarbons(HC) = Average Concentration Hydrocarbons(HC) X Soil Density X Soil Volume

$$\text{Total} = \frac{5000 \text{ lbs. HC}}{1\text{X}10^6 \text{ lbs. Soil}} \times \frac{100 \text{ lbs. Soil}}{\text{ft}^3} \times 100 \text{ yd}^3 \text{ Soil} \times \frac{27 \text{ ft}^3}{\text{yd.}^3} \text{ Hydrocarbons}$$

= 1350 lbs. Hydrocarbons (See Table 1 for amount of hydrocarbons to be treated for varying levels of contamination and soil volume.)

Step 2. Write the appropriate half reactions and the equation for cell growth using the yield fractions, f_e and f_s.

For $C_aH_bO_cN_d$, $e = 4a + b - 2c - 3d$

for $C_{10}H_8$; $a = 10, b = 8, c = 0, d = 0$

Answer: $e = 4(10) + 8 = 48$

Half Reaction of Electron Donor (H_D):

H_D: $1/e\ (C_aH_bO_cN_d) + 2(a\text{-}c)/e\ (H_2O) = a/e\ (CO_2) + (d/e)\ (NH_3) + H^+ + e^-$

$$H_D: 1/48\ C_{10}H_8 + 20/48\ H_2O = 10/48\ CO_2 + H^+ + e^-$$

Half Reaction of Electron Acceptor (H_A) for Aerobic Reaction:

$f_e = .5$ H_A: $1/4\ O_2 + H^+ + e^- = 1/2\ H_2O$

$$f_eH_a: 1/8\ O_2 + 1/2\ H^+ + 1/2\ e^- = 1/4\ H_2O$$

Cell Synthesis Equation (Cs) for Ammonia as Nitrogen Source:

$f_e = .5$ Cs: $1/4\ CO_2 + 1/20\ NH_3 + H^+ + e^- = 1/20\ C_5H_7O_2N + 2/5\ H_2O$

$$\text{feCs}: 1/8\ CO_2 + 1/40\ NH_3 + 1/2\ H^+ + 1/2e^- = 1/40\ C_5H_7O_2N + 1/5\ H_2O$$

Step 3. Write the overall reaction by summation of half reactions and cell growth equation.

Answer: $1/48\ C_8H_{10} + 1/8\ 0_2 + 1/40\ NH_3 = 1/40\ C_5H_70_2N + 1/12\ CO_2 + 1/30\ H_20$

Simplifying, one obtains the overall stoichiometric redox equation as:

$$5\ C_8H_{10} + 30\ O_2 + 6\ NH_3 = 6\ C_5H_7O_2N + 20\ CO_2 + 8\ H_2O$$

for 1 lb. HC, the overall stoichiometric redox equation for fuel oil (represented as $C_{10}H_8$) is:

$$C_{10}H_8 + 6\,O_2 + 1.2\,NH_3 = 1.2\,C_5H_7O_2N + 4\,CO_2 + 1.6\,H_2O$$

Step 4. Calculate molecular weights to establish stoichiometric mass ratios.

Answer: MW: $C_{10}H_8$ = 128
$6\,O_2$ = 192
$1.2\,NH_3$ = 20.4

Step 5. Calculate the number of pounds of oxygen, ammonia, and phosphorus necessary to degrade the hydrocarbons to be treated.

Answer: **Oxygen:** $1350 \text{ lbs. hydrocarbons (step 1)} \times \dfrac{192 \text{ lbs. } O_2 \text{ required}}{128 \text{ lbs. hydrocarbons}}$ (step 4)

= **2025 lbs. oxygen** (See Table 4 for oxygen requirements for varying levels of contamination and soil volume. See Table 2 for air flow rates which will satisfy these oxygen requirements.)

Ammonia: $1350 \text{ lbs. hydrocarbons} \times \dfrac{20.4 \text{ lbs. } NH_3 \text{ required}}{128 \text{ lbs. hydrocarbons}}$

= **215 lbs. (as ammonia)**

or **215 lbs. ammonia X (14 lbs. nitrogen/17 lbs. ammonia)**

= **177 lbs. (as nitrogen)** (See Table 6 for nitrogen requirements for varying levels of contamination and soil volume.)

Phosphorus: $\dfrac{1 \text{ lb. phosphorous required}}{6 \text{ lbs. nitrogen required}} \times 177 \text{ lbs. nitrogen required}$

= **30 lbs. phosphorous** (See Table 8 for phosphorous requirements for varying levels of contamination and soil volume.)

A site contaminated with 1350 pounds of hydrocarbons, having an having an average composition of $C_{10}H_8$, will require 2025 lbs. of oxygen. The nutrient needs are 177 pounds of nitrogen and 30 pounds of phosphorus.

Step 6. Calculate the number of pounds of fertilizer necessary to degrade 1350 pounds of hydrocarbons.

Answer: **Based on the requirement for a 6:1 nitrogen:phosphorous ratio, and the prepackaged fertilizers which are available, 19:3:3 fertilizer is chosen.**

$$\text{Amount Fertilizer Required (lbs.)} = \text{Amount Nitrogen Required} \times \frac{\text{100 lbs. 19:3:3 fertilizer}}{\text{19 lbs. nitrogen}}$$

$$\text{Amount Fertilizer Required (lbs.)} = \text{177 lbs. Nitrogen Required} \times \frac{\text{100 lbs. 19:3:3 fertilizer}}{\text{19 lbs. nitrogen}}$$

= **932 lbs. 19:3:3 fertilizer** (See Table 1 in Appendix B for fertilizer requirements for varying levels of contamination and soil volume.)

Hydrocarbon Loads

Table 21.C1 lists the amounts of hycrocarbons to be treated for varying levels of contamination and amounts of soil. This information is used to calculate nutrient needs for degradation of petroleum projects. Soil density is assumed to be 100 lb/ft^3, and total hydrocarbons are calculated as follows:

$$Total\ HC's\ (lbs.) = TPH\ (ppm)\ x\ Soil\ Density\ (\frac{lb}{ft^3})\ x\ Soil\ Volume\ (ft^3)\ x\ 27\ \frac{ft^3}{yd^3} \quad (6)$$

Table 21.C1: Amount of Hydrocarbons to be Treated (lbs.)

		Volume of Contaminated Soil (yd.^{3})							
		30	40	50	60	70	80	90	100
Total Petroleum Hydrocarbons (TPH) (ppm)	1000	81	108	135	162	189	216	243	270
	2000	162	216	270	324	378	432	486	540
	3000	243	324	405	486	567	648	729	810
	4000	324	432	540	648	756	864	972	1080
	5000	405	540	675	810	945	1080	1215	1350
	6000	486	648	810	972	1134	1296	1458	1620
	7000	567	756	945	1134	1323	1512	1701	1890
	8000	648	864	1080	1296	1512	1728	1944	2160
	9000	729	972	1215	1458	1701	1944	2187	2430
	10000	810	1080	1350	1620	1890	2160	2430	2700
	12500	1013	1350	1688	2025	2363	2700	3038	3375
	15000	1215	1620	2025	2430	2835	3240	3645	4050
	17500	1418	1890	2363	2835	3308	3780	4253	4725
	20000	1620	2160	270	3240	3780	4320	4860	5400

Oxygen Requirements and Flow Rates

Table 21.C2 represents the amount of oxygen delivered for various pump flow rates. Based on the oxygen requirements found in Tables 21.C-3 and 21.C-4, and the operating capabilities of a 1 hp pump, a 1 hp pump can be operated at a low flow rate to meet the oxygen requirements.

Table 21.C2: Oxygen Supplied by Pump System

Gas Flow ($scfm_{air}$)	Oxygen Delivered (lbs/day)
1	23
5	117
10	233
20	467
50	1170
100	2330

Source: Brown, R.A. and Crosbie, J.R. (1989)

Table 21.C3 lists the amounts of oxygen required for the bioremediation of varying levels of gasoline oil contamination and varying amounts of soil to be treated. Assumptions include: soil density = 100 lb/ft^3, and average composition for gasoline is C_8H_{10}.

$$Amount\ O_2 = Amount\ HC's\ x\ \left(\frac{168\ lbs.\ O_2\ Required}{106\ lbs.\ HC's}\right) \tag{7}$$

Table 21.C3: Amount of Oxygen Required to Treat Gasoline-Contaminated Soil (lbs.)

		Volume of Soil (yd.^{3})							
		30	40	50	60	70	80	90	100
Total Petroleum Hydrocarbons (TPH) (ppm)	1000	128	171	214	257	300	342	385	428
	2000	257	342	428	514	599	685	770	856
	3000	385	514	642	770	899	1027	1155	1284
	4000	514	685	856	1027	1198	1369	1541	1712
	5000	642	856	1070	1284	1498	1712	1926	2140
	6000	770	1027	1284	1541	1797	2054	2311	2568
	7000	899	1198	1498	1797	2097	2396	2696	2995
	8000	1027	1369	1712	2054	2396	2739	3081	3423
	9000	1155	1541	1926	2311	2696	3081	3466	3851
	10000	1284	1712	2140	2568	2995	3423	3851	4279
	12500	1605	2140	2675	3209	3744	4279	4814	5349
	15000	1926	2568	3209	3851	4493	5135	5777	6419
	17500	2247	2995	3744	4493	5242	5991	6740	7489
	20000	2568	3423	4279	5135	5991	6847	7703	8558

Table 21.C4 lists the amounts of oxygen required for the bioremediation of varying levels of fuel oil contamination and varying amounts of soil to be treated. Assumptions include: soil density = 100 lb/ft^3, and average composition for fuel oil is $C_{10}H_8$.

$$Amount\ O_2 = Amount\ HC's\ x\ (\frac{192\ lbs.\ O_2\ Required}{128\ lbs.\ HC's}) \tag{8}$$

Table 21.C4: Amount of Oxygen Required to Treat Fuel Oil-Contaminated Soil (lbs.)

		Volume of Soil (yd.^{3})							
		30	40	50	60	70	80	90	100
Total Petroleum Hydrocarbons (TPH) (ppm)	1000	122	162	203	243	284	324	365	405
	2000	243	324	405	486	567	648	720	810
	3000	365	486	608	729	851	972	1094	1215
	4000	486	648	810	972	1134	1296	1458	1620
	5000	608	810	1013	1215	1418	1620	1823	2025
	6000	729	972	1215	1458	1701	1944	2187	2430
	7000	851	1134	1418	1701	1985	2268	2552	2835
	8000	972	1296	1620	1944	2268	2592	2916	3240
	9000	1094	1458	1823	2187	2552	2916	3281	3645
	10000	1215	1620	2025	2430	2835	3240	3645	4050
	12500	1519	2025	2531	3038	3544	4050	4556	5063
	15000	1823	2430	3038	3645	4253	4860	5468	6075
	17500	2126	2835	3544	4253	4961	5670	6379	7088
	20000	2430	3240	4050	4860	5670	6480	7290	8100

Nitrogen Requirements

Table 21.C5 lists the amounts of nitrogen required for the bioremedation of varying levels of gasoline contamination and varying amounts of soil to be treated. Assumptions include soil density = 100 lb/ft^3, and average compositon for gasoline is C_8H_{10}.

$$Amount\ N_2 = Amount\ HC's\ x\ (\frac{14\ lbs.\ N_2}{17\ lbs.\ NH_3})\ x\ (\frac{17.85\ lbs.\ NH_3\ Required}{106\ lbs.\ HC's}) \quad (9)$$

Table 21.C5: Amount of Nitrogen Required to Treat Gasoline-Contaminated Soil (lbs.)

		Volume of Contaminated Soil (yd.^{3})							
		30	40	50	60	70	80	90	100
Total Petroleum Hydrocarbons (TPH) (ppm)	1000	11	15	19	22	26	30	34	37
	2000	22	30	37	45	52	60	67	75
	3000	34	45	56	67	79	90	101	112
	4000	45	60	75	90	105	120	135	150
	5000	56	75	94	112	131	150	168	187
	6000	67	90	112	135	157	180	202	225
	7000	79	105	131	157	183	210	236	262
	8000	90	120	150	180	210	240	270	300
	9000	101	135	168	202	236	270	303	337
	10000	112	150	187	225	262	300	337	374
	12500	140	187	234	281	328	374	421	468
	15000	168	225	281	337	393	449	505	562
	17500	197	262	328	393	459	524	590	655
	20000	225	300	374	449	524	599	674	749

Table 21.C6 lists the amounts of nitrogen required for the bioremediation of varying levels of fuel oil contamination and varying amounts of soil to be treated. Assumptions include soil density = 100 lb/ft^3, and average composition for fuel oil is $C_{10}H_8$.

Table 21.C6: Amount of Nitrogen Required to Treat Fuel Oil-Contaminated Soil (lbs.)

		Volume of Soil (yd.^{3})							
		30	40	50	60	70	80	90	100
Total Petroleum Hydrocarbons (TPH) (ppm)	1000	11	14	18	21	25	28	32	35
	2000	21	28	35	43	50	57	64	71
	3000	32	43	53	64	74	85	96	106
	4000	43	57	71	85	99	113	128	142
	5000	53	71	89	106	124	142	159	177
	6000	64	85	106	128	149	170	191	213
	7000	74	99	124	149	174	198	223	248
	8000	85	113	142	170	198	227	255	284
	9000	96	128	159	191	223	255	287	319
	10000	106	142	177	213	248	284	319	354
	12500	133	177	221	266	310	354	399	443
	15000	159	213	266	319	372	425	478	532
	17500	186	248	310	372	434	496	558	620
	20000	213	284	354	425	496	567	638	709

$$Amount\ P = \frac{Amount\ N_2}{6} \tag{11}$$

Phosphorous Requirements

Table 21.C7 lists the amounts of phosphorous required for the bioremediation of varying levels of gasoline contamination and varying amounts of soil to be treated. Assumptions include soil density = 110 lb/ft^3, and average composition for gasoline is C_8H_{10}.

Table 21.C7: Amount of Phosphorous Required to Treat Gasoline-Contaminated Soil (lbs.)

		Volume of Soil (yd.^{3})							
		30	40	50	60	70	80	90	100
Total Petroleum Hydrocarbons (TPH) (ppm)	1000	2	2	3	4	4	5	6	6
	2000	4	5	6	7	9	10	11	12
	3000	6	7	9	11	13	15	17	19
	4000	7	10	12	15	17	20	22	25
	5000	9	12	16	19	22	25	28	31
	6000	11	15	19	22	26	30	34	37
	7000	13	17	22	26	31	35	39	44
	8000	15	20	25	30	35	40	45	50
	9000	17	22	28	34	39	45	51	56
	10000	19	25	31	37	44	50	56	62
	12500	23	31	39	47	55	62	70	78
	15000	28	37	47	56	66	75	84	94
	17500	33	44	55	66	76	87	98	109
	20000	37	50	62	75	87	100	112	125

Table 21.C8 lists the amounts of phosphorous required for the bioremediation of varying levels of contamination and varying amounts of soil to be treated.

Assumptions include soil density = 100 lb/ft^3, and average composition for fuel oil is $C_{10}H_8$.

$$Amount\ P = \frac{Amount\ N_2}{6} \tag{12}$$

Table 21.C8: Amount of Phosphorous Required to Treat Fuel Oil-Contaminated Soil (lbs.)									
		Volume of Soil (yd.^{3})							
		30	40	50	60	70	80	90	100
Total Petroleum Hydrocarbons (TPH) (ppm)	1000	2	2	3	4	4	5	5	6
	2000	4	5	6	7	8	9	11	12
	3000	5	7	9	11	12	14	16	18
	4000	7	9	12	14	17	19	21	24
	5000	9	12	15	18	21	24	27	30
	6000	11	14	18	21	25	28	32	35
	7000	12	17	21	25	29	33	37	41
	8000	14	19	24	28	33	38	43	47
	9000	16	21	27	32	37	43	48	53
	10000	18	24	30	35	41	47	53	59
	12500	22	30	37	44	52	59	66	74
	15000	27	35	44	53	62	71	80	89
	17500	31	41	52	62	72	83	93	103
	20000	35	47	59	71	83	95	106	118

Field Moisture Capacities

Table 21.C9 lists field moisture capacities for various soil types. Moisture content in soil should be maintained at 50-60% of field moisture capacity for bioremediation. Although this can be calculated, a qualitative approach to proper moisture content involves maintaining the soil at a wet, not puddly, state.

Table 21.C9: Average Field Capacities

Soil Texture	Field Capacity
Clay	22.3
Silty Clay	39.4
Sandy Clay	30.2
Silty Clay Loam	25.3
Clay Loam	12.6
Sandy Clay Loam	14.4
Silty Loam	24.2
Loam	22.2
Silt	24.3
Sandy Loam	17.2
Loamy Sand	9.0
Sand	5.2

Source: McDole, Robert E. and McMaster, G.M., Idaho Cooperative Extension Service, Published and Distributed in Furtherance of the Acts of May 8 and June 30, 1914.

APPENDIX D

Small-Scale Bioremediation
Chemical Composition of Petroleum Products

Calculating Overall Chemical Composition for Gasoline

Nutrient requirements are estimated based on balancing a redox stoichiometric equation which includes a hydrocarbon which best represents the overall chemical composition of the contaminant to be remediated. The overall chemical composition can be estimated by calculating the weighted average of all components of the contaminant with a mass fraction of 5% or more. Using the weighted average, a hydrocarbon with similar molecular weight and structure as these components is chosen to represent the overall chemical composition of the contaminant.

$$\text{Weighted Average} = \frac{\text{Total [Percent by Weight X Molecular Weight] for Components} \geq 5\%}{\text{Total Percent by Weight}}$$

Overall Chemical Composition is selected based on weighted average and structure of components used in weighted average calculation.

The following calculations were performed to estimate overall chemical composition for regular and unleaded gasoline. Compositions of these substances are tabulated on the following page. Because compositions are given as ranges, calculations were performed based on high range and mid-range for components with a mass fraction of 5% or more.

Regular Gasoline:

Weighted Average (Based on Average Component Compositions)

$$= \frac{(6.7)(92.1) \quad + \quad (8.2)(106.2)}{14.9} = 99.9$$

Based on the weighted average and structure of these components, Xylene is chosen to represent the overall composition of regular gasoline.

Weighted Average (Based on High Component Compositions)

$$= \frac{(10)(92.1) \quad + \quad (11)(106.2)}{21} = 99.5$$

Based on the weighted average and structure of these components, Xylene is chosen to represent the overall composition of regular gasoline.

Unleaded Gasoline:

Weighted Average (Based on Average Component)

$$= \frac{(8.2)(92.1) \quad + \quad (11.7)(106.2)}{19.9} = 100.4$$

Based on the weighted average and structure of these components, Xylene is chosen to represent the overall composition of unleaded gasoline.

Weighted Average (Based on Average Component Compositions)

$$= \frac{(12)(92.1) + (16)(106.2)}{28} = 100.16$$

Based on the weighted average and structure of these components, Xylene is chosen to represent the overall composition of unleaded gasoline.

Overall Chemical Composition for Fuel Oil

Based on EPA Method 8270 results of many fuel oil samples, naphthalene is a semi-volatile component found in significant concentrations on a regular basis. There are many other heavier straight-chain compounds which would require greater amounts of nutrients; however, there are no specific analytical tests for these compounds. Therefore, naphthalene ($C_{10}H_8$) is chosen to represent the overall composition of fuel oil for the purpose of calculating nutrient needs for biodegradation.

Table 21.D1: Characteristic Components of Five Petroleum Fuels

Component	Molecular Weight	Regular Gasoline (Six Samples) percent by weight			Unleaded Gasoline (Three Samples) percent by weight			Aviation Gasoline (One Sample) percent by weight	Kerosene (Three Samples) percent by weight	Diesel No. 2 (Three Samples) percent by weight
		high	low avg.		high avg.	low				
Benzene	78.11	0.47	3.6		<0.2	3.2		<0.2	<0.2	<0.2
Toluene	92.10	3.40	10.0	6.7	4.4	12		17	0.23 - 0.44	<0.2
Ethylbenzene	106.17	1.50	3.1		1.8	4.7	8.2	0.77	0.36 - 0.38	<0.2
Xylenes	106.20	5.40	11.0	8.2	7.4	16		1.6	0.62 - 1.30	<0.2
n-Propyl benzene	120.20	0.64	1.0		0.87	1.0		<0.2	0.25 - 0.35	<0.2
1,3,5-Trimethylbenzene	120.19	1.10	1.5		1.3	3.9	11.7	<0.2	0.51 - 1.00	<0.2
Naphthalene	128.17	0.10	0.6		0.2	0.5		0.006	0.30 - 0.60	0.140 - 0.17
Fluorene	166.22	<0.0003	0.02		<0.0003	0.007		0.0005	0.006 - 0.03	0.070 - 0.10
Phenanthrene	178.23	<0.0003	0.06		<0.0003	0.004		0.0004	0.02 - 0.03	0.260 - 0.30
Anthracene	178.23	<0.0001			<0.0001	0.00-		0.00002	<0.0001	0.013 - 0.17
Ethylene dibromide	187.86	0.015	0.02			06		0.054		
Lead	267.20	0.03	0.43					0.056		

Source: New York State Department of Environmental Conservation, Division of Water, Bureau of Spill Prevention and Response, Albany, New York, "Sampling Guidelines & Protocols: Technical Background and Quality Control/Quality Assurance For NYS DEC Spill Response Program," March 1991.

CHAPTER 22

Enhancing Site Remediation Through Radio Frequency Heating

Stephen L. Price, KAI Technologies, Inc., Woburn, Massachusetts, **Raymond S. Kasevich,** KAI Technologies, Inc., Woburn, Massachusetts, **Michael C. Marley,** VAPEX Environmental Technologies, Inc., Canton, Massachusetts

INTRODUCTION

Radio Frequency (RF) heating systems can be used *in-situ* to increase the recovery rates of oil and other environmental contaminants when combined with standard remediation techniques. RF heating provides controlled, efficient heating by directing RF energy into contaminated soil where it is efficiently converted into thermal energy. The basic components and theory of operation of an RF heating system are discussed and its usage in a recent pilot study in combination with soil vapor extraction (SVE) to enhance the recovery rate of #2 fuel oil in silty soil at a depth of 20 feet is described.

THEORY

The heating process begins by coupling RF energy, provided by a generator, into a flexible coaxial transmission line connected to a site-specific, designed antenna system. The antenna system consists of one or more RF applicators, placed into boreholes located within the contaminated region. The RF energy radiated by these applicators is then absorbed by the contaminated soil resulting in a temperature rise. This phenomenon is called dielectric heating and is the principal process used by a microwave oven for cooking food, but on a much larger scale.

The RF energy is efficiently coupled into the soil by taking the soil's dielectric properties into account in the design of the antenna system and by employing an impedance matching network. A matching network allows energy to be coupled from the generator to the antenna system by adjusting the impedance of the antenna system to correspond to that of the generator. Maintaining this match is accomplished by a computerized diagnostic and control system which responds automatically to changes in the impedance of the antenna system by retuning the matching network. The impedance variations are caused by changes in the soil's electrical properties due to heating and the removal of liquid contaminants and water. A typical single applicator RF heating system located in a vertical borehole is shown in Figure 22.1.

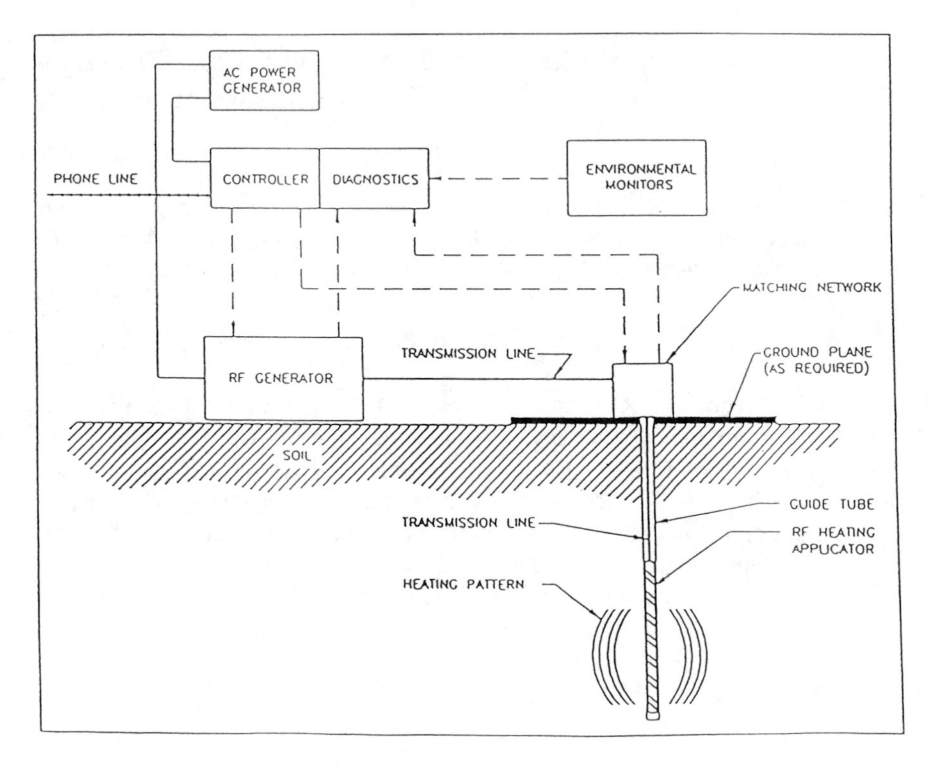

Figure 22.1. Radio frequency heating system.

The RF heating system is located in a mobile shelter and consists of a generator and equipment for control of the heating process. Power for the system is provided either by 208 or 240 volt AC utility lines or a diesel-fueled generator. Transmission lines, which feed power to applicators in the borehole, can be either rigid or flexible with diameters of 7/8-inch or 1 5/8-inch. Typically, applicators range in diameter from one to six inches, radiating element lengths from less than five feet to fifty feet long. Heating systems operate on authorized frequencies (within the ISM range) located between 6 and 40 MHz with radiated power levels of up to 25,000 watts per applicator.

Borehole diameters typically range from four to nine inches and often accommodate both an applicator and a non-metallic vapor/liquid extraction tube. These boreholes can be spaced from 10 to 50 feet apart horizontally or vertically and have lengths of up to 1,000 feet.

At sites where applicators are located near the earth's surface, shielding is employed. The metallic shielding provides for RF emission levels in compliance with OSHA (Occupational Safety and Health Administration) and FCC (Federal Communications Commission) limits.

The RF energy radiated by an applicator produces both a pattern of electromagnetic energy and a corresponding pattern of thermal energy which extends radially away from the applicator into the contaminated soil. This pattern is a function of the operating frequency, the length of the applicator and the effective dielectric constant and conductivity of the soil and its contaminants.

In an application where water is converted to steam during the RF heating, the steam plays a significant role by increasing the extent of penetration of the heating pattern from the borehole. Dielectric losses which govern how much RF energy is absorbed decrease as the water is driven out of the soil. This then allows the heating pattern to effect a greater soil volume while the steam produced increases the flow of thermal energy radially away from the borehole. Thus the presence of water in the contaminated soil has a dynamically beneficial effect on the heating pattern.

When more than one applicator is employed in the antenna system, the pattern can be adjusted to heat preferential areas within the volume. This is possible when phased array, beam steering technology, common in advanced military radar systems is applied to RF heating. With this capability, energy can be controlled to heat regions vigorously in timed sequences and create effects such as thermal stirring whereby the heating pattern is moved in time through the soils. This can be especially useful in the application of RF heating to enhance *in-situ* biodegradation through relatively low but controlled temperature rises.

Once the contaminated region has been heated from the absorption of RF energy, liquids and vapors flow toward the recovery wells because of the pressure gradients maintained by a vacuum extraction system. The volume in the immediate vicinity of the applicator becomes cooler than the surrounding volume because of heating and the removal of liquid contaminants. The heating and water removal causes a change in the electrical properties of this region, making the soil less lossy or less able to absorb the RF energy than at the beginning of heating. Numerous designs for remediation can be developed based on these principles, and site specifics will dictate the appropriate design.

Figure 22.2, shows the theoretical heating rate (°C per hour) versus the electrical field intensity (volts per meter) for several soil conductivities. The conductivity of a soil is a measure of its ability to absorb RF energy and thereby convert it to heat. This property and the relative dielectric constant of the soil is affected by the amount of water located in the soil, shown in Figure 22.3 for several different soil types and volumetric water contents. Figure 22.4 is a 3-D plot of the underground electric field distribution truncated to 100 volts per meter of an applicator located deep within a homogeneous soil.

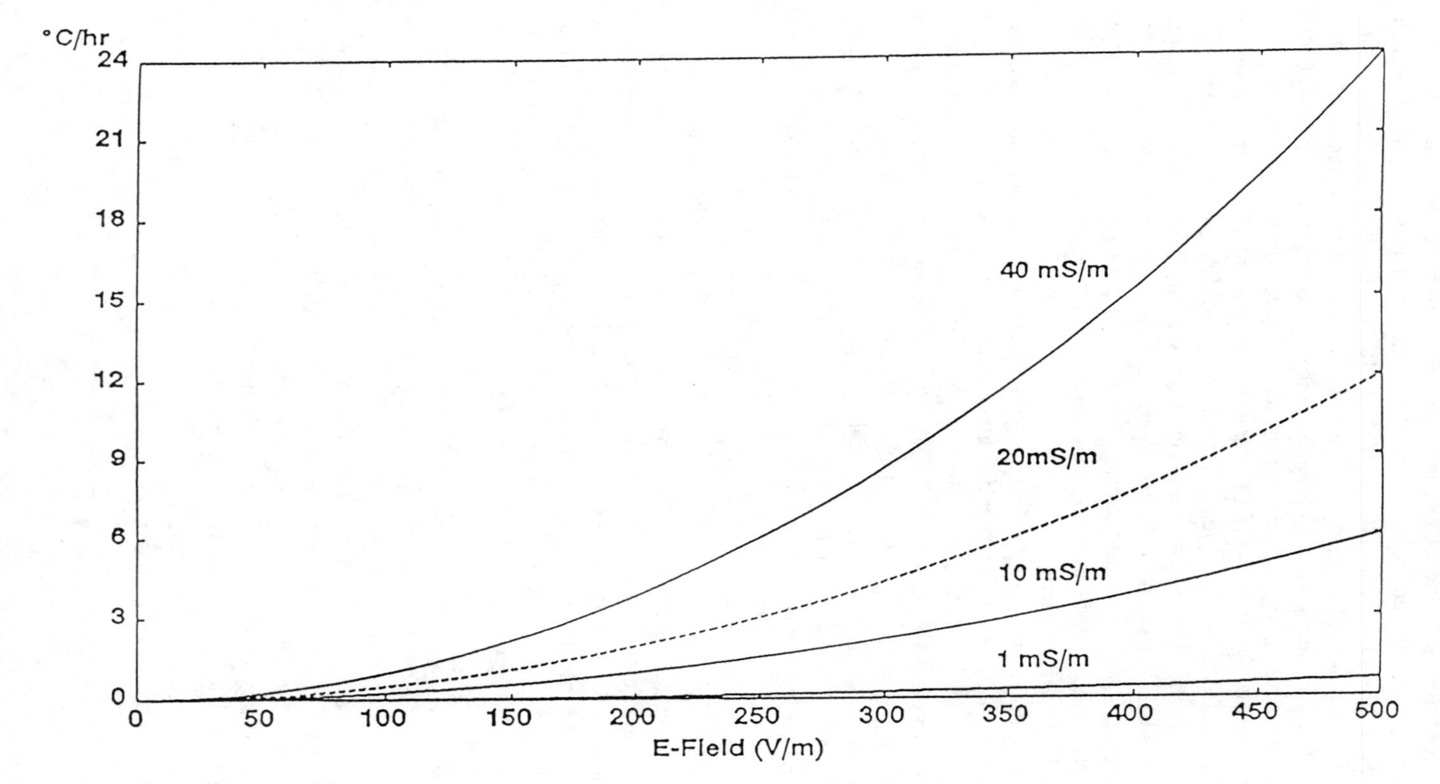

Figure 22.2. Theoretical heating rates.

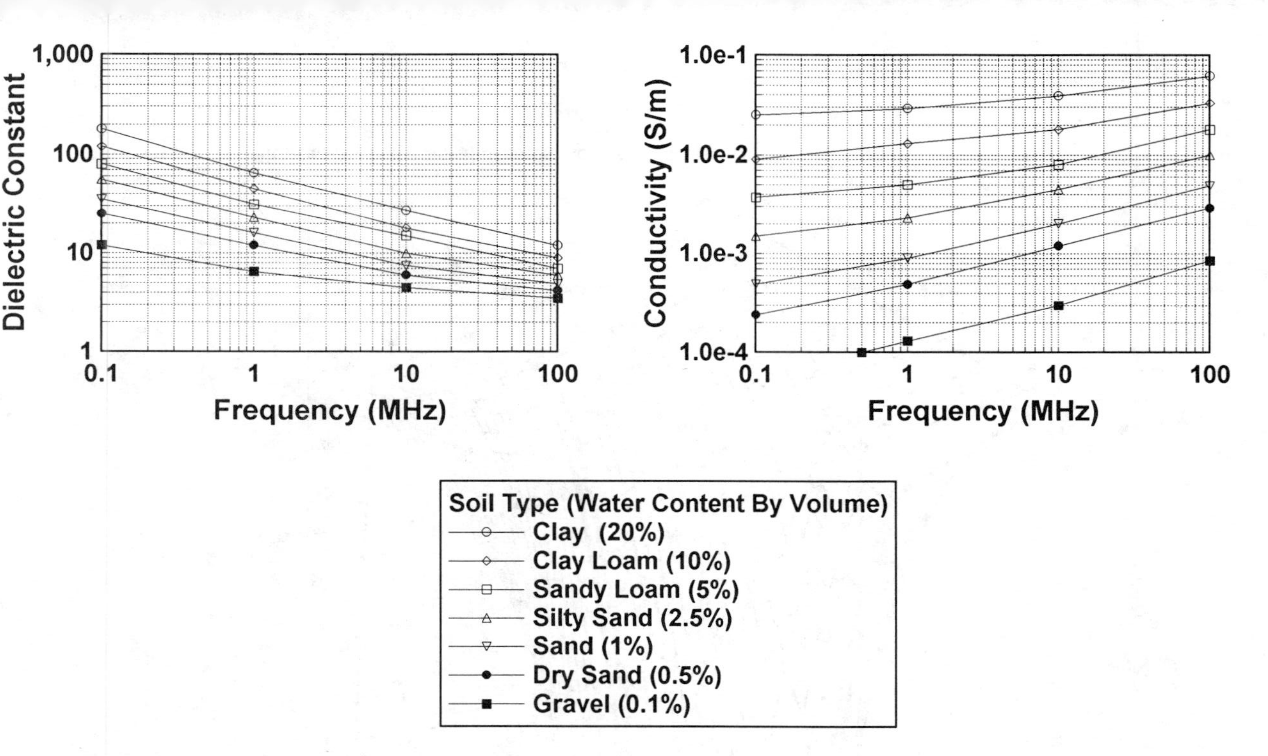

Figure 22.3. Dielectric constant and conductivity vs. frequency and water content.

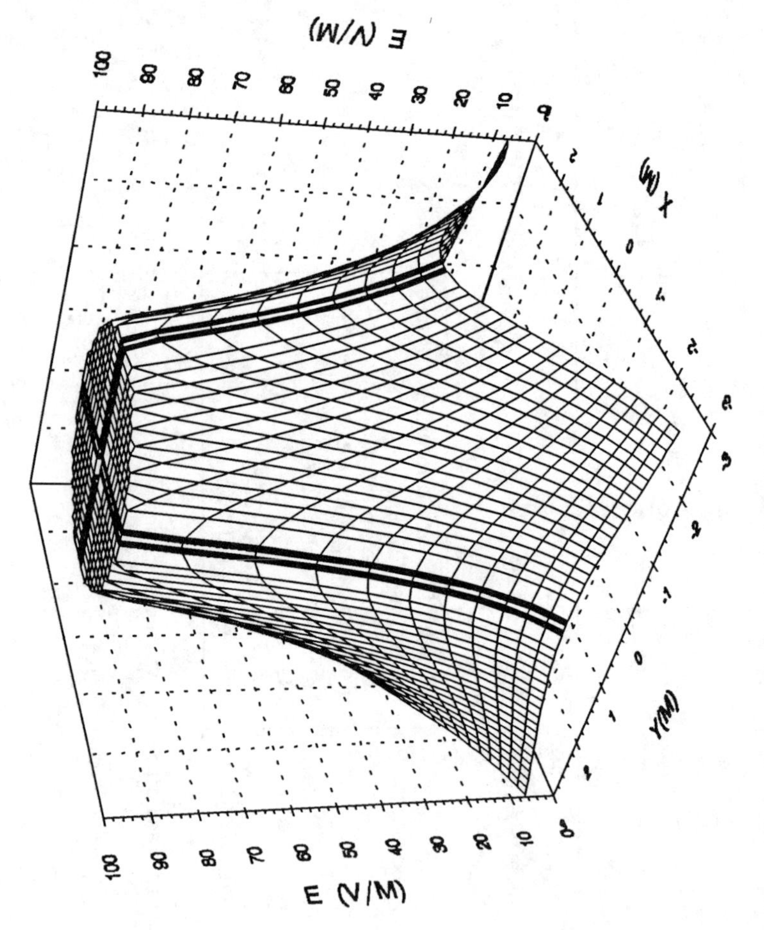

Figure 22.4. Single applicator electric field distribution.

For example, if 25 kW is delivered into soil by a single applicator with a conductivity of 10-20 mS/m at 13.56 MHz, it will cause the temperature within a radial distance of 9 m to increase although the rate of temperature change will vary and be inversely proportional to the radial distance from the applicator. In this example maximum temperature rates of 12°C per hour are achieved at radial distances of up to one meter, 3°C per hour at three meters, 0.8°C per hour at 6 meters, and 0.2°C at 9 meters during two to three weeks of continuous heating.

The above example using a single applicator does not produce uniform heating in the volume, but a system employing an array of applicators spaced three to six meters apart can achieve nearly uniform heating of a soil volume. It is estimated that a four applicator system using 100 kW at 13.56 MHz could heat a volume of 150 cubic yards of sand, with 25% water by volume, to temperatures in excess of 100°C after three weeks of operation.

The following lists the energy and time required to heat one cubic yard of representative materials using a 25 kW system at 100% efficiency.

1) Sand	- 25 kwh (from 20°C - 100°C)	1 hour
2) Water	- 100 kwh (from 20°C - 100°C)	4 hours
3) Water	- 750 kwh (to vaporize at 100°C)	30 hours
4) Heavy Oil	- 44 kwh (from 20°C - 100°C)	1.75 hours

PILOT TEST STUDY (EAST COAST)

A 25-kW, 13.56 MHz mobile RF heating system was used in a pilot test to enhance remediation by soil vapor extraction (SVE) on a #2 fuel oil plume in soil. At this site recovery rates had dropped from a thousands of gallons per hour under several feet of product head to the low hundreds of gallons per month. Given this low oil recovery rate it was uncertain how much longer the present gravitational product recovery system would be in operation before shutdown. As a result the client became interested in RF heating combined with a soil vapor recovery system to enhance the product recovery rates.

The pilot study involved three phases: bench-scale tests, low power RF heating and oil vapor recovery tests, and high-power RF heating with vapor recovery tests. The bench-scale laboratory tests determined the rate of recovery of #2 fuel oil from representative site soil samples, during RF heating system. Bench-scale testing also determined that the temperature of the contaminated soil must be 130°C for substantial oil recovery. *In-situ* low-power RF heating tests were employed to characterize the proposed high-power test area and for gaining knowledge of the electrical properties of the soils. This data was then used in the site specific design of the applicator so that it would efficiently couple RF energy into the contaminated soil located in a 5-10 feet band above the water table. Heating profiles in Figures 22.5 and 22.6 show the field measured temperature profiles at the site at the completion of high power testing.

Before installing the applicator, a four inch diameter, high temperature fiberglass borehole liner and two inch Teflon dual phase extraction tube were installed into a ten inch borehole located at the site. The Teflon extraction tube was screened from 16 to 26.5 feet below grade. The soil layer contaminated with oil was located in an approximately five foot thick region on top of the water table, which was located at 22.5 feet below grade.

Heating was controlled during the high-power tests by integrating "real time" temperature data, provided by a fiber optic temperature probe system, into the computer control system that operated the 25-kW generator. Fiber optic probes were used because the probes are not affected by the RF fields, as they have no metal parts. The control system allowed an on-board computer to monitor continuously and operate the generator and diagnostic equipment. This allowed the RF heating system to be cycled on and off to maintain a temperature of 150°C in the borehole, preventing damage to the liner. This capability also saves on labor costs.

During the two weeks of high-power testing, a total of 8000 kwh was applied to the contaminated oil region, resulting in surface recovery of oil and water. Heated soil samples (70 to 80°C) collected towards the end of the test from boreholes located at two and four feet away from the applicator had a jar headspace analysis performed on them which yielded non-detectable readings to within one or two feet from the water table. The results of this headspace analysis are shown in Table 22.1. Measurements of the permeability, porosity, and fluid saturation of the soil samples were made prior to heating (Table 22.2) and after heating (Table 22.3). When compared, they show significant reductions in the percentages of water and low levels of oil in the pore volume after heating. This water level reduced below its residual saturation value, is a strong indication that this water was converted to steam during the RF heating process.

CONCLUSION

Radio frequency (RF) heating is an efficient method of applying energy to the subsurface to heat soil. The RF can overcome many of the problems associated with the more conventional heating techniques of hot air and steam injection.

There are other potential candidates for *in-situ* RF heating which include hazardous wastes and sludges containing coal tar or fuel oil. Other applications involve reducing the viscosity of hydrocarbons in lagoons and tanks, and separating out non-nuclear wastes from mixed wastes. Furthermore, the recovery of other compounds such as gasoline, diesel fuel, hexane, benzene, toluene, ethylbenzene, carbon tetrachloride, chloroform, acetone, and methanol can be enhanced when a focused beam of RF energy is applied to the matrix. Currently, the use of RF heating for these applications is being actively pursued.

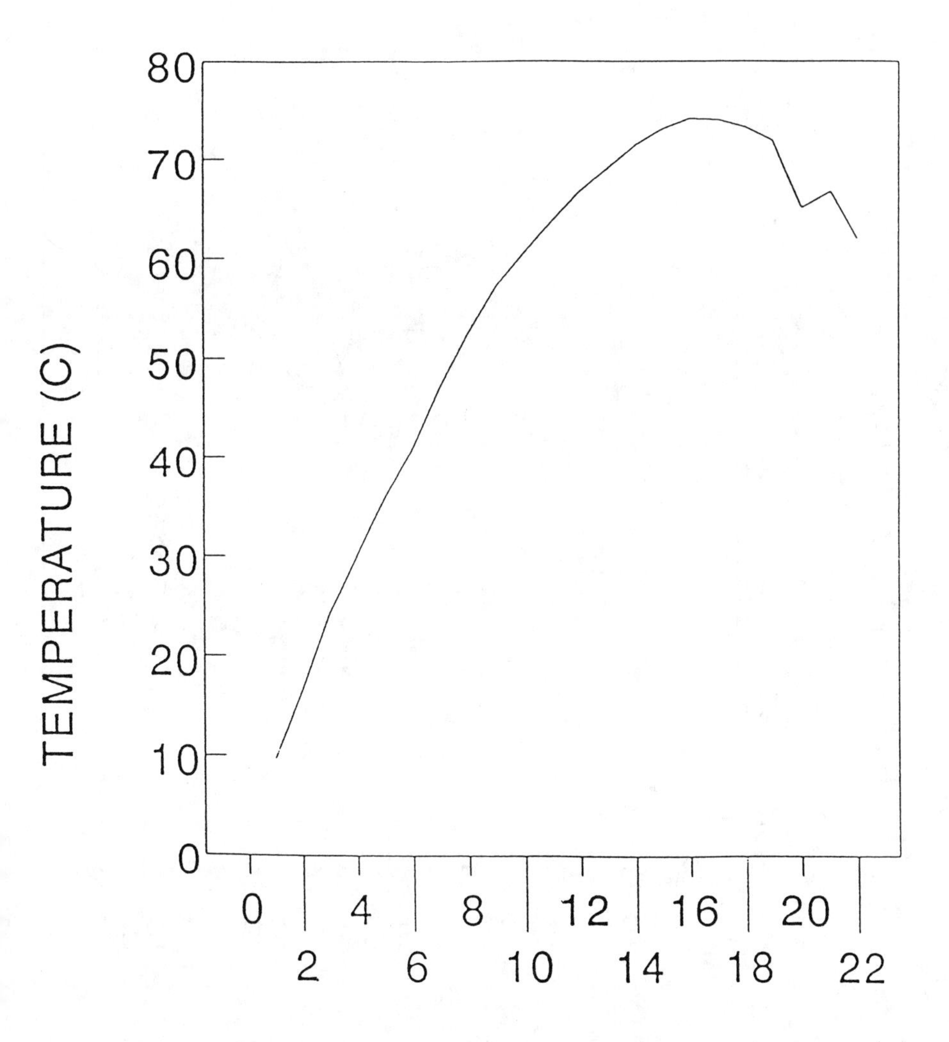

Figure 22.5. Temperature profile at RF-6 3.5 hours after test H.

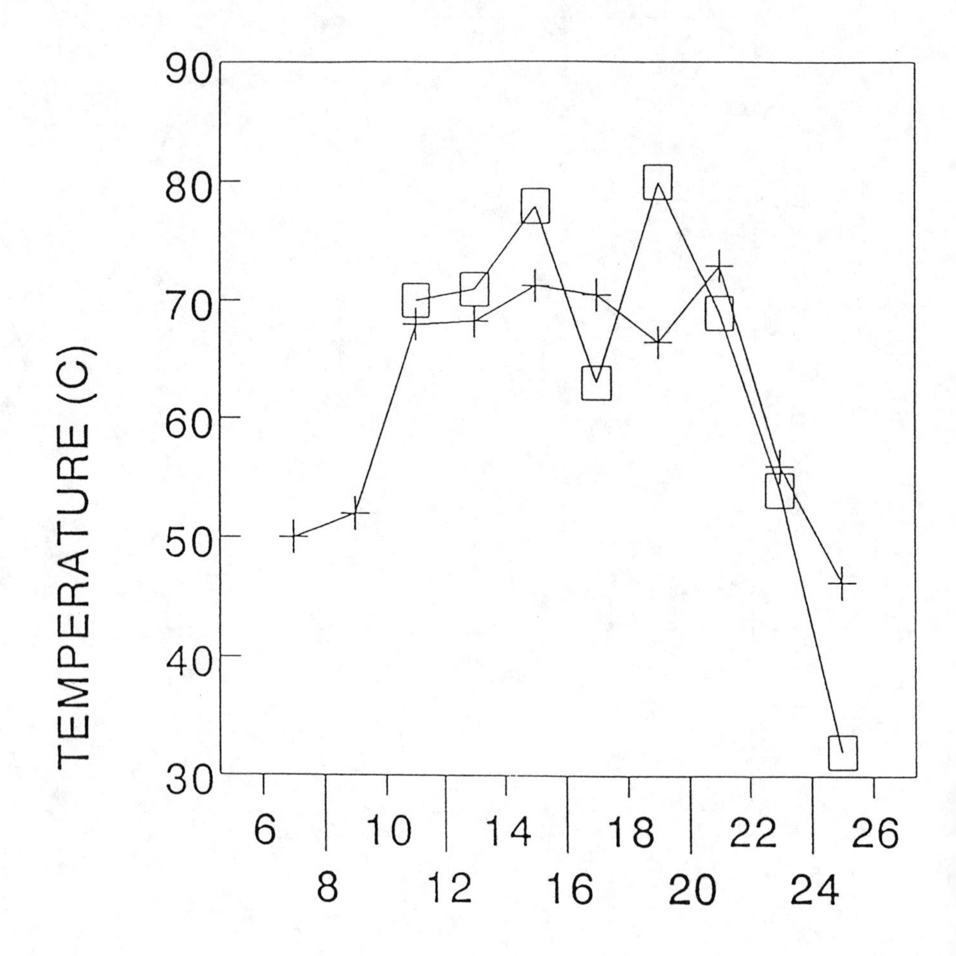

Figure 22.6. Temperature profiles at RF-6 following high power test F.

Table 22.1. Soil sample headspace analysis (from post-heating soil borings).

B1 (2 FEET FROM ANTENNA)

DEPTH (feet)	HEADSPACE** (ppmv as Benzene)
7	ND
9	ND
11	ND
13	ND
15	ND
17	ND
19	ND
21	70
23	150
25	90
Water table at 23 feet	

B2 (4 FEET FROM ANTENNA)

DEPTH (feet)	HEADSPACE** (ppmv as Benzene)
7	ND
9	ND
11	ND
13	ND
15	ND
17	ND
19	20
21	50
22	90
23	300
23	200
Water table at 22.5 feet	

Note: Analysis performed utilizing a model HW101 HNU with a 10.2ev Photo–ionization detector, calibrated to benzene.

** Headspace analysis was performed on soil samples at approximately 70 to 80 degrees celsius.

Table 22.2. Pre-test soil characteristics.

Sample	Depth	Perm	Por	Residual Sat. Percent Pore		O/W	Total	Grain	
Number	Feet	KA md	%P.V.	Oil	Water	Ratio	Liquid	Den	Description
1	22'	5665.4	33.1	6.5	31.1	0.21	37.6	2.69	Sd tan vf–mgr slslty mstn dyel flu
2	23'	1140.3	35.7	36.5	53.1	0.69	89.5	2.68	Sd tan vf–fgr/gran slty mstn dyel flu
3	24	468.5	34.3	9.6	77.3	0.12	86.9	2.68	Sd tan vfgr slty mstn dyel flu
4	25	442.9	37.3	17.9	66.5	0.27	84.4	2.68	Same

Table 22.3. Post-test soil characteristics.

Sample Number	Depth Feet	Perm KA md	Por %P.V.	Residual Sat. Percent Pore		O/W Ratio	Total Liquid	Grain Den	Description
				Oil	Water				
1	19'	14635.9	29.8	3.5	4.7	0.75	8.2	2.72	Sd tan f–vegr/pbls 1 stn dyel flu
2	21'	13234.2	35.6	5.3	6.7	0.79	11.9	2.68	Sd tan f–mgr/vegrs 1 stu dyel flu
3	23	2213.1	39.4	13.4	85.4	0.16	98.8	2.68	Sd tan vf–fgr alslty 1 stu dyel flu
4	25'	2003.1	37.7	1.6	92.4	0.02	94.0	2.68	Same
5	17'	17215.6	31.3	1.0	16.6	0.06	17.5	2.69	Sd tan f–vegr/pbls 1 stu dyel sp flu
6	21'	7814.4	35.9	7.9	11.2	0.70	19.1	2.69	Sd tan f–mgr/vegrs 1 stu dyel flu
7	22'	13255.5	28.9	6.7	3.0	2.26	9.6	2.69	Sd tan f–vegr/pbls 1 stu dyel flu
8	23'	8656.7	40.3	29.5	54.5	0.54	84.0	2.67	Sd tan vf–fgr alslty 1 stu dyel flu

CHAPTER 23

Extensive Review of Treatment Technologies For the Removal of Hydrocarbons From Soil

Dennis I. Rubin, Woodward-Clyde Consultants, Wayne, New Jersey, **Gonzalo J. Mon,** Public Service Electric and Gas Company, Newark, New Jersey

INTRODUCTION

During the past several years, the number of innovative technologies for the treatment of hydrocarbons in soils has been steadily increasing. While several of these technologies have matured to the point of regulatory acceptance and commercial viability, the number of emerging technologies continues to rise at an ever increasing rate. With conflicting assertions and claims of success, the private regulated community continues to struggle to determine an appropriate strategy for the remediation of contaminated sites.

In 1990, Public Service Electric and Gas Company of New Jersey confronted with the obligation to remediate former manufactured gas plants began an analysis of technologies suitable for the treatment of hydrocarbon contaminated soils. It was established, during Remedial Investigations, that both volatile organic compounds (VOCs) and semi volatile compounds (SVOCs) were contaminants of concern. However, based upon the results of these investigations, it became evident that, because of their carcinogen potential, the treatment of four, five, and six ring polynuclear aromatic hydrocarbons (PAHs) would drive the remediation of the site. It was additionally recognized that any technology that could treat SVOC contamination would logically treat VOC contamination as well.

INITIAL SCREENING CRITERIA

In order to establish an initial methodology to screen potential technologies, five fundamental criteria were applied:

- Technical Feasibility;
- Assessment of Risk Reducing Capability;
- Assessment of Regulatory Requirements;
- Commercial Viability; and,
- Cost Effectiveness.

Technical Feasibility

Technical feasibility, simply stated, determines if the alternative under consideration relies on demonstrated or experimental technologies, and have prior demonstrations of the technology involving similar wastes. It should be noted that, while a specific technology may be patented, or in some form use a proprietary process, there are often direct competing technologies using the same basic concepts. An example of this is thermal desorption. Several vendors now offer this basic technology, even though parts of their individual processes may be protected by patents. In the case of thermal desorption, these patents often relate to the flue gas discharge or the thermal input design of the unit.

In context of this study, the ability of a technology to achieve a specific cleanup level became of predominant importance.

When evaluating the effectiveness of any technology, the site-specific cleanup standard determines the acceptability of the technology. Cleanup standards are regulatory compliance end points, and their derivation varies considerably from jurisdiction to jurisdiction. For example, The New Jersey Department of Environmental Protection and Energy has recently promulgated soil cleanup criteria for all environmental programs within the State. These criteria are risk based numeric standards (Table 23.1). Outside of New Jersey, other states have adopted the philosophy of site-specific health-based risk analyses to determine cleanup standards. Similarly, other states allow for the negotiation of a cleanup standard based upon the removal of a percentage of the contamination (i.e., 95% or 99.9999%), or simply utilize perceived standards that purport to be protective of human health and the environment. This divergence in cleanup standards leads to the situation where what is "clean" in one jurisdiction requires remediation in another and, consequently, a technology that may be totally appropriate in one state is completely unsuitable in another. However, regardless of the cleanup standard, it is almost a universal truth that the lower the cleanup standard, the fewer the treatment options available to meet that criteria.

Coupled with different state standards, many innovative technologies have had limited field applications, and it is often difficult for a vendor to accept that, while their technology was successful in one application, it is inappropriate in another.

For our evaluation, our basis for determining technical feasibility was compliance with the soil cleanup criteria used within the State of New Jersey. Therefore, our evaluation of vendor claims of successful projects or demonstrations were often divergent with their assertions.

Assessment of Risk Reducing Capability

A technology was also evaluated to determine to what extent the alternative reduces the potential public health or environmental risks *or generates new risks*. In several instances, technologies generate, through concentration or reformation of contaminants, waste streams that are hazardous wastes or are more contaminated than the source feed stock. In these instances, the technology was considered a volume reduction technology rather than a treatment technology.

Table 23.1. Selected New Jersey soil cleanup criteria.

Volatile Organic Compounds		
Benzene	3	mg/kg
Xylenes (Total)	410	mg/kg
Semi-Volatile Organic Compounds		
Benzo (a) anthracene	0.9	mg/kg
Benzo (a) pyrene	0.66	mg/kg
Benzo (b) fluoranthene	0.9	mg/kg
Dibenz (a,h) anthracene	0.66	mg/kg

Assessment of Regulatory Requirements

A technology must also be assessed in light of federal, state, or local laws that might delay or block the implementation of the technology. A common denominator in many of the technologies evaluated was the necessity, or expectation, of obtaining an air quality permit or variance from local land use ordinances.

The assessment of regulatory requirements should not be confused with the issue of public acceptance, although they may be closely related. Many, but not all, permit processes legally require public hearings or public notice. In these forums, issues not directly related to the permit in question may be raised and take on a controlling or dominant role in the permitting process. The effectiveness of a public outreach program, when warranted, is subjective and was not used in our evaluation of technologies.

Commercial Viability

When technical feasibility is verified, the question of "commercially available" must be evaluated. The authors wish to note that our assessment of commercially available may differ from what the technology vendors may claim. A technology that no one is using, or at least pilot testing, would not meet our definition of commercially available.

Emerging technologies, by definition, are not commercially available. Innovative technologies may be commercially available, but, in several instances, were found to be undercapitalized and had neither the financial nor the technical resources to achieve commercial acceptance.

This phenomena has manifested itself with the genesis of technologies that the authors have concluded are in the business of "treatability studies". The authors agree that treatability studies are often necessary for the determination of process operating parameters, or to determine treatment costs; however, when a large investment in treatability studies is required to demonstrate the technical feasibility of a technology, serious questions concerning the economic long-term viability of the process must be raised.

Accepted technologies are those that, by common business standards, are economically viable. Often this means that competitive bids or competitive negotiations can be obtained from more than one vendor.

Cost Effectiveness

Many treatment alternatives are simply not cost effective. During early development and testing, a number of thermal processes (i.e., plasma technologies) clearly demonstrated the ability to destroy or otherwise treat the contaminants of concern. However, the cost of these treatment technologies is simply too expensive on an absolute or comparative basis; thus, they remain an emerging or innovative technology.

EVALUATION PROCESS

After identification of VOCs and SVOCs as the contaminants of concern, background information on various soil treatment technologies was assembled. This information came principally from professional and trade journals, as well as information exchanges with other environmental consultants and public utilities. It became apparent, at this point in time (1990), that there was a lack of specific information concerning the treatment of multi-ring PAH compounds, although several successful remediation projects were reported where SVOCs were the contaminants of concern. Unfortunately, much of the information gathered was not detailed enough to determine if the reported application would be appropriate for soils where treatment of PAHs was required.

Based upon published information and recommendations, vendors were contacted. Chemical and site-specific data obtained from the Remedial Investigation were provided as part of our request for a Statement of Qualifications (SOQ). In this SOQ, specific technical information concerning their technology was requested. Surprisingly, and in retrospect, now understanding the differences in defining what is "clean", many vendors claimed success in the treatment of multi-ring PAHs. Based upon this initial positive result of our inquiry, selected vendors were invited to make formal presentations of their technologies. These presentations encompassed the domain from "black boxes" to concepts in search of financing, to potential technologies that possibly could treat multi-ring PAHs.

In an attempt to determine the most promising technology, the authors visited either full-scale field applications or pilot study laboratories. For several technologies, multiple visits to alternative sites were performed. The technologies discussed below do not include a report of all technologies visited. The authors quickly discovered that, to obtain sufficient accurate information, discussions directly with the originator or operator of the technology was necessary, rather than speaking with a technical (i.e., sales) representative.

Field visits quickly disclosed the flaws in accepting vendors claims of success, as well as revealing the subtle nuances of a technology that had a substantial impact on their claimed successes. An example of these nuances came during an inspection of a bio-reactor. The contamination under remediation was VOCs, as well as light SVOCs. While the feed stock was not classified as a hazardous waste, after treatment the bio-mass used for treatment became a Resource Conservation Recovery Act (RCRA) characteristic waste. This experience, as well as similar incidents, illustrated the value and need to witness the technology at work in a milieu similar to that under investigation.

TECHNOLOGY EVALUATION

Predominantly, treatment technologies tended to be categorized into four major groups, with variation leading to subgroups. These groupings are:

- Biological;
- Chemical;
- Physical; and,
- Thermal.

Biological

Bioremediation has demonstrated technical feasibility, commercial viability, and cost effectiveness in numerous remediation projects. Bioremediation can be performed either *in-situ* or *ex-situ.* Biodegradation of organics, being a relatively mature technology, is more cost sensitive within its own technological realm and, therefore, the majority of projects investigated used a form of *in-situ*, rather than *ex-situ*, treatment. Regardless of the details of each bio-system, the basic underlying technology relies on the use of microorganisms to degrade organic compounds. These microorganisms fall into two, and possibly three, major classifications:

- Indigenous;
- Designer; and,
- Genetically Altered.

The use of indigenous microorganisms to destroy contaminants is well documented, especially in the remediation of VOCs. There is evidence that biodegradation of up to four ring PAHs has been achieved in certain conditions. There are reported successful remediation projects, generally within the pulp and paper industry, where multi-ring PAHs have been treated. These successes are predominantly based upon a reduction in total PAHs rather than in achieving a specific end point. There is a growing consensus that substantial biodegradation of five and more ring PAHs cannot be achieved with this technology, except under certain unique circumstances.

In an attempt to improve the performance of biodegradation, some vendors are producing microorganisms specifically adapted to environments containing high concentrations of PAHs. These "designer" bugs often have an ancestral heritage based in the wood treating or manufactured gas industry. Problems associated with this category of microorganisms are that of uniquely identifying the microorganisms that are apparently degrading the larger (greater than four ring) PAH compounds and then reproducing the environment necessary for their continued microbial action are still in the formative stage. We were unable to clearly document any remediations where designer microorganisms alone could be shown to have been successfully used to degrade the larger PAH compounds.

No specific vendors claimed to have developed genetically altered microorganisms to degrade multi-ring PAHs. However, in one case, outside of the United States, the authors were shown data that indicated that bioremediation of multi-ring PAHs was being achieved. Regrettably, verification of these data could not be obtained. The vendor indicated that "a high incidence of small mammal mortality at the site still needed to be addressed". This, combined with extraordinary laboratory procedures and protocols, lead the authors to believe that, in fact, genetically altered microorganisms are being used at this site.

Based upon the examination of available evidence, the authors have concluded that, at this time, bioremediation, while somewhat promising, has yet to clearly demonstrate its effectiveness in the treatment of multi-ring PAH compounds to the levels required in New Jersey.

Chemical

There are several technologies that utilize chemical processes for the reduction or treatment of soil contamination. Technologies that use a chemical-based process range from those that are considered innovative to those that are commercially available, albeit not widely accessible. Technologies that use treatment with acids or bases were considered to be emerging technologies and not proven technically feasible. The chemical technologies included in this review include:

- Solvent Extraction; and,
- Supercritical Fluid Extraction.

Solvent Extraction

This technology fundamentally uses a leaching solvent that is blended with the contaminated soils to extract the contaminants. The extraction fluid is subsequently reclaimed for recycling to the process, and the contaminant waste stream is treated or otherwise disposed. Two of the processes investigated used proprietary solvents and/or chemical reagents to remove organic contamination. Solvent extraction processes have been used in the petroleum refining industry since the mid-1980s; however, they have yet to demonstrate a wide acceptance within the remediation industry.

Supercritical Fluid Extraction

The use of a solvent gas, often carbon dioxide, at supercritical conditions has been used for the treatment of contaminated sludges. In supercritical fluid extraction, small changes in system pressure or temperature cause large changes in solvent density and its ability to solubilize VOC and SVOC contaminants. When the pressure is reduced below the critical pressure, contaminant precipitation occurs. The precipitate contaminant waste stream is further treated.

The primary use of solvent extraction processes, as well as supercritical fluid extraction, appears to be within the petroleum refining industry for the treatment of refinery sludges and wastes. The degree of acceptance of these technologies within the petroleum refinery industry may simply be the familiarity of this industry with similar chemical processes.

Physical

This group of technologies does not treat or otherwise destroy contaminants, but rather separates contaminants from the soil or encapsulates the contaminants to prevent leaching to the environment. They are normally not considered "treatment" technologies, but rather source reduction, source concentration, or containment technologies. These include:

- Soil Washing;
- Froth Flotation;
- Stabilization;
    - Lime / Flyash
    - Cement; and,
- Coal Tar Agglomeration.

Soil Washing

Soil washing technologies include both *ex-situ* soil washing and *in-situ* soil flushing. Soil washing and flushing is an aqueous-based technology that may use chemical surfactants or leaching agents combined (*ex-situ*) with mechanical agitation to separate contaminants from soil. These technologies are site specific in that they are most effective in sand and gravel soils. Contaminants in silts and clays are difficult, if not impossible, to remove by soil washing or flushing because of the high adsorptive capacity of these soils for organics.

Ex-situ soil washing appears to be primarily directed towards the treatment of inorganics, although several pilot studies have indicated that organic contamination can also be removed from the soil matrix under certain unique conditions. The resulting waste stream requires further treatment for recovery, destruction, or disposal. Several vendors commercially offer this technology using various designs. By the end of 1992, this technology had been selected in a Record of Decision (ROD) for approximately 20 Operable Units at USEPA Superfund Sites. The authors are unaware of the results of any of these remediations.

Where *in-situ* soil flushing is employed, hydraulic control of the site in both the saturated and unsaturated zones is necessary to recover the aqueous solution, as well as any additives. The resulting waste stream requires further treatment for recovery, destruction, or disposal. By the end of 1992, this technology had been selected in a ROD for approximately 15 Operable Units at USEPA Superfund Sites. The authors are unaware of the detailed results of any of these remediations.

Froth Flotation

This technology utilizes techniques developed in the mineral processing industry. Gravity separation is also often employed with this technology. This technology is akin to soils washing technologies in that the contaminants are not destroyed. To the best of the authors knowledge, this technology is not presently being used in the remediation field.

Stabilization / Solidification

Stabilization and solidification technologies commonly employ the use of lime, flyash, or cement, and occasionally a cement/bentonite mixture, to form a fixed blend of the native soil matrix and contaminants that will not leach into the environment. It can be performed either *in-situ* or *ex-situ*. This technology is not considered a treatment technology per se, but is often classified as a containment technology.

When performed *ex-situ*, a pug mill or conventional equipment employed in the construction of slurry walls is commonly used. For *ex-situ* applications, air permitting issues must be addressed during the permitting process.

Several vendors offer this technology *in-situ*, and it has been successfully employed to contain the movement of contaminants. Its success depends on specific site conditions and the clear identification of the contaminants of concern. There are data that suggests that chemical reactions between certain admixtures employed and some organic contaminants is not fully understood.

Coal Tar Agglomeration

The AGLOFOAT coal-oil agglomeration process, developed by The Alberta Research Council (ARC) with EPRI sponsorship, is an example of an extraction process that uses a solid sorbent rather than a liquid sorbent to remove contaminants from waste. The process operates on the principle that oily waste constituents are strongly adsorbed on the surface of fine coal particles and that the coal-organic agglomeration thus formed can be separated from the soil in an aqueous slurry. The recovered agglomerates can be used as fuel in boilers.

Thermal

Thermal technologies encompass numerous variations of a basic principle; that is, as heat is applied to a soil matrix containing the contamination, volatilization of VOCs and SVOCs occurs. As the contaminants vaporize, they are desorbed and separated from the soil matrix. Depending on the technology, the contaminants are either destroyed in the primary treatment chamber or they are collected in a separate device, condensed and recovered, or incinerated. Thermal processes may be either *in-situ* or *ex-situ*, as well as being conducted on or off site. Presently, *ex-situ/on site* and *ex-situ*/off-site treatment are the prevalent technologies. To the best of the authors knowledge, no *in-situ* thermal technologies have been commercially viable. Thermal technologies have been classified as follows:

- Thermal Desorption;
  - Low temperature 350 - 500°F
  - Medium temperature 500 - 900°F
  - High Temperature >1200°F
- Asphalt Batching;
- Cement Kilns;
- Incineration;
- Pyrolysis;
- Vitrification; and,
- Co-Burning.

Thermal Desorption

Ex-situ thermal desorption processes have been commercially successful for several reasons:

- The concept is relatively simple;
- Thermal desorption systems are relatively simple in design, construction, and operation;
- Contaminated soils are very abundant;
- Thermal desorption can treat a variety of wastes including VOCs, SVOCs, and volatile inorganics; and,
- Thermal desorption is cost effective.

In-situ thermal desorption has not gained widespread acceptance because:

- *In-situ* thermal desorption, being very site specific, causes it to be more difficult to design, monitor, and evaluate results; and,

- The cost effectiveness of *in-situ* thermal processes is questionable, as such a technology is energy intensive and soils are a superior heat sink.

Low-temperature *ex-situ* thermal desorbers have been successfully used in numerous applications to remediate VOC contamination. This technology has attained the status where technical feasibility, regulatory acceptance, and commercial cost effectiveness is no longer in question. Several vendors offer desorber units that can be used on site. Except in rare circumstances, these units are not used to treat RCRA hazardous wastes. Low-temperature thermal desorbers are not suitable for the remediation of SVOCs because the unit's temperature is insufficient to desorb the multi-ring PAHs.

Medium-temperature desorbers share the same degree of acceptance as low-temperature units. Although several vendors offer modular units that can be erected at the site, the most common thermal units in this temperature range are fixed based. This market developed regionally to serve the underground storage tank removal programs and, as such, required higher temperatures to thermally desorb fuel oil and diesel contamination. At higher temperatures (above 800°F), effective desorption of multi-ring PAHs has been proven. This effectiveness varies between individual thermal units depending upon the geometry and material handling portion of the process. It is believed that, at the higher temperatures, steam stripping may play a role in the treatment process.

High-temperature thermal desorbers predominantly seem to have been constructed with a specific contaminated feed stock as the basic design premise. Due the capital cost involved in constructing these units, they appear to be generally used where RCRA hazardous wastes are encountered. At the high temperatures at which these units operate, all organic contaminants are desorbed. At the extreme end of the temperature scale, thermal cracking may also occur. Two units were evaluated in detail. The first unit was successfully used on two polychlorinated biphenyls (PCB) cleanups. The second unit was treating oil refinery wastes and sludges (KO-48 and KO-52 listed wastes). In both instances, non-detect levels of contaminants after treatment were achieved. While both units treated their respective waste streams, they varied radically in process design.

Asphalt Batching

Setting aside the potential issues of end product liability the use of contaminated soils as a feedstock for asphaltic products appears to satisfy the screening criteria assembled above. The requirements for asphalt recycling necessitate a specific soil matrix as well as identification of the contaminant source. The use of contaminated soils in an asphalt batch plant does not destroy or treat the contamination; instead, it generally incorporates the heavier PAHs into the basic asphalt product. Because the temperatures used in the production of asphalt products tend to be that used in low temperature thermal desorption, this technology lends itself to VOC and to the three-ring PAH compound remediation. There is some evidence that compounds such as methyl-naphthalene may leach over time from asphaltic mixtures.

Cement Kilns

The use of contaminated soils as a partial replacement feed stock for cement kilns is well documented. At the temperatures (over 2500° F) and residence time within the kiln all organic contamination is destroyed. Acceptance criteria as a feedstock varies widely across this industry. Some facilities require a certain BTU content while others may not accept any soil or rock fragments larger than 2 inches in size. One cement kiln evaluated introduced the contaminated soils into the central portion of the kiln in five gallon pails. Several of the facilities inspected were operating under temporary RCRA Part B permits and were modifying their physical plant to comply with the new Boiler Industrial Furnace Regulations. Regardless of the facility, changing Federal and State standards permitting a facility to accept wastes is dynamic and is currently under review by the Federal Government as well as several State entities.

Incineration

Incineration is a proven process for the destruction of organics. Because incineration is predominantly reserved for the treatment of hazardous wastes, the costs associated with this technology generally prove too expensive when compared to thermal desorption.

Pyrolysis

Several technology developers have attempted to commercialize plasma technologies. Although there has been considerable interest in this technology to the best of the authors knowledge, outside of the SITE program, there is little activity that would indicate that this technology is advancing towards technical or economic feasibility.

Vitrification

This technology would seem to be an inclusive method to treat contaminated wastes containing both organics and inorganics. Vitrification can be performed either *in-situ* or *ex-situ.* To the best of the authors knowledge no current technology is being offered for *ex-situ* vitrification.

In the past ten years over 150 *in-situ* vitrification tests at various scales have been conducted on a variety of wastes. By early 1992 this technology had been selected in a ROD at three Superfund sites. However, to the best of our knowledge none of these remedial actions has been implemented. In 1991, EPA Region VIII raised concern about this technology at the Rocky Mountain Arsenal Superfund site in Colorado.

There appear to be serious technical problems concerning offgassing of contamination associated with this technology. Coupled with this technical issue is the unambiguous energy and capital costs associated with this technology. This combination of technical complexity, high costs and permitting issues may prevent this technology from reaching commercial viability.

Co-Burning

This technology uses existing coal fired utility boilers where the contaminated waste is mixed with coal and burned as part of the fuel requirements to generate electric power. This technology is highly site specific and is being tried at two utilities in the mid-west and one utility in the northeast. It is a captive technology and not commercially available.

CONCLUSION

The resources required for screening of technologies including vendor discussions, information interchange with colleagues, analysis of pilot studies, and site visits of applied technologies is dwarfed by the cost of the remediation itself. In the authors case, it was proven that the time and effort dedicated to this process was successful.

The authors conclude that, at the present time, generically, thermal applications provide the most viable treatment technology for the remediation of multi-ring PAH compounds. Of the seven thermal technologies reviewed, thermal desorption surpasses other thermal technologies in satisfying the basic five screening criteria used in this study.

Bioremediation continues to be a viable option, although its effectiveness seems limited in achieving the degradation of multi-ring PAHs.

Chemical technologies, while commercially available, have not demonstrated widespread acceptance within the remediation community.

Physical technologies, specifically soil washing and flushing, have been increasingly selected in RODs at USEPA Superfund Sites. These technologies appear to be primarily directed towards the treatment of inorganics. Soil washing was not considered by the authors to be a treatment technology, but rather a source reduction technology.

CHAPTER 24

Remediation of Contaminated Soil and Sediment Using the Biogenesis^{SM} Washing Process

Mohsen C. Amiran, Ph.D., Physical Organic Chemistry, BioGenesis Enterprises, Inc., Des Plaines, Illinois,
Charles L. Wilde, M.S., BioGenesis Enterprises, Inc., Springfield, Virginia

INTRODUCTION

BioGenesis Enterprises, Inc. has developed a soil and sediment washing process capable of cleaning heavy hydrocarbon pollutants (including crude oil, PAHs, fuel oils, and diesel) from most matrices. The process is applicable to a broad range of hazardous organics and metals, including harbor sediments. The company has demonstrated its large particle technology in the U.S. EPA Superfund Innovative Technology Evaluation (SITE) program and tested its sediment washing technology under the auspices of Environment Canada's Great Lakes Cleanup Fund and Wastewater Technology Centre's Contaminated Sediment Treatment Technology Program.

BioGenesis^{SM} washing technology advances the state of the remediation art by solving three obstacles to widespread implementation of washing technology--inability to handle heavy pollutants, inability to wash small sediments, and the capital cost and relative immobility of large processing plants. Additionally BioGenesis^{SM} technology incorporates the use of synthetic biosurfactant chemicals that provide continuing remediation action after washing is completed. This chapter describes the technology and reports the results of U.S. and Canadian evaluation programs.

PROCESS DESCRIPTION

The BioGenesis^{SM} washing process is an *ex-situ*, on-site, extraction technology for organic pollutants and metals. Figure 24.1 gives an overview of the total system. The process uses complex bioremediating surfactant blends, water, heat, mixing, and friction to clean soil and sediment. Two types of mobile equipment wash different particle sizes. A truck mounted batch unit processing 40 yards per hour washes soil particles 0.5 mm and larger. A mobile, continuous flow unit can clean over 80 yards per hour for sediment particles smaller than 0.5 mm. Auxiliary equipment includes particle sizing equipment, tanks, dewatering and water treatment equipment, and a bioreactor. Extraction efficiencies range from 85 to 99% depending on the pollutant type, initial concentration, and soil/sediment type. Figure 24.2 illustrates the sediment washing process for small particles and Figure 24.3, the soil washing process for larger particles.

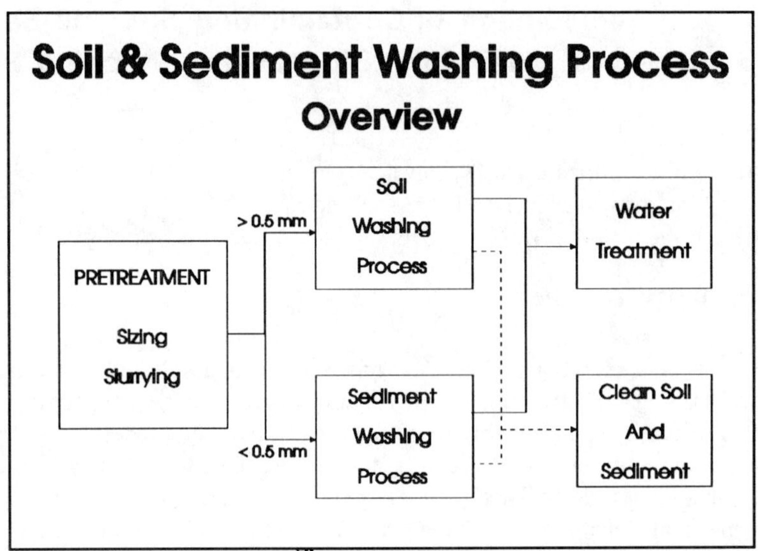

Figure 24.1 BioGenesis[SM] soil and sediment washing system overview.

Sediment Subsystem

The sediment washing machine is a continuous flow unit. Capacities of up to 80-100 cubic yards per hour are possible using parallel processing and multiple equipments.

Sediment is pretreated via grizzlies to separate debris not suitable for shredding. These oversize materials are diverted to the large particle washer for treatment. Material passing the grizzly flows to a shredder and thence to pretreatment tanks. The shredded material is blended, heated, and mixed with water and biosurfactant chemicals. This forms a slurry.

The slurry then passes to a shaker screen separator that sizes particles into two streams. Material greater than 0.5 mm diameter is diverted to the large particle soil washer. Material 0.5 mm and smaller continues to the sediment washer's feed hopper. From there the slurry is injected to the sediment collision chamber where it collides with water and cleaning chemical at 10,000 to 15,000 psi pressure. This accomplishes primary loosening of the bonds between the pollutant and the particle.

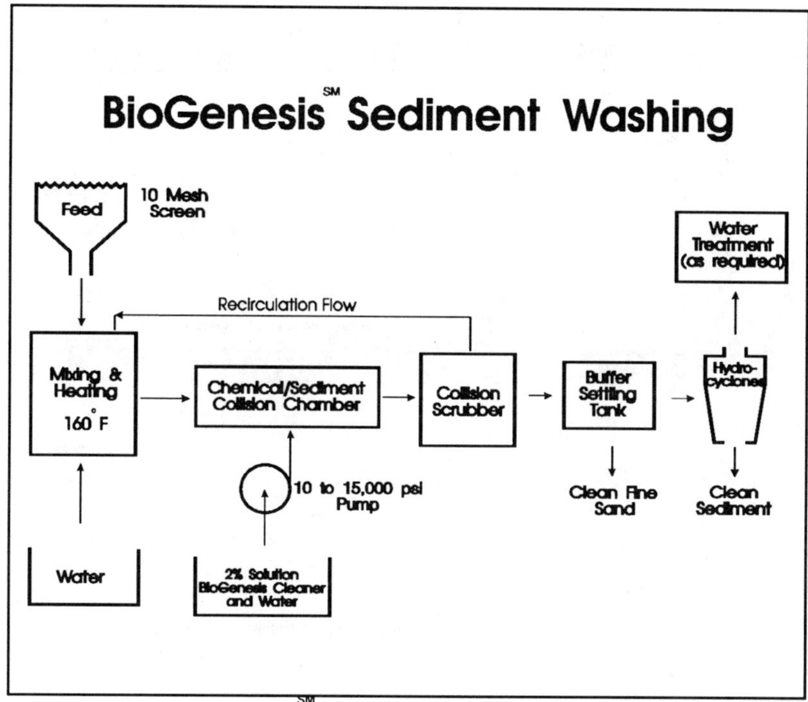

Figure 24.2. BioGenesis SM small particle sediment washing system flow.

After the collision chamber, the slurry flows to the collision scrubber which ensures that the particles are thoroughly wetted. The scrubbing process further weakens the bonds between contaminant and particle. Normally three collision chamber/collision scrubber sets are connected in series to accomplish successive washings. Following the last scrubber, the slurry passes through a buffer tank where any large particles separate by gravity. The slurry then flows through hydrocyclone banks to separate solids down to 5-10 microns in size. The free liquid routes to a centrifuge for final solid-liquid separation.

All solids go to the clean soil pile whereas all liquid is routed to wastewater treatment to remove organic and inorganic contaminants. Decontaminated water is recycled back through the process.

Soil Subsystem

The soil washing system for larger particles is a batch process with throughput capacity of up to 40 yards per hour. The system consists of a trailer mounted gondola plumbed for air mixing, water/chemical addition, oil skimming, and liquid drainage. Water, BioGenesis SM cleaning chemicals, and soil are loaded into the gondola. Aeration nozzles in the bottom of the gondola feed compressed air to create the effect of a fluidized bed. The resulting slurry is agitated by the aerators for about 30 minutes to release organic and inorganic contaminants from

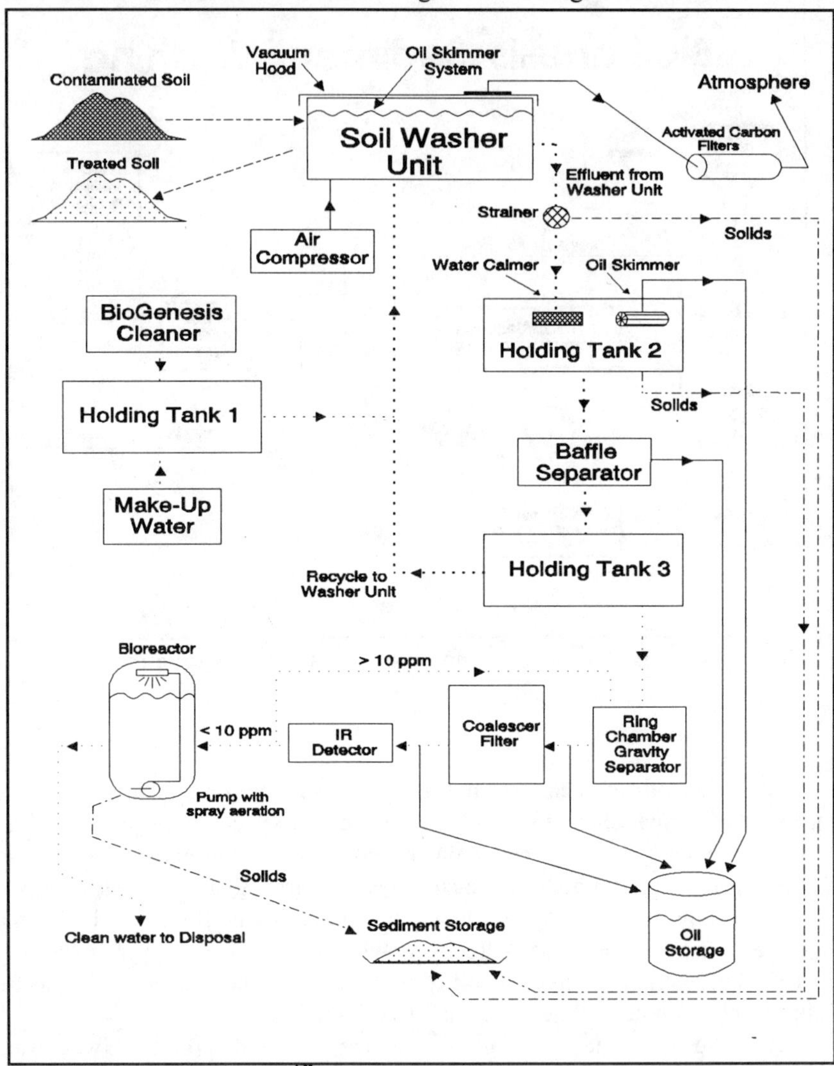

Figure 24.3. BioGenesis[SM] large particle soil washing system flow.

the soil particles. After mixing, a short settling period allows the soil particles to sink and the oil removed to rise to the water surface where it is skimmed for reclamation or disposal. Following drainage of the wash water, the clean soil is evacuated by raising the unit's dump mechanism. Processed soil contains a moisture level of 20-30% depending on the soil matrix.

The gondola is equipped with an emission control system to trap VOCs if a volatile contaminant is being cleaned. Process air passes first through the slurry, and then through a chilling unit. This traps VOC's in a collection tank.

Carbon filter beds provide a final polishing effect before the air is released to the atmosphere.

SEDIMENT PROCESS TESTING

Under the auspices of Wastewater Technology Centre's (WTC) Contaminated Sediment Treatment Technology Program, BioGenesis contracted to test its washing technology on sediment from a former wood preserving site at Thunder Bay, Ontario. This site containing 20,000 cubic meters is one of 43 "Areas of Concern" identified by the International Joint Commission, a joint U.S.-Canada body tasked to administer the Great Lakes Water Quality Agreement. The major contaminants on the site are PAHs, with low levels of PCBs, phenols, and several metals. The PAHs were determined to be the primary target of the washing test. Typical sediment grain sizes were as depicted in Figure 24.4 with 81% being less than 38 microns in size.

Test sediment was selected from the worst contaminated areas of Thunder Bay as determined by surveys in 1984, 1988, and 1992. In early June 1993, BioGenesis performed the testing under the audit of a Canadian representative of WTC. Split-sample procedures were followed to maintain testing integrity. Independent testing of all samples was conducted for BioGenesis by Galson Laboratories, Inc. of Syracuse, N.Y. The testing was originally planned as a bench scale test. However, due to the high pressures involved and inability to effectively model the process parameters in bench scale equipment, the testing used pilot-scale equipment capable of processing 1½ to 2 cubic yards per hour. Table 24.1 shows the cumulative reduction of contamination levels with each wash cycle for PAHs (Cycle 1 - 16%, Cycle 2 - 84%, and Cycle 3 - 90%). There appear to be no technical obstacles to fine tuning the scrubbers to increase removal effectiveness per cycle by up to 20% and also no obstacle to adding additional scrub cycles without diminishing the throughput rate. Predicted process efficiency with these changes is 98%+. Despite relatively high organic content, PAH extraction efficiencies were consistent with testing results for oil & grease and semi-volatile hydrocarbons. Figure 24.5 illustrates this correlation. Figures 24.6 and 24.7 show individual compound results for the PAHs which were the primary extraction target. Note that the pattern of removal effectiveness was consistent among the 16 PAHs. The extraction level averaged 90% with negligible variation in extraction efficiencies among different contaminants.

BioGenesis Sediment Washing, 6/1/93
Pilot testing for Environment Canada, Wastewater Technology Centre, Great Lakes Cleanup Program
Thunder Bay Harbour, Ontario Sediment

TEST		SOLIDS (Parts per Million) UNTREATED	CYCLE 1	CYCLE 2	CYCLE 3	LIQUID (Parts per Million) WASTEWATER
Oil & Grease		91,600	NR	NR	3,940	NR
Semi-volatile Petroleum HC		21,000	NR	NR	2,200	NR
Total Petroleum Hydrocarbon		4,770	4,840	1,670	400	NR
Total Organic Content		11.5%	NR	NR	2.9%	NR
CAS No.	**COMPOUND**					
91-20-3	Naphthalene	1,400	1,000	170	73	14
85-01-8	Phenanthrene	770	700	130	88	2.2
206-44-0	Fluoranthene	460	430	83	59	1.0
83-32-9	Acenaphthene	340	290	55	34	1.2
129-0-0	Pyrene	320	300	59	44	0.8
86-73-7	Fluorene	260	230	45	30	0.8
56-55-3	Benzo(a)anthracene	110	100	23	19	0.2E
120-12-7	Anthracene	97 E	90 E	21	16	0.2E
205-99-2	Benzo(b)fluoranthene	97 E	88 E	24	19	ND
50-32-8	Benzo(a)pyrene	78 E	61 E	15	12	ND
218-01-9	Chrysene	69 E	68 E	15	12	0.1
207-08-9	Benzo(k)fluoranthene	42 E	40 E	6.5 E	6.1	ND
191-24-2	Benzo(g,h,i)perylene	36 E	32 E	5 E	3.9 E	ND
193-39-5	Indeno(1,2,3-cd)pyrene	33 E	30 E	5.9 E	5 E	ND
208-96-8	Acenaphthylene	15 E	ND	2.4 E	1.5 E	ND
53-70-3	Dibenzo(a,h)anthracene	ND	ND	ND	1.4 E	ND
	16 PAHs	**4,079**	**3,429**	**652**	**416**	**21**
	CUMULATIVE REMOVAL PERCENTAGE		**15.9%**	**84.0%**	**89.8%**	**NA**

ND = Below detection limits
E = Estimated concentration
NA = Not applicable
NR = Not requested
Note: Removed oils floated on the wastewater surface. Testing not designed for mass balance determination.

Table 24.1. Washing test data, Thunder Bay Harbour, Ontario, sediment.

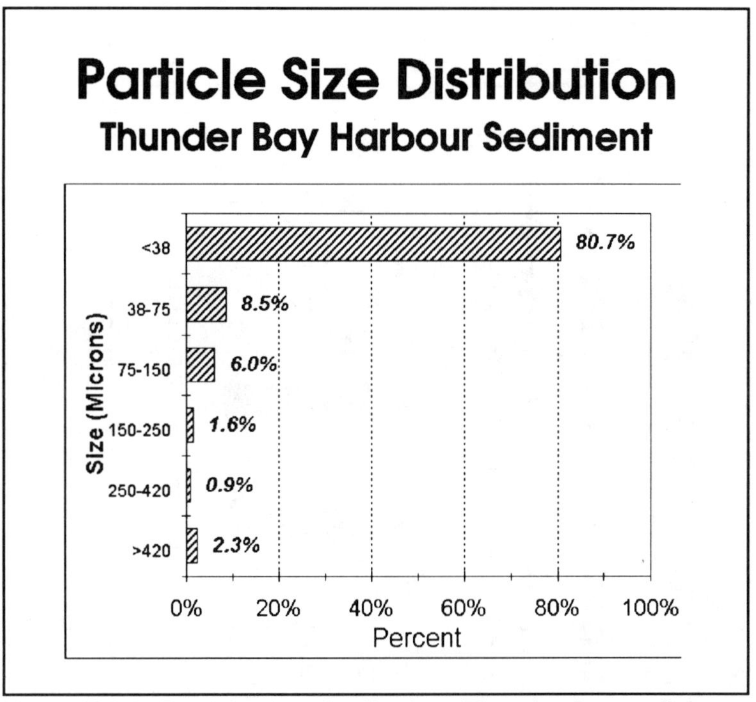

Figure 24.4. Particle size distribution, Thunder Bay sediment.

SOIL WASHING PROCESS TESTING

To efficiently wash soils with grain sizes larger than approximately 0.5 mm, the BioGenesis[SM] process uses equipment that takes advantage of the lower bonding energy of organics and inorganics on larger particles. This equipment uses heat, water, cleaner, and air mixing to remove and float hydrophobic pollutants or to solubilize compounds which are heavier than water.

The soil washing equipment was demonstrated in the U.S. EPA SITE program during November 1992. About 3,800 tons of soil was contaminated with up to 3% heavy crude oil at a refinery. Due to extended weathering, the soil contained only trace levels of benzene, toluene, ethylbenzene, and xylene. Total recoverable petroleum hydrocarbons (TRPH) was selected as the contaminant group of concern. Figure 24.8 shows the particle size distribution of the soil. Effective grain size was approximately 50 microns (10% smaller and 90% larger).

Based on an initial contamination level of 30,800 ppm, extraction effectiveness for washing alone was 85-90% with subsequent biodegradation raising that to an overall effectiveness of 95-98%. These results are illustrated in Figure 24.9. Results were tabulated for soil fractions greater than, and less than, 300 microns. As was expected, after the initial washing, greater extraction

Overall Removal Effectiveness

Pilot Testing on Thunder Bay Harbour, Ontario, Sediment

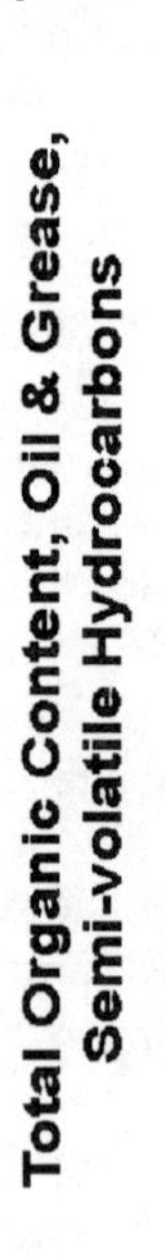

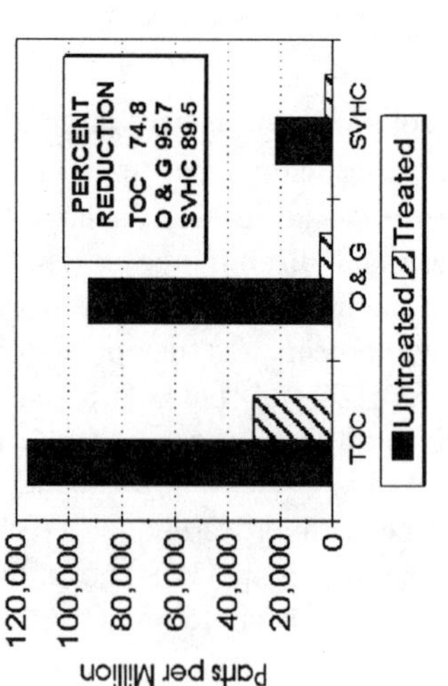

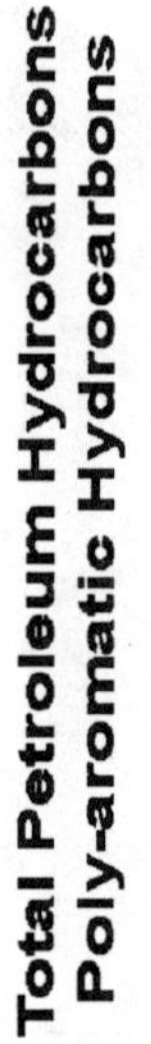

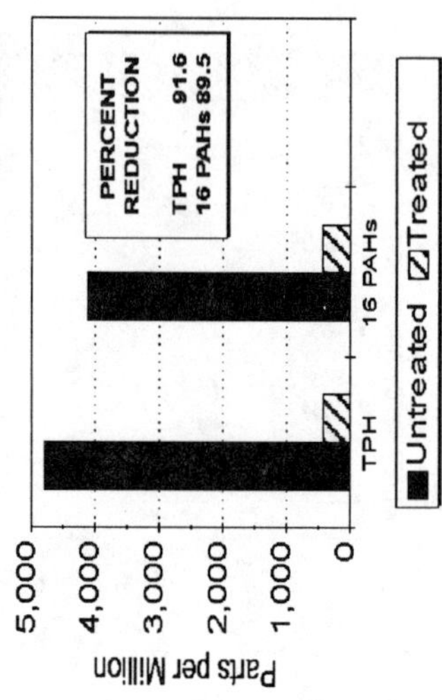

Figure 24.5. Overview of washing results, Thunder Bay Harbour

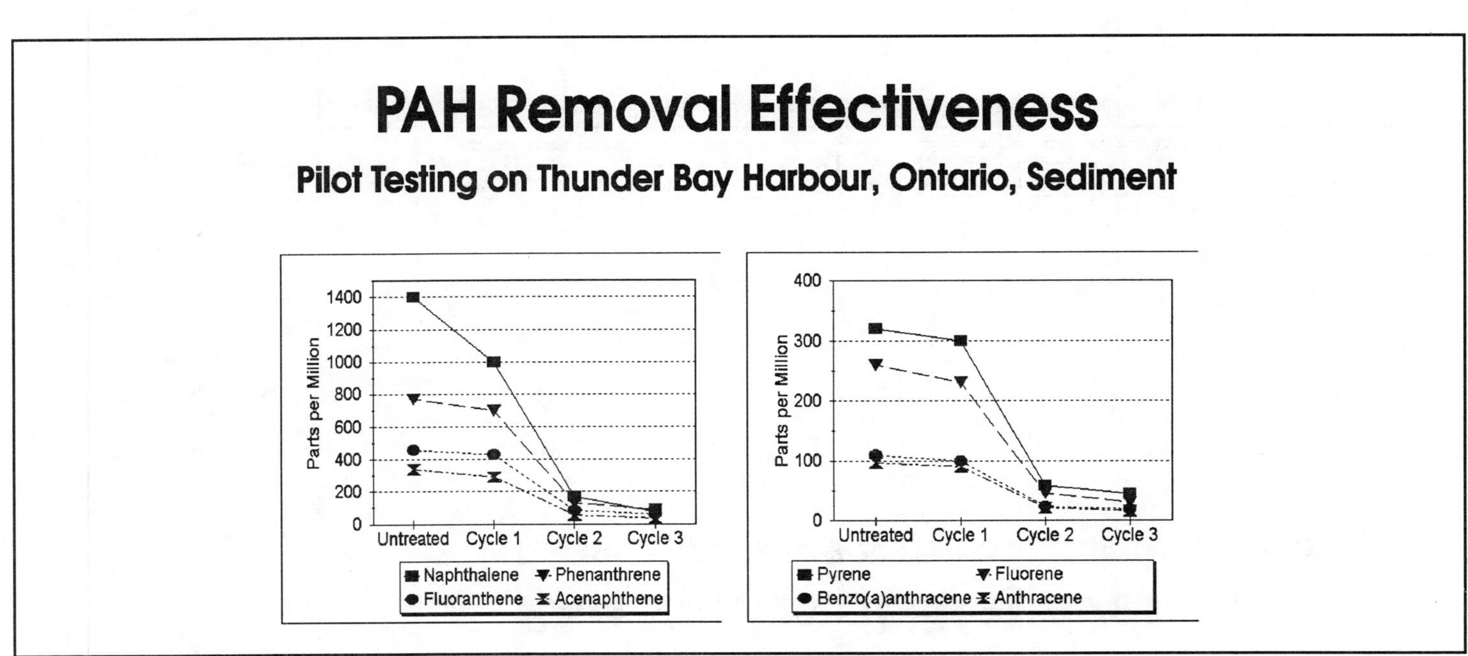

Figure 24.6. PAH removal effectiveness, higher concentration pollutants

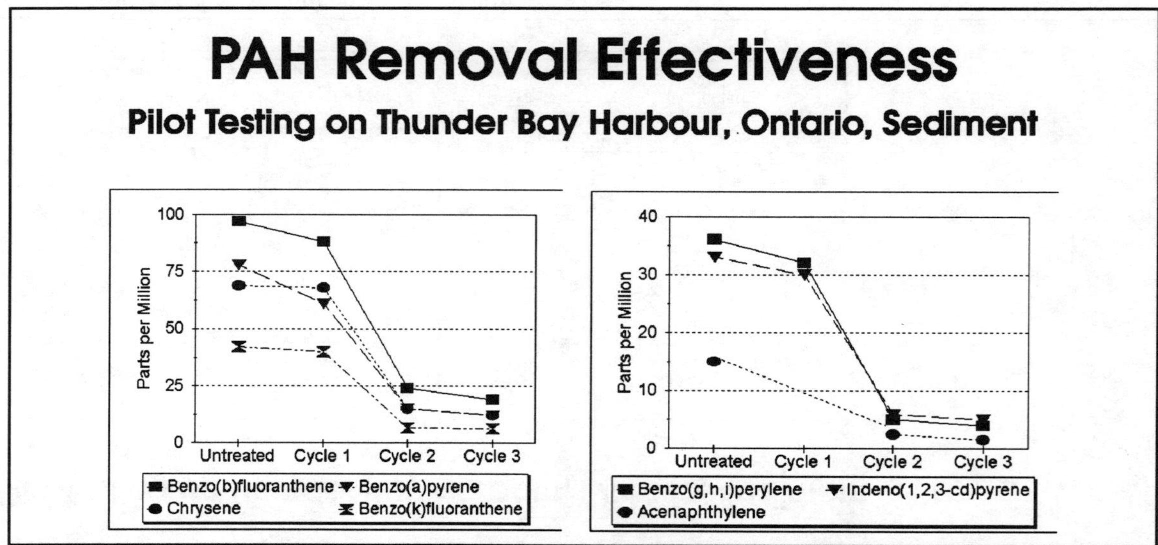

Figure 24.7. PAH removal effectiveness, lower concentration pollutants

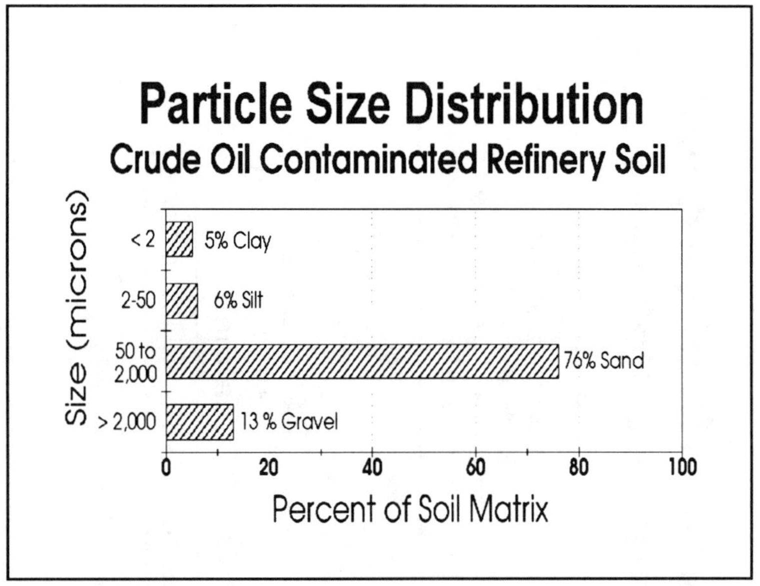

Figure 24.8. Particle size distribution, crude oil soil washing

(91%) was achieved on the larger fraction than on the smaller particle sizes. Noteworthy though is that even on the fines fraction, 85% extraction resulted.

Both the larger and smaller fractions were then monitored for biodegradation of residual contamination not removed in the washing. This monitoring was to ascertain the degree to which the BioGenesis^{SM} washing chemicals enhanced and facilitated biodegradation. As shown in Figure 24.9, on the fines fraction, rapid biodegradation was observed during the succeeding two weeks, with a reduction of the "after washing" level of 52% after seven days and a cumulative reduction of the "after washing" level by 71% at the end of two weeks. Biodegradation of the larger size fraction representing over 85% of the soil was monitored for 31 days. At the 7, 14, 21, and 31 day points, cumulative reductions from the "after washing" level were tested as 7%, 14%, 64%, and 75% respectively. After washing and one month of biodegradation, washing and biodegradation had removed 95-98% of the crude oil contamination in both the coarse and fines fractions. EPA testing verified the reproducibility of washing results at constant operating conditions.

Direct conclusions drawn from the SITE demonstration include a general range of washing effectiveness from 85% to 95%, the validity of considering biodegradation induced by washing with BioGenesis^{SM} chemicals in overall effectiveness, and the ability of the BioGenesis^{SM} process to consistently remove weathered, heavy oils from soil which has an effective grain size of 50 microns. Significant inferences from the SITE demonstration are that the process will have higher effectiveness on pollutant structures less complex than weathered crude

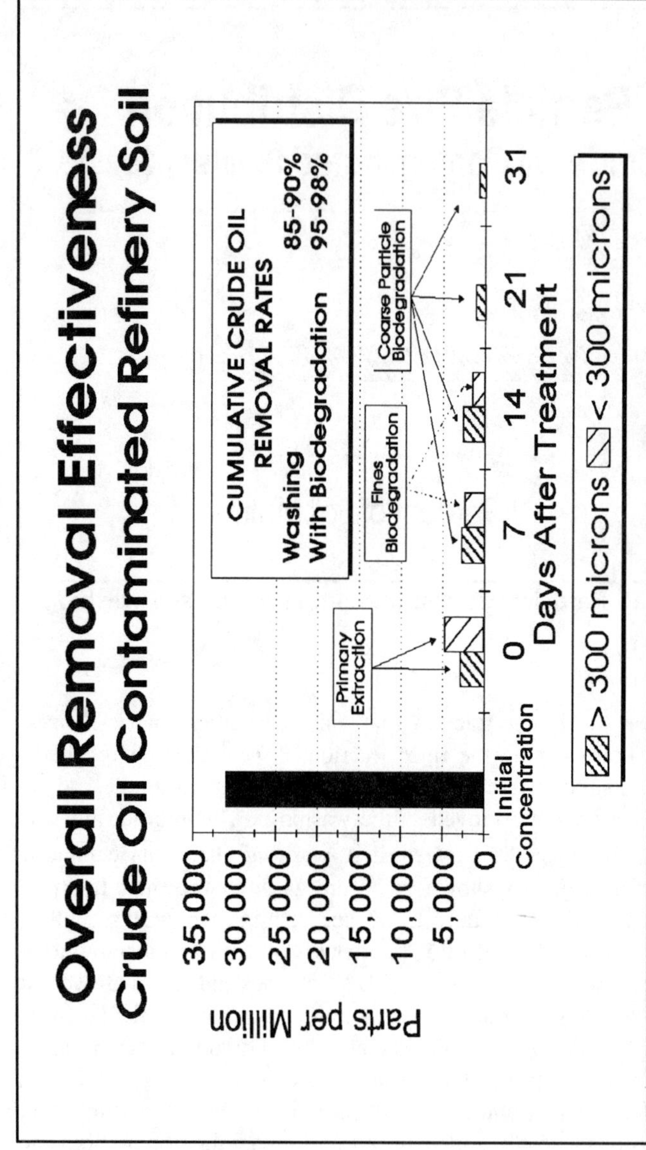

Figure 24.9. Removal effectiveness, soil washing and biodegradation

oil, e.g. diesel fuel, and that it can also be applied successfully to other types of organic contaminants such as PCBs, dioxins, and pesticides.

SUMMARY

BioGenesis^{SM} soil and sediment washing combines equipment design factors (temperature, pressure, friction, duration) with proprietary chemical blends tailored to specific site conditions. The process achieves high extraction levels on oils, and, by extension, on most organic pollutants in both large and small grain soils. Additionally, the relatively small size of the equipment and its mobility promises economic treatment for the large number of sites below the economic threshold of conventional soil washing. Finally, negligible undesirable by-products, high processing rates, the absence of air pollution, and elimination of the necessity to transport contaminated material offsite all point to reduced cost and acceptability of this technology both by regulatory authorities and public interest and environmental groups.

CHAPTER 25

Regulatory Aspects of Hydrocarbon Contaminated Soil and Groundwater Remediation at a Building Construction Site

Suresh R. Kikkeri and Edward P. Hagarty, P.E., Woodward-Clyde Federal Services, Rockville, Maryland
Jimmy L. Wilcher, U.S. Army Corps of Engineers, Baltimore, Maryland

INTRODUCTION

When Cameron Station, a U.S. Army Military installation in Alexandria, Virginia, closes in 1995 under the Base Realignment and Closure (BRAC) initiative, the Military District of Washington (MDW) logistics activities and other operations are scheduled to be moved to the proposed logistics Warehouse and Administrative Building at Fort Myer, another U.S. Army Military installation located in Arlington, Virginia, (Figures 25.1 and 25.2). The proposed Logistics Complex includes the construction of a vehicle maintenance building and vehicle storage area and a warehouse and administration building. The vehicle maintenance building and vehicle storage areas are planned to be located in the areas including and surrounding existing Building 323 (Figure 25.3). The warehouse/administration building is planned to be located in the areas currently occupied by the motor pool and buildings 206-209 (Figure 25.4).

In order to clear the areas where the construction is proposed, underground storage tanks (USTs) that were not in service were removed. During the time of removal, it was noticed that petroleum products remained in some USTs; some USTs had holes; free product was noticed in the excavation pits; and soil stains were observed. All these visual observations triggered an immediate follow up investigation to examine the extent of contamination and subsequent remediation. During the same period, one of the USTs which is still in service (Tank 15) was pressure tested for leaks. It was found out that this system was leaking. The leak was corrected and the system was placed back in service. However, this tank is now targeted for removal. The details of these USTs are presented in Table 25.1. Further field investigations and immediate corrective measures carried out at the site included:

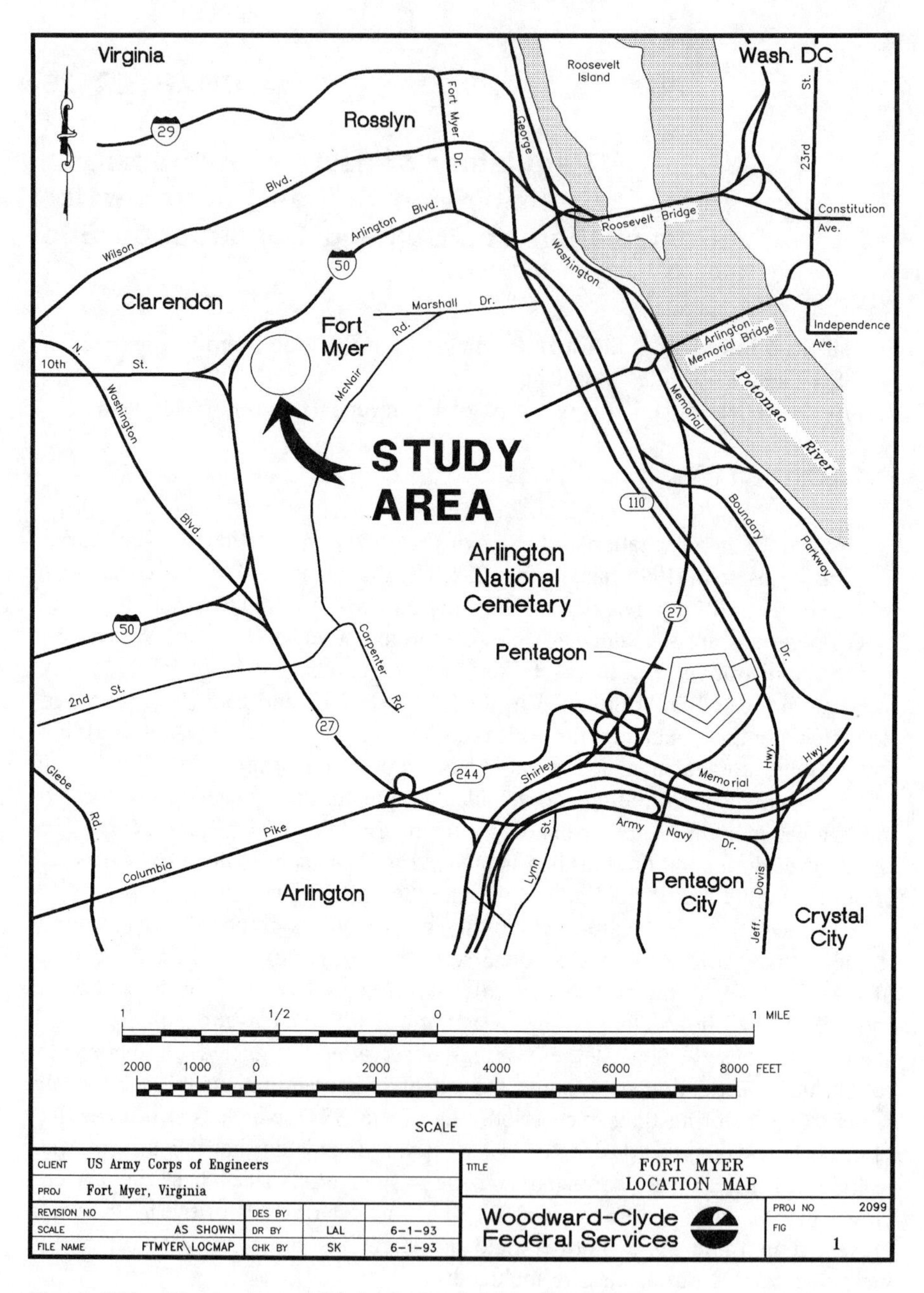

Figure 25.1. Warehouse and Administrative Building, Fort Myer.

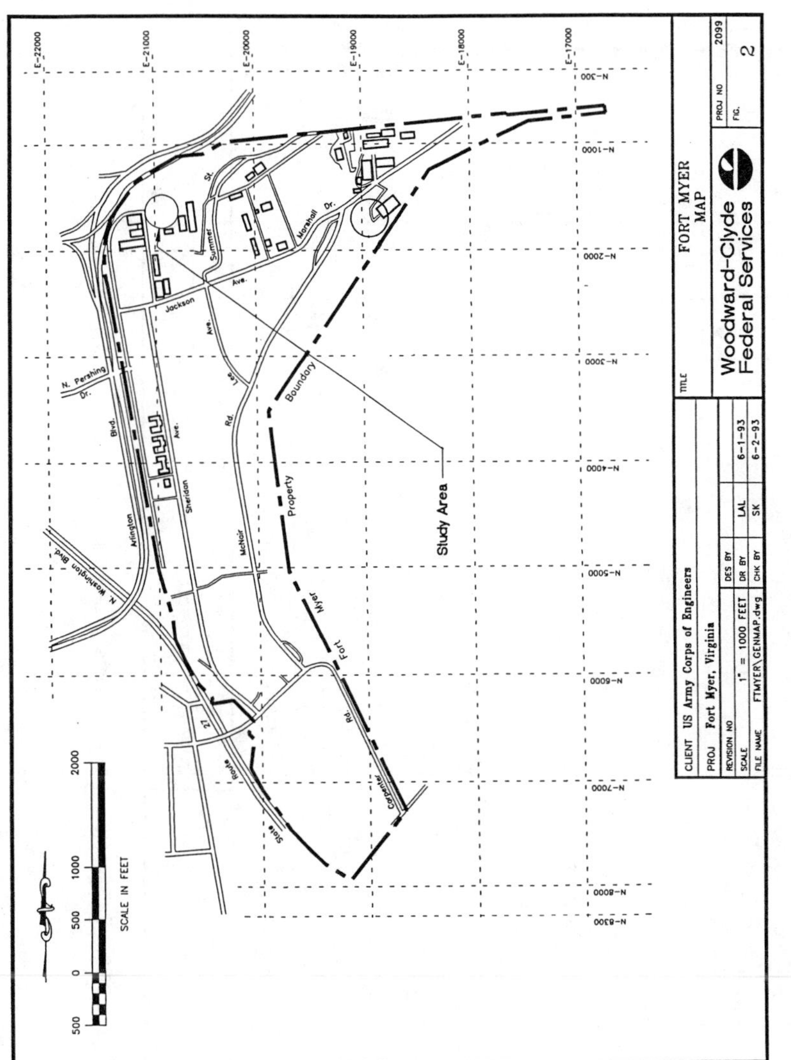

Figure 25.2. Warehouse and Administrative Building, Fort Myer.

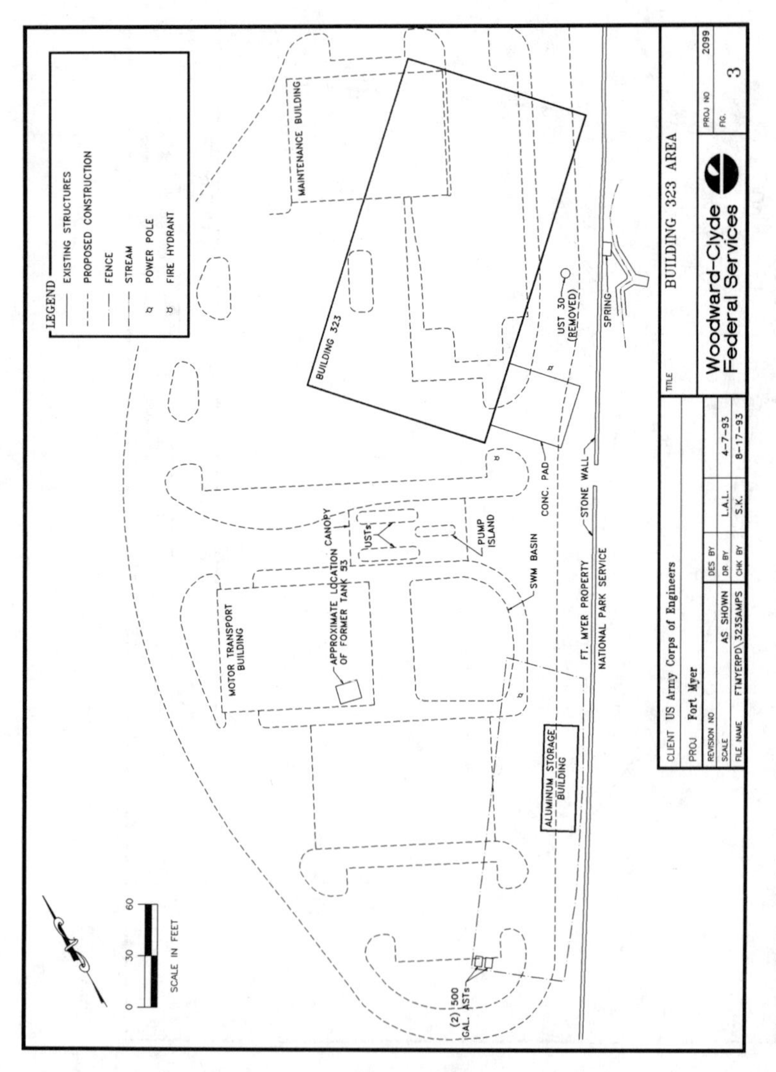

Figure 25.3. Building 323—Vehicle Maintenance Building and Vehicle Storage Areas.

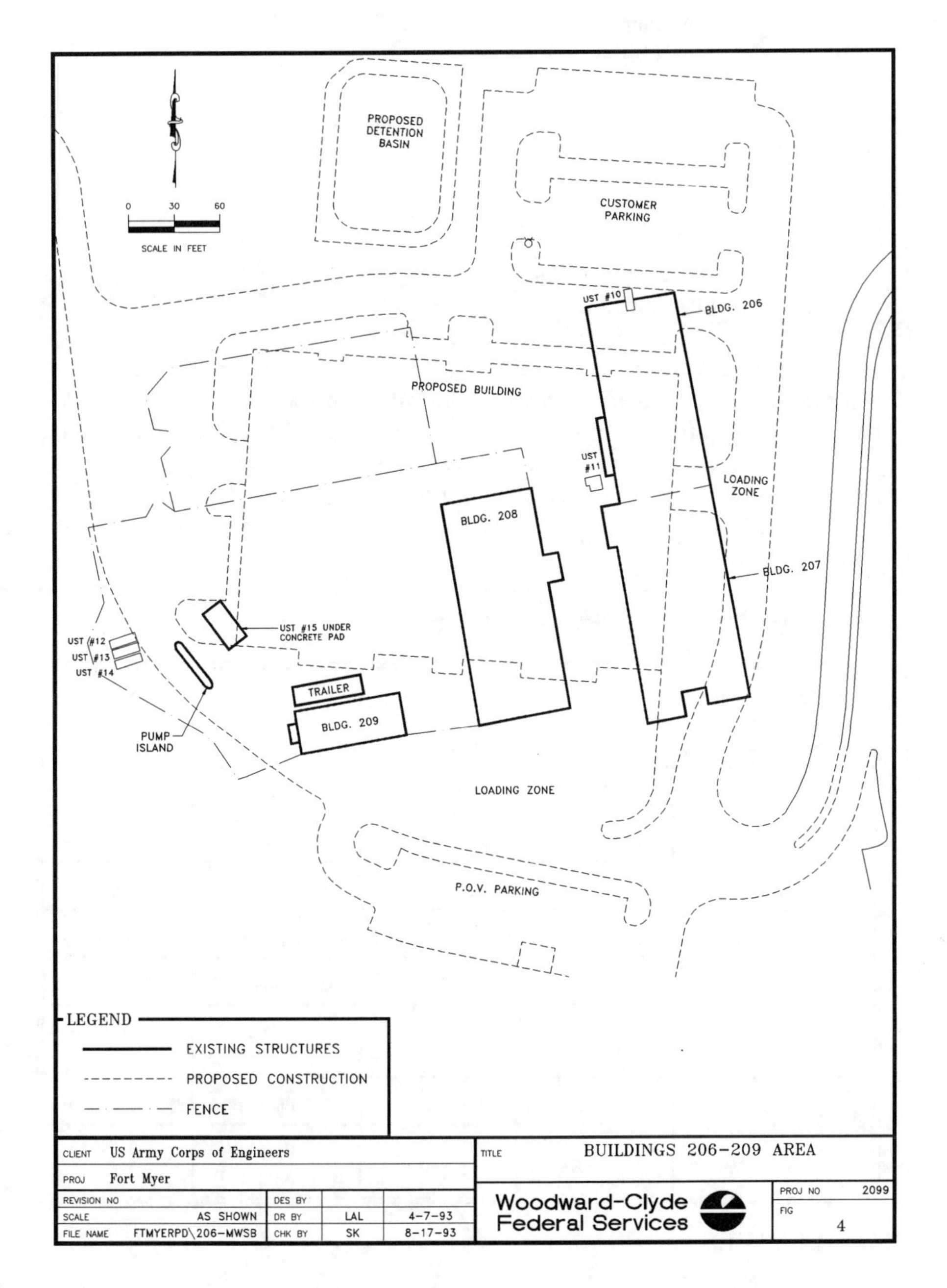

Figure 25.4. Warehouse/Administration Building.

- Initial abatement and site check
- Site characterization
- Free product recovery

Based on the above mentioned investigations, the following reports were subsequently prepared:

- Site Characterization Report
- Risk Assessment Report
- Corrective Action Plan
- Site Clearance Report

The field investigations were conducted in an accelerated schedule to expedite the actual remedial actions at the site. The schedule was accelerated because, in accordance with the BRAC schedule, the construction of the proposed Logistics Complex was planned to begin in September 1993. Upon completion of the field investigations, a Risk Assessment was performed, the results of which were used in preparing the Corrective Action Plan (CAP) and Site Clearance Report (SCLR).

Table 25.1: Underground storage tank information.

Building Nos. near the Location of UST	UST No.	Capacity (gallons)	Contents	Status
206-209	10	1,000	No.2 Fuel Oil	Removed
	11	2,000	No.2 Fuel Oil	Removed
	12	5,000	Gasoline	Removed
	13	5,000	Gasoline	Removed
	14	5,000	Diesel Fuel	Removed
	15	6,000	Diesel Fuel	Targeted for removal
323	30	1,000	No.2 Fuel Oil	Removed
	53	3,000	No.2 Fuel Oil (not confirmed)	Removed

OBJECTIVES

The objectives of this chapter are to illustrate the various field activities performed in an accelerated schedule and explain briefly how the performance of each of the activities was required in order to be in compliance with various regulations. These regulations include US Environmental Protection Agency's regulations under Resource Conservation and Recovery Act (RCRA), US Army regulations, regulations administered by the Department of Labor under Occupational Safety and Health Act (OSHA), regulations enforced by the Department of Environmental Quality (DEQ) of the Commonwealth of Virginia and other regulations.

APPLICABLE REGULATIONS

The various activities performed on the site and off the site needed the consideration of the following regulations.

Resource Conservation and Recovery Act (RCRA)

The Hazardous and Solid Waste Amendments (HSWA) of 1984 added Subtitle I to RCRA, authorizing the Environmental Protection Agency (EPA) to develop and implement a new regulatory program for Underground Storage Tanks (USTs) containing petroleum and other regulated substances. Technical standards required for release detection, prevention, and correction as necessary to protect human health and the environment were promulgated in 53 Federal Register 37082 (September 23, 1988). As per 40 CFR 280 (Subpart F), release response and corrective action for USTs containing petroleum products include initial abatement, initial site characterization, free product removal, investigations for soil and groundwater cleanup and corrective action plans.

Occupational Safety and Health Act (OSHA)

OSHA was promulgated in 1970 and requires employers throughout the U.S. and its territories to provide safe working conditions for their employees. Corrective actions involving cleanup operations at sites covered by RCRA have to meet all health and safety regulations as described in 29 CFR 1910.120. Safety and health regulations for construction (29 CFR 1926), promulgated by the Department of Labor under section 107 of the Contract Work Hours and Safety Standards Act are also be applicable. These regulations were considered before any field activity commenced.

US Army Regulations

On military installation sites, prior to the commencement of any construction activity, a Site Clearance Report is required to meet the criteria specified in the U.S. Army Corps of Engineers Guidance Documents and Army Regulations (in particular AR 415-15).

Corps of Engineers activities and operations must also meet safety and health requirements mentioned in the manual published by the U.S. Army Corps of Engineers (EM 385-1-1).

DEQ Regulations, Commonwealth of Virginia

Virginia State Regulations VR 680-13-02 and VR 680-13-03 under the Article 9 of the Virginia State Act require that a detailed process be followed as shown in Figure 25.5 for releases from USTs. VR 680-13-02 deals with technical standards and corrective action requirements for USTs and VR 680-13-03 deals with the financial responsibility requirements of UST owners/operators. Under VR 680-13-02, USTs used for storing heating oil with a capacity of more than 5,000 gallons are regulated. If USTs have capacity of less than 5,000 gallons and have been used for on -site heating oil storage, they are exempt from the requirements of VR 680-13-02 and VR 680-13-03. Releases from leaking USTs that are exempt and the subsequent contamination of the media must be addressed under Article 11 (Discharge of Oil into Waters, Virginia State Water Control Law, Title 62.1, Chapter 3.1). The term *underground storage tank* means anyone or combination of tanks (including underground pipes connected thereto) that is used to contain an accumulation of regulated substances, and the volume of which is 10% or more beneath the surface of the ground. This term does not include any tank used for storing heating oil for consumption on the premises where stored, except for tanks having a capacity of more than 5,000 gallons and used for storing heating oil.

When the above-mentioned definitions were applied to the Fort Myer project, only four tanks (Tanks 12 through 15), were required to be considered as regulated tanks under VR 680-13-02. Prior to the implementation of remediation plans, the UST regulations require that a Site Characterization Report (SCR) and a CAP be submitted to the state authorities. Among various remedial alternatives considered, excavation and off-site disposal was considered more feasible for soil; and pump and treat (air stripping or carbon adsorption) was considered more feasible for groundwater. Remediation goals should be based on risk based cleanup standards.

The regulations require that a Corrective action permit must be received before the remediation of the contaminated soil and groundwater can begin. The SCR and the CAP mentioned above must be approved by the state before the permit application can be submitted. However, the state was very interested in getting the contaminated media cleaned up as soon as possible, and did not want to wait for the six to ten months normally required for the permit to be approved. Accordingly, in order to expedite the process, upon the submission of an SCR that meets all the required criteria, the state will grant "interim authorization" to begin remediation. The SCR is to include risk based cleanup goals, technologies proposed to remediate the contaminated media, duration of remediation and other necessary details. Interim authorization would allow the responsible parties to initiate the remediation.

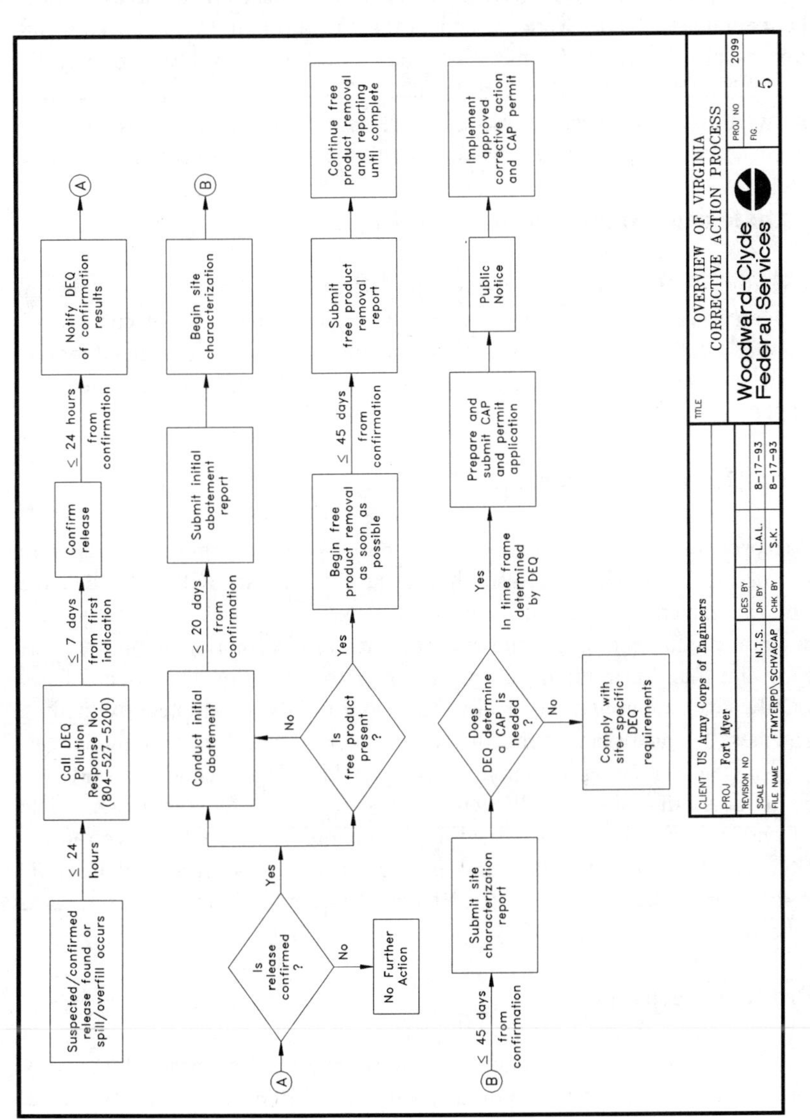

Figure 25.5. Virginia State Regulations VR 680-13-02 and VR 680-13-03.

Compliance with the Regulations

Since the field related activities had to be completed in the proposed construction area efficiently in a short time, a conservative approach was adopted by considering all the USTs as regulated tanks for the purpose of immediate remedial response. Therefore, in accordance with VR 680-13-02, initial abatement measures and free product recovery operations were conducted at all the tank areas. Soil and groundwater samples were taken at numerous points by installing monitoring wells, drilling soil borings and Hydropunches^{TM}. These samples were analyzed for total petroleum hydrocarbons (TPH); benzene, toluene, ethylbenzene, and total xylenes (BTEX) in almost all the areas. In the area where regulated USTs were located (Tanks 12 through 15), environmental samples were also analyzed for methyl-tertiary butyl ether (MTBE), polycyclic aromatic hydrocarbons (PAHs) and metals. The results of these chemical analyses were used to derive risk-based remedial end points. Regulatory compliance activities conducted on and off-site are briefly discussed below.

Initial Abatement Measures and Site Check

In accordance with 40 CFR 280.62 and VR 680-13-02, Section 6.3, initial abatement measures and site checks were conducted at the areas of concern by emptying the UST systems and subsequently the "Initial Abatement Reports" were prepared. Upon the removal of the USTs, free product was encountered at certain UST areas. Free product removal commenced immediately.

Site Characterization Report

In accordance with CFR 280.63 and VR 680-13-02, Section 6.4, SCRs were prepared for the areas where releases had occurred. These SCRs included the details of the materials released from USTs, extent of contamination of the environmental media, geological and hydrogeological information about the areas of concern and their surrounding areas. In order to determine the extent of soil and groundwater contamination, a fast-track approach was adopted by drilling Hydropunches^{TM} and by analyzing the samples on the site by an immunoassay technique (a field screening technique). A detailed risk assessment report was prepared to determine the remedial end points of various contaminants. The remedial end points were compared with the maximum detected concentrations at the UST locations and their surroundings. These findings (presented in Table 25.2. were incorporated into the SCR. Remedial alternatives were developed as part of the SCR.

Free Product Recovery

In the areas where free product was encountered, free product recovery operations were carried out as required by 40 CFR 280.64 and VR 680-13-02,

Section 6.5. Free product was recovered until the remaining free product was less than 0.125 inches (in accordance with the state's requirement).

Table 25.2: Summary of Risk-Based PRGs[1] and Maximum Concentrations

(Maximum concentrations were detected only in Tanks 12-15 area. The concentrations in other areas were either "non-detect" or far below than PRGs)

CHEMICAL	SOIL		GROUNDWATER	
	PRG† mg/kg	Max. detected conc. mg/kg	PRG† mg/l	Max Conc mg/l
Benzene	0.25	1.8	15.0	19.7
Ethylbenzene	2.00	4.0	15.0	3.6
Toluene	1.20	5.6	36.0	33.8
Xylenes	55.00	15.8	260.0	17.3
Anthracene	2,000	0.09		ND
Benzo(a)anthracene	1,500	0.12		ND
Benzo(a)pyrene	200	0.20		ND
Benzo(b)fluoranthene	1,500	0.18		ND
Benzo(k)fluoranthene	3,200	0.13		ND
Benzo(ghi)perylene	9,700	0.30		ND
Fluoranthene	270,000	0.54		ND
Indeno(1,2,3-cd)pyrene	900	0.12		ND
Naphthalene	ND	ND	12	0.12
Phenanthrene	330	0.28	35	0.01
Pyrene	200,000	0.42		ND
MTBE	3.00	0.02	30.0	0.04

†Preliminary remedial goals are based on construction worker exposure

[1]Presented Preliminary Remediation Goals (PRGs) are based upon a chemical-specific carcinogenic risk level of 1×10^{-4} and a total Hazard Index of 1.0, considering the inhalation exposure pathway for future Logistics Complex workers, and the inhalation and groundwater dermal contact exposure pathways for construction workers (other pathways not significant).

Corrective Action Plan

Discharges to surface waters from the groundwater treatment system is to have a corrective action permit. In order to obtain this permit, the CAP has to be submitted. The CAP was prepared for the regulated tanks (Tanks 12-15) in accordance with 40 CFR 280.66 and VR-680-13-02, Section 6.6. The CAP consisted of an SCR, a detailed conceptual design, remediation endpoints, a schedule, a monitoring plan (during and after remediation), plans for obtaining permits and authorizations for waste disposal and discharge, and public notification plans.

Site Clearance Report

Prior to the construction of any building in a U.S. Army installation, an SCLR must be prepared in accordance with AR 415-15. Sites to be evaluated for potential site contamination are categorized into one of three groups (see Appendix A). The sites in question at Fort Myer were placed in Category III. Category III sites are those located in areas currently known or suspected to be contaminated. The SCLR, which included the site history, information about the risk assessment, and a detailed description of the extent of contamination, was prepared for both regulated and non-regulated tanks.

CONCLUSION

Implementation of applicable regulations for this project is summarized in Table 25.3. In order to begin construction of the Logistics Complex, the sites have to be remediated. The remedial activities can begin upon the approval of the CAP or upon granting interim authorization from the State of Virginia.

Table 25.3. Use of Different Regulations at Various Stages

Activities	Major Components of Activities	Regulations				
		RCRA	OSHA	US Army	State	Local
Initial Abatement	Free Product Removal	X	X	X	X	
Site Characterization Report and Corrective Action Plan	Work Plan	X	X	X	X	X
	Field Activities (Drilling/Surveying/Sampling)					X
	Lab Analysis and Results					
	Risk Analysis			X		
	Design of Remedial				X	
	Technologies	X			X	X
Risk Assessment	Developing Preliminary Remedial Goals				X	
Site Clearance Report	Similar to Site Assessment of hydrocarbon contaminated area (regulated and non-regulated UST)			X		

APPENDIX A

EXCERPT FROM DRAFT AR 415-15

A. All proposed sites will be evaluated for potential site contamination and categorized as one of the following:

(1) Category I. This site is located in a traditional non-hazardous location, such as in an administrative, recreation, or housing area. The installation has no reason to suspect contamination.

(2) Category II. Current and former industrial sites or other hazard-producing activity sites will fit into this category. This site category consists of a perceived clean location, which, due to former industrial or other activities within or near the site, have the potential for contamination. Site survey will be accomplished by IAW USATHAMA guidance. Assistance may be requested from: CDR, USA Toxic and Hazardous Materials Agency, ATTN: CETHA-IR, Aberdeen Proving Ground, MD 21010-5401, commercial phone, 301-671-3921/2828, autovon, 584-3921/2828.

(3) Category III. Sites located in areas currently known or suspected to be contaminated are included within this category. Contamination will vary: i.e., known disposal site as identified in previous studies; unexploded ordnance at former range, etc. Site survey will be accomplished IAW USATHAMA guidance.

B. Actions required for evaluation, mitigation, and verification of site contamination are below. The statement following each action will be inserted as a separate sub-paragraph in paragraph D9, Summary of environmental consequences, in the DD Form 1391 Processor, to highlight this issue.

(1) Category I sites require surface and records survey as shown below. A physical inspection (walk of the site IAW USATHAMA guidance) will be conducted for evidence of possible contamination and the results will be recorded in Detailed Justification Paragraph D9. A review of the following documents will be conducted and the findings recorded in Block D9:

(a) Aerial photography from the Environmental Protection Agency, Environmental Photographic Interpretation Center (EPIC), P.O. Box 1587, Vint Hill Farms Station, Warrenton, VA 22186, Commercial phone 703-349-8970, FTS, 557-3110.

(b) Initial Installation Assessment and any updates available prepared by USATHAMA.

(c) Installation historical records.

(d) If a Category I site investigation discovers contaminated conditions (or the possibility thereof) the site will be reclassified as Category II or II as appropriate and those procedures followed.

CHAPTER 26

Bioremediation of Soils Contaminated with Petroleum: Comparative Studies Using Conventional Techniques and Solid Peroxygen

Sarah C. Tremaine, Ph. D., and Pamela E. Bell, Ph. D., Environmental Protection Systems, Inc., Charlottesville, Virginia, **Nancy B. Matolak, P.E.,** and **Alexis A. Hartz** formerly of Hydrosystems, Inc., Sterling, Virginia

INTRODUCTION

Bioremediation is effective at causing the degradation of many complex petroleum contaminants from soils.[1-4] Two such soil contaminants are creosote and kerosene. Creosote is a tar-like product produced during the distillation of petroleum. It is composed of a complex mixture of polynuclear aromatic hydrocarbons (PNAs), that can be degraded under aerobic conditions. The degradation rate of creosote is limited by cleavage of the benzene rings (which requires oxygen), so that higher oxygen concentrations promote higher biodegradation rates. Kerosene is a mixture of cyclic, straight-chain, and branched-chain hydrocarbons that are more easily degraded by bacteria than are PNAs. High oxygen availability also promotes higher biodegradation rates of kerosene.

There are a variety of bioremediation technologies available to treat contaminated soils which focus on enhancing biodegradation by naturally occurring bacteria. Biodegradation of complex organic compounds is generally inhibited by a lack of oxygen, nutrients, or water, acidic pH, or sorption of the contaminant so that it is unavailable to the bacteria. Most treatment technologies focus on adding oxygen (or other alternate electron acceptors), nutrients, water, alkaline chemicals and/or desorption agents to alleviate the inhospitable conditions.

The single most important factor limiting the biodegradation of petroleum compounds in contaminated soils is oxygen. Many strategies for overcoming this mass transfer limitation have been devised: mechanical aeration (tilling with a variety of devises including giant augers and specially designed tillers), soil ventilation (using blowers and vacuum pumps to move air or enriched oxygen mixtures through pipes running through soil piles), and chemical oxygenation (addition of hydrogen peroxide has been used for *in-situ* remediation). Chemical oxygenation of surface soils (the top 1 to 2 meters) has been limited by the rapid dissipation of hydrogen peroxide at the surface; however, solid peroxygen, dissolves slowly so that the oxygen released is primarily retained in the soil. Solid peroxygen is easy to apply along with nutrients or lime and has the potential of accelerating remediation significantly by greatly increasing soil oxygen concentrations.

Chemical oxygenation (Permeox^{TM}) was tested in two investigations: 1) a pilot-scale remediation study of creosote contaminated soil and 2) a bench-scale study of kerosene contaminated soils.

CASE STUDY #1: CREOSOTE CONTAMINATED SOILS

Materials and Methods

A pilot-scale bioremediation experiment of creosote contaminated soils was conducted during the summer of 1992. The test area was in the vicinity of drip tracks associated with two creosoting autoclaves at the site of a former railroad tie creosoting plant. The area was divided into 11 test plots: 8 treatment plots and 3 control plots (Figure 26.1). Two treatments were examined: mechanical aeration (plowed with lime and nutrients added, plots A, E, G, and I); and oxygen addition (Permeox^{TM}, lime, and nutrients added, plots B, D, H, and J). Two controls were included: lime addition (plots C and F) and a no treatment control (plot K). The nutrient fertilizers used in the study were a proprietary mixture. Ten randomly located soil samples were taken from each plot at each time step during the twelve week experiment and were analyzed to determine the concentrations of the creosote target compounds, nutrients, and heterotrophic bacteria.

Target compounds were measured using two different methods: a total polynuclear aromatic hydrocarbon (TPNA) method[5] and the contract laboratory procedure for polynuclear aromatic hydrocarbons (CLP-PNA; data presented elsewhere).[6] The results presented here will include only the TPNA data. The TPNA method is a screening technique developed by HS to determine total PNA concentrations. This method is very useful for examining large areas of contaminated soil or for monitoring experiments because it is rapid, costs approximately 1/10th of the price of the conventional CLP-PNA method, and has a correlation coefficient of 0.94 with the CLP-PNA method, which is linear over a five order of magnitude concentration range. The CLP-PNA method was performed on 10% of the samples as part of the quality assurance/quality control requirements for the site.

Results and Discussion

Creosote contaminant concentrations and biodegradation rates varied considerably across the plots (Figure 26.1). Average initial TPNA concentrations varied with both the treatment designation and block position (Table 26.1). Initial TPNA concentrations were generally higher in the southern block (H, J, G, and I) than in the northern block (B, D, A, and E) and the values for the

Permeox^{TM} treated soils (H and J) were significantly higher than the plowed soils (Figure 26.2; G and I). Therefore, inherent spacial heterogeneity was a confounding factor in evaluating the relative treatment effectiveness. To overcome this problem, we included initial contaminant concentration as a co-variant in the statistical analyses.

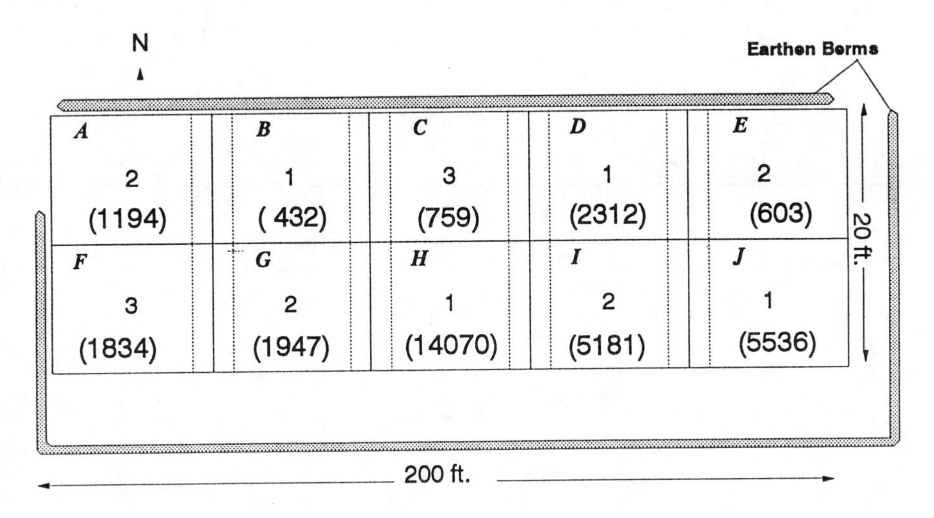

Figure 26.1. Plan of pilot-scale land treatment plots. Letters A-K denote the individual plots. The numbers (1-4) denote the treatments applied to each plot: 1= Permeox^{TM}, 2=Plowed, 3=Limed control, and 4=Untreated control. Numbers in parentheses are the mean initial total polynuclear hydrocarbon (TPNA) concentrations (mg/kg dry weight of soil) for ten samples for the plots at the beginning of the experiment. The dashed lines indicate buffer zones between the treatment plots where samples were not taken.

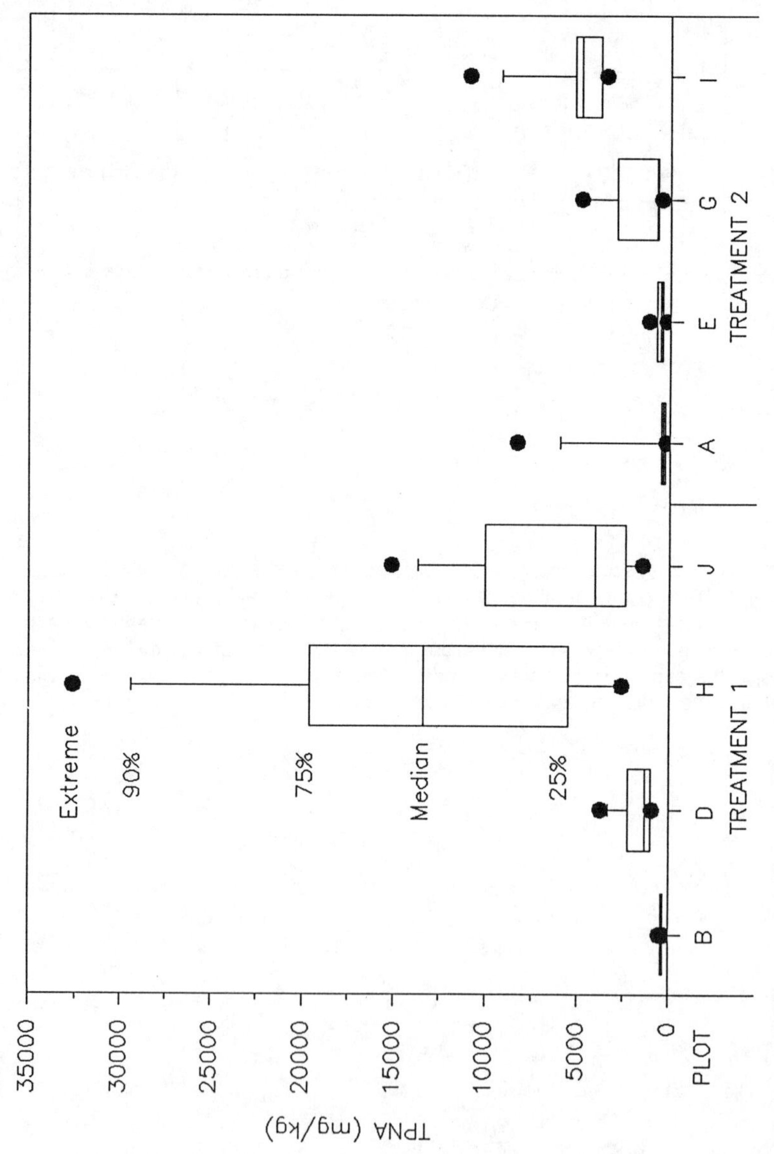

Figure 26.2. Box plots of initial TPNA concentrations (mg/kg dry weight soil) showing medians, 25th and 75th percentiles in the boxes. The error bars show the 10th and 90th percentiles. Extreme values are indicated by filled circles.

Table 26.1. Analysis of variance in the initial concentration of TPNAs (probability level = 0.05; F is the calculated F statistic).

Source of Variation	Sum of Squared Errors	Degrees of Freedom	Mean Squared Error	F Statistic	Probability Level
Within Plots	1125174373	72	15627422		
Constant	1221969078	1	1221969078	78.19	0.000
Treatment	224939366	1	224939366	14.39	0.000
Block	616161005	1	616161005	39.43	0.000
Plots within Blocks	20032012	1	20032012	1.28	0.261
Treatment by Block	166418343	1	166418343	10.65	0.002

TPNA concentrations generally decreased in the study plots over the twelve week experiment (Figures 26.3 and 26.4); however concentrations remained approximately the same in the two control plots (K and F) and two of the mechanical aeration treatment plots (B and I). TPNA concentration increases were observed in many of the plots during weeks five to seven. These increases coincided with saturated soil conditions (data not shown), which may have inhibited bacterial degradation of dissolved TPNAs due to oxygen and nutrient limitation (the saturated soils prevented nutrient augmentation). When drier conditions resumed, after week six, TPNA concentrations began to decline again.

To determine whether significant biodegradation had occurred, and to evaluate the relative effectiveness of the treatments, the initial TPNA concentration was included as a co-variate in a repeated measures analysis of variance (ANOVA) (Table 2)[7, 8]. The treatment by block interaction term was not significant ($F=1.33$, $p>0.05$), meaning that since there were no joint effects, the main effects could be examined. TPNA concentrations decreased significantly over the 12 week study (Regression:$F=180.4$, $p<0.05$). The treatments did not appear to produce significantly different losses of TPNAs when the data from all the plots were considered together (treatment effect). North and south blocks, however, had significantly different effects on TPNA concentrations (Block effect) so that data from the two blocks were considered separately. TPNA concentrations decreased significantly over time in each block ($F= 264.35$ and 92.93, $p< 0.05$ for north and south blocks, respectively). In the northern block, where lower TPNA concentrations were present, the treatment factor accounted for a significant portion of the variance ($F=8.71$, $p<0.05$), indicating that the treatments were significantly different in their ability to stimulate the degradation the TPNAs. In the southern block, where there were higher contaminant concentrations, the treatments were not significantly different ($F=0.87$, $p>0.05$). Graphs of changes in TPNA concentrations suggest that the

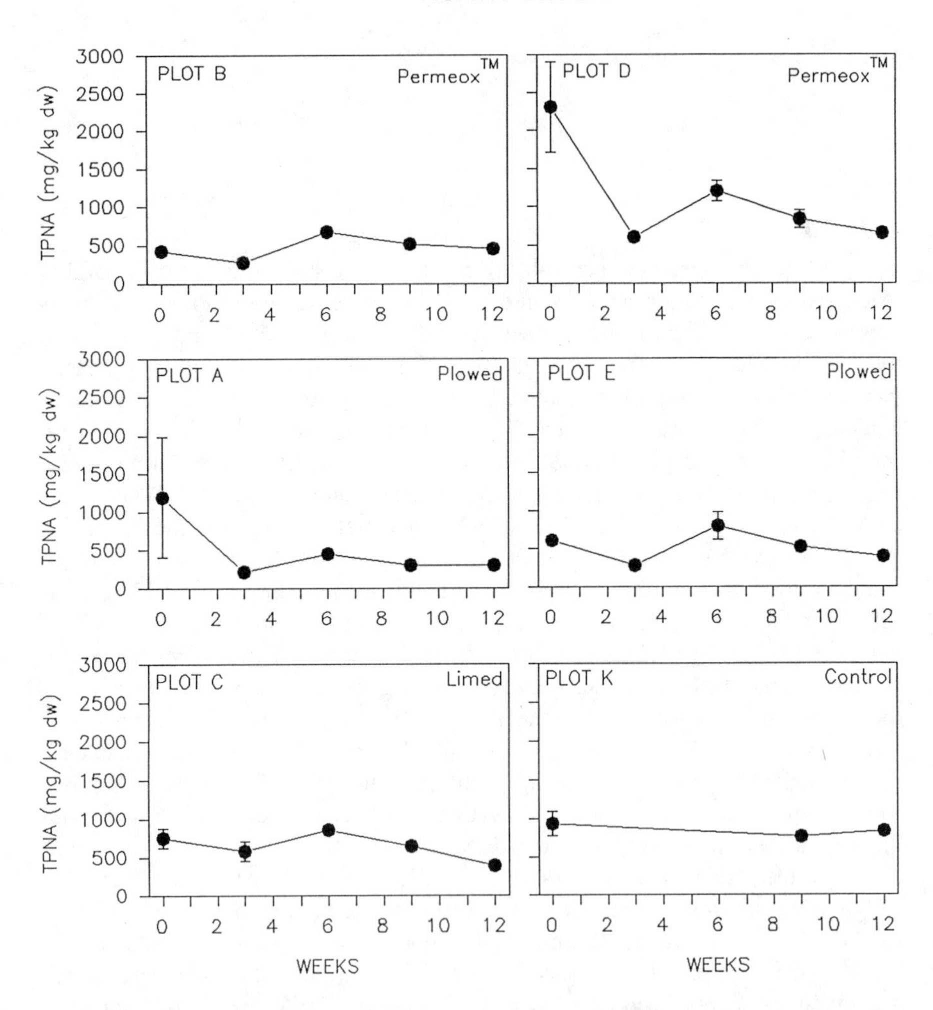

Figure 26.3. Mean soil TPNA concentrations with standard errors, measured in plots in the northern block of the land treatment area during the 12-week experiment. Concentrations in the control plot (K) are included for comparison.

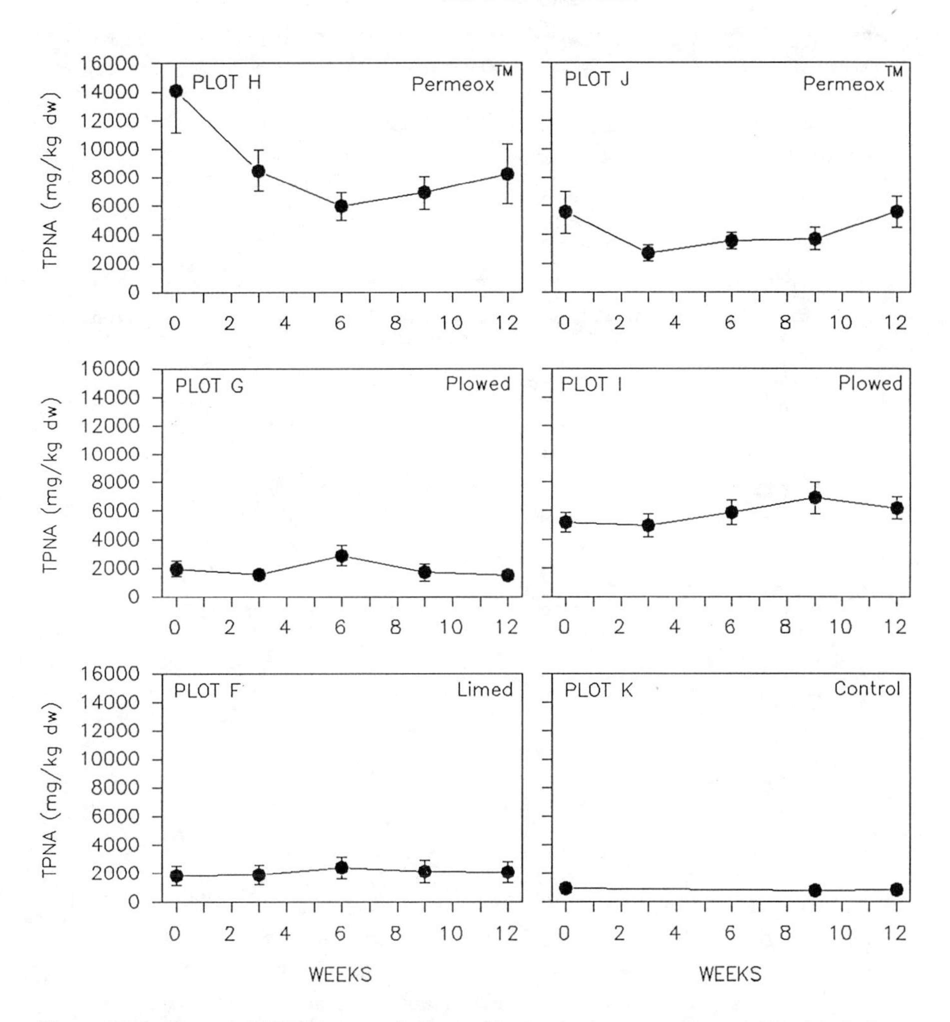

Figure 26.4. Mean soil TPNA concentrations with standard errors, measured in plots in the southern block of the land treatment area during the 12-week experiment. Concentrations in the control plot (K) are included for comparison.

treatments actually had very different effects on TPNA concentrations in the highly contaminated southern block (Figure 26.4); however the large variability in TPNA concentrations associated with the large values caused extremely high within treatment variance so that between treatment differences were not statistically significant.

Table 26.2. Repeated measures analysis of variance of the concentration of TPNAs using initial TPNA concentration as a co-variate (probability level = 0.05).

Table 2. Repeated measures analysis of variance of the concentration of TPNAs using initial TPNA concentration as a co−variate (alpha = 0.05).

All Data Source of Variation	Sum of Squared Errors	Degrees of Freedom	Mean Squared Error	F Statistic	Probability Level
Within Cells	855829845	93	9202471		
Regression	1660118205	1	1660118205	180.40	0.000
Constant	302598567	1	302598567	32.88	0.000
Treatment	10607806	2	5303903	0.58	0.564
Block	244291403	1	244291403	26.55	0.000
Treatment by Block	24526800	2	12263400	1.33	0.269

Northern Block Source of Variation	Sum of Squared Errors	Degrees of Freedom	Mean Squared Error	F Statistic	Probability Level
Within Cells	5138601	46	111709		
Regression	29530304	1	29530304	264.35	0.000
Constant	27592382	1	27592382	247.00	0.000
Treatment	1945301	2	972651	8.71	0.001

Southern Block Source of Variation	Sum of Squared Errors	Degrees of Freedom	Mean Squared Error	F Statistic	Probability Level
Within Cells	821560523	46	17860011		
Regression	1659718622	1	1659718622	92.93	0.000
Constant	386608631	1	386608631	21.65	0.000
Treatment	31193063	2	15596532	0.87	0.424

To determine which of the treatments produced the highest degradation rates, two different sets of degradation rate calculations were performed (Table 26.3). Examination of plots of TPNA concentration with time (Figures 26.3 and 26.4) indicated that there were two biodegradation phases: an initial rapid decline of contaminants between weeks zero and three, followed by an increase in concentration when soils were saturated and nutrients were depleted (data to be presented elsewhere). Following these wet conditions in week six, contaminant levels generally decreased, but more slowly than during the initial period. The graphs suggested that degradation processes during the initial three weeks (unaffected by the period of saturated soil conditions) might be different from those observed during most of the study period. Therefore, two sets of linear degradation rate calculations were performed: one for the entire study period and one for the first three weeks (Table 26.3). Rates could not be computed for the unamended control plot (K) due to insufficient data.

Table 26.3. Mean total polynuclear hydrocarbon (TPNA) degradation rates for weeks zero to three and zero to twelve with the standard error of the mean (SEM). Rates computed as the difference in mean TPNA concentration divided by the number of days elapsed.

TREATMENT	PLOT	BLOCK	BIODEGRADATION RATE			
			WEEKS 0−3 (ppm/day)		WEEKS 0−12 (ppm/day)	
			Mean	SEM	Mean	SEM
1−Permeox	B	N	−7.3	1.9	0.3	1.3
	D	N	−81.4	28.5	−19.9	7.0
	H	S	−265.9	135.9	−70.6	39.4
	J	S	−133.7	45.5	0.4	9.5
	Mean		−122.1	47.2	−22.5	10.9
2−Plowed	A	N	−46.8	38.0	−10.8	9.5
	E	N	−15.3	3.7	−2.5	0.5
	G	S	−20.0	18.4	−5.5	5.3
	I	S	−10.9	30.8	11.9	8.0
	Mean		−23.3	7.0	−1.7	3.5
3−Limed	F	N	−8.2	8.9	−4.3	1.5
	C	S	−3.1	32.2	3.0	9.9
	Mean		−2.5	4.0	−0.7	4.9

During the first three weeks of the experiment, the Permeox™ treatment produced mean biodegradation rates that were greater (122 ppm/day) than those seen in either the plowed or limed treatments (23 and 2.5 ppm/day, respectively). This relationship holds true for the entire study period with the Permeox™ - treated soils having a mean biodegradation rate of 22 ppm/day versus 12 and 1 ppm/day in the plowed and limed soils, respectively.

Overall there was significant biodegradation of creosote (Table 26.2) and the Permeox™ treatment produced faster degradation rates than the mechanically aerated treated or limed soils (Table 26.3). The effect this has on overall site remediation can be seen by extrapolating the degradation rates into the future. Since we have seen that biodegradation rate changes with time (Figures 3 and 4), we have used mean initial and final concentrations from the experiment to fit an exponential curve and thereby solve for the exponential decay constant. We consider the exponential model a more realistic estimate of biodegradation rates for long time periods than a linear model. We then took the rate constants and applied them to two contaminant levels: low (4,000 ppm) and high (16,000 ppm). This exercise assumes constantly warm environmental conditions, so that in temperate locations, the total bioremediation time would be lengthened proportional to the "growing season" (unless a soil heating source is used). Additionally, we have assumed that all of the TPNAs are degradable and that there are not any significant quantities of recalcitrant compounds.

With oxygen addition and in the case where sites have soil contamination in the range of 4,000 ppm TPNAs (as in the northern block) it would take 25 to 42 weeks to degrade the contamination to 50 ppm TPNAs (the target cleanup level) depending on the treatment used (Figure 26.5). In the case where there is higher contamination of 16,000 ppm TPNA as in the southern block, remediation would take twice as long (50 to 80 weeks) (Figure 26.6).

CASE STUDY #2: KEROSENE-CONTAMINATED SOILS

Materials and Methods

Kerosene is a diverse mixture of aromatic, straight chain and branched hydrocarbons similar to diesel fuel, that biodegrades more rapidly than PNAs. Contaminated soils having total petroleum hydrocarbon (TPH) concentrations greater than 1500 ppm must be disposed of in a hazardous waste landfill, be incinerated, or be bioremediated. To evaluate the effectiveness of bioremediation of kerosene contaminated soils, several treatments were tested in a bench-scale experiment. Lime was added initially to all of the soil to adjust the pH to near neutral. The effectiveness of chemical oxygenation was tested using Permeox™ in the presence of added nutrients. Four treatments were tested: (1) lime, (2) lime and fertilizer; (3) lime, fertilizer, and 0.1% (by mass) Permeox™; (4) lime, fertilizer, 0.2% Permeox™. The fertilizer used in the study is a proprietary mixture that has been developed for use with Permeox™. Samples were collected weekly over the six week experiment and were analyzed to determine total petroleum hydrocarbon (TPH using EPA method 418.1), kerosene degrading bacteria (using the most probable number method with kerosene as a carbon source), and nutrient concentration (nitrate and ortho-phosphate by colorimetric methods and ammonia using an ion specific electrode).

Results and Discussion

Kerosene degradation rate was highest in the 0.1% Permeox™ treatment (Figure 26.7; Table 26.4) though due to the low number of replicate samples (two) the standard errors were high, resulting in an inability to discern any significant differences between the treatments. Generally, bacterial populations were in the range of 10^8 CFU/g soil (Figure 26.8). Numbers of kerosene degrading bacteria increased in the Permeox™ treatments, but by week three all of the treatments had similar though variable bacterial abundances. The losses of kerosene were modeled using non-linear parameter estimation[7,8], to compute degradation rate

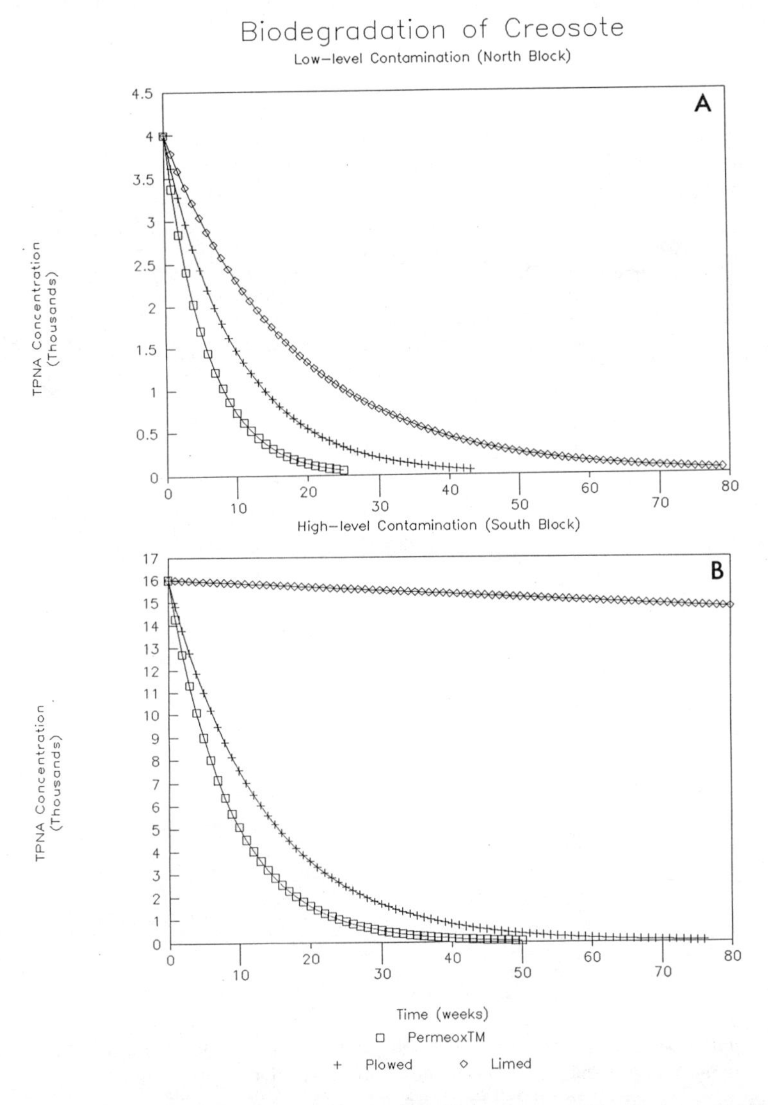

Figure 26.5. Biodegradation of creosote in the presence of low level contamination in soils. Rates are based on the mean concentration values observed in the experiment. Rates were modeled using an exponential decay relationship and an initial contaminant concentration of 4,000 ppm. Rate constants computed from the model used to generate this graph were 0.17, 0.10, and 0.055 for Permeox™, plowed and limed treatments, respectively.

Figure 26.6. Biodegradation rate of creosote in the presence of high-level contamination in soils. Rates were modeled using an exponential decay relationship and an initial contaminant concentration of 16,000 ppm. Rate constants computed by the model used to generate this graph were 0.115, 0.075, and 0.001 for Permeox™, plowed and limed treatments, respectively.

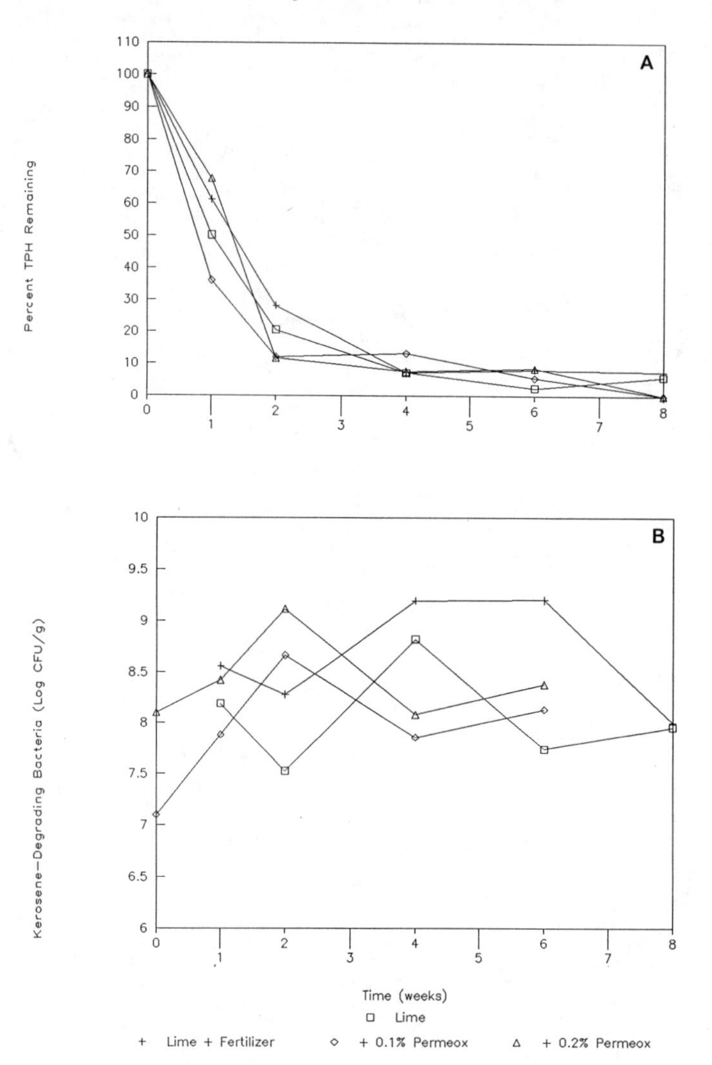

Figure 26.7. Change in concentration of TPH with time in the kerosene bench-scale experiment. Treatments are as follows: Lime, Lime and fertilizer, Lime, fertilizer, and 0.1% Permeox™, and Lime, fertilizer, and 0.2% Permeox™.

Figure 26.8. Change in abundance of kerosene-degrading bacteria with time in the kerosene biodegradation bench experiment. Treatments as described for Figure 26.7.

constants. These rate constants ranged between 0.141 and 0.083, with the Permeox™ treatment having the fastest rate constant (Table 26.4). Overall rates were also computed and used to predict the time required to achieve target cleanup levels of 50 ppm TPH. The results of this study suggest that in soils contaminated with 10,000 mg TPH/ kg soil (the concentration of contaminants in this study) the 0.1% Permeox™ treatment would degrade the contaminant kerosene to 50 ppm in about 38 days, 11 to 23 days more quickly than the other two treatments and the control (Table 26.4). If one assumes similar degradation rates at lower contaminant concentrations (2,000 ppm), biodegradation would achieve the 50 ppm target in 26 days. Results from this study also indicate: (1) a higher concentration of Permeox™ (0.2%) may have inhibited bacterial contaminant degradation since that treatment had a lower degradation rate; and (2) that lime in the absence of fertilizer may have been more effective than lime with fertilizer (Table 26.4). Biological remediation is significantly more cost effective than hazardous waste land fill disposal or incineration. Given a decision to proceed with bioremediation, the critical decision concerning the use of Permeox™ then, remains one of considering the cost effectiveness of slightly higher chemical costs versus the added time for the remediation without Permeox™.

Table 26.4. Biodegradation rate constant for kerosene in soils computed using non-linear regression, the standard error and r^2 for the regression. Biodegradation rates based on rates computed in the bench-scale study. The number of days to achieve "clean" soil (50 ppm) are noted.

Treatment	Rate Constant	Asymtotic Standard Error	r2	Rate (ppm/day)	Number of days to achieve 50 ppm TPH Given initial concentration of:	
					10,000	2,000
Lime	−0.104	0.013	0.96	−1040	51	36
Lime + Fertilizer	−0.083	0.006	0.99	−830	64	44
Lime + 0.1% Permeox	−0.141	0.032	0.88	−1410	38	26
Lime + 0.2% Permeox	−0.095	0.026	0.84	−950	56	39

CONCLUSIONS

The results presented here concern the biodegradation of two very different organic contaminants, and shows that with moderate to high creosote and kerosene levels, the treatments using Permeox^{TM} with lime and nutrient additions were the most effective at stimulating biodegradation. Biodegradation rate constants were similar in the creosote experiment (0.001 to 0.17; Figures 26.5 and 26.6) as compared to the kerosene study (0.08 to 0.14; Table 26.4). The highest rate constant (0.17) was for the Permeox^{TM} treatment at low concentrations (4000 ppm) of creosote. The numbers of days for remediation to target cleanup levels varied based on the initial contaminant concentration and the treatment used. In the cases described, remediation was achieved in less than a year for creosote using Permeox^{TM} and in one to two months for kerosene.

The results from these studies demonstrate that these petroleum based compounds are readily degraded. The question arises in biodegradation studies as to whether the losses are due to biological activity or due to mechanical or chemical losses. The only way to prove biological activity is to conduct studies using radiolabeled contaminant materials. Short of that, contaminant losses attributable to biological activity can be inferred in these experiments based on two lines of evidence. First, the plowed treatment in the creosote experiment, where mechanical mixing was maximized, showed less loss than the chemically oxygenated (Permeox^{TM}) plots. Secondly, bacterial abundance was higher in the treatments than in the unamended control and the bacterial community in the Permeox^{TM} plots was more diverse than either the control or the plowed-treated soil communities.[9] Therefore, the abundant and diverse bacterial community is the likely cause of the observed TPNA losses.

This study supports the use of Permeox^{TM} as not only is it easy to use and involves less maintenance; but it stimulated higher biodegradation rates cutting remediation 25 to 40%. Its use should be considered for near surface soils, contaminated with petroleum based compounds.

REFERENCES

1. Mueller, J.G., S.E. Lantz, B.O. Blattmann, and P.J. Chapman. Bench-Scale evaluation of alternative biological treatment processes for the remediation of pentachlorophenol- and creosote- contaminated materials: slurry-phase bioremediation. *Hazardous Waste & Hazardous Materials.* 8, 115, 1991.
2. Baker K.H., D.S. Herson, and D.A. Buniski. Bioremediation of soils contaminated with a mixture of hydrocarbon wastes: A case study. *Proc. of the 9th National Superfund Conference.* 490, 1988.
3. Block, R.N., T.P. Clark, M. Bishop. Biological remediation of petroleum hydrocarbons. In: *Sixth National Conference on Hazardous Wastes and Hazardous Materials.* HMCRI Eds., New Orleans, HMCRI, 315, 1989.
4. Sims, J.L., R.C. Sims, and J.E. Matthews. Approach to bioremediation of contaminated soil. *Hazardous Waste & Hazardous Materials.* 7, 117, 1990.

5. Tremaine S.C., P.E. McIntire, P.E. Bell, A.K. Siler, N.B. Matolak, T.W. Payne, and N.A. Nimo. Bioremediation of water and soils contaminated with creosote: suspension and fixed-film bioreactors vs. constructed wetlands and plowing vs. solid peroxygen treatment. *Bioremediation of Chlorinated and Polycyclic Aromatic Hydrocarbons.* Hinchee R.E., A. Leeson, L. Semprini, and S.K. Ong, Eds., Lewis Publishers, Boca Raton, FL, pp. 172-187, 1994.
6. Beach, R.B., K.M. West, L. Silka, M.D. Albertson, and A. Gilchenok. A screening method for total polynuclear aromatics. In: *Proceedings of the 14th Annual EPA Conference on Analysis of Pollutants in the Environment.* Norfolk, VA., 1990.
7. Tabachnick, B.G., L.S. Fidell. *Using Mutivariate Statistics.* New York: Harper & Row, 1983.
8. SPSS Inc. *SPSS/PC+ Advanced Statistics V2.0.* Chicago: SPSS Inc., 1985.
9. Bell, P.E. and S. C. Tremaine. Biodegradation: The effect of chemical oxygenation on soil microbial community structure. In preparation.

Glossary of Acronyms

AB	Absorption efficiency
ABS	Absorption factor
ACL	Alternate concentration limit
ADEC	Alaska Department of Environmental Conservation
AF	Soil to skin adherence factor
AFB	Air Force Base
Al	Aluminum
ANOVA	Analysis of variance
API	American Petroleum Institute
ARC	The Alberta Research Council
ASTM	American Society Testing Material
AT	Averaging time
ATSDR	Agency for Toxic Substances and Disease Registry
AUC	Area under plasma concentration time curve
Ba	Barium
BHA	Bottom hole assembly
BHRAs	Baseline health risk assessments
BLS	Below land surface
BRAC	Base Realignment and Closure
BSA	Bovine serum albumin
BSF	Biokinetic slope factor
BTEX	Benzene, toluene, ethylbenzene, xylenes
BTU	British thermal unit
BTX	Benzene, toluene and xylenes
BW	Body weight
C	Exposure concentration
CAD	Computer aided design
CAP	Corrective action plan
CBC	Construction Battalion Center
CDC	Centers for Disease Control
CERCLA	Comprehensive Environmental Response, Compensation and Liability Act
CF	Conversion factor
CFUs	Colony forming units
CHESS	Council for the Health and Environmental Safety of Soils
CLP	Contract laboratory procedure
CNS	Central nervous system
COCs	Chemicals of concern
CPFs	Cancer potency factors
CR	Cancer risk
CRJ	United Church of Christ's Commission on Racial Justice

CS	Chemical concentration in soil
CSF	Inhalation cancer slope factor
DA	Diffusion coefficient in air
DCAs	Dichloroethane
DCEs	Dichloroethene
DEC	Department of Environmental Conservation
DEQ	Department of Environmental Quality
DNAPL	Dense nonaqueous phase liquid
DOD	Department of Defense
DQO	Data quality objective
DSM	Division of Spills Management
DTSC	Department of Toxic Substance Control
ED	Exposure duration
EF	Exposure frequency
EFDs	Engineering field divisions
EIA	Enzyme immunoassay format
EJAPs	Environmental Justice Advisory Panels
ELISA	Enzyme linked immunoassay
EPA	Environmental Protection Agency
EPA/RREL	Environmental Protection Agency/Risk Reduction Engineering Laboratory
EPRI	Electric Power Research Institute
EPTFE	Expanded polytetrafluoroethylene
ESE	Environmental Science & Engineering
F	Flux
F&T	Fate and transport
FCC	Federal Communications Commission
FI	Fraction ingested from contaminated source
FID	Flame ionization detector
FPR	Free product recovery
FTP	Former tank pit
GAC	Granular activated carbon
GAO	General Accounting Office
GC	Gas chromatography
GC/MSD	Gas chromatography/mass selective detection
GC/FID	Gas chromatography/flame ionization detector
GC-MS	Gas chromatography-mass spectrometer
GIS	Geographic information systems
GRO	Gasoline range organics
H	Henry's Law constant
HAP	Hazardous air pollution
HASS	Hot air/steam stripping
HBCLs	Health based cleanup levels
HCl	Hydrochloric acid
HDPE	High density polyethylene
HEAST	Health effects assessment summary tables

HI	Sum of HQs
HPLC	High pressure liquid chromatography
HPLC	High performance liquid chromatography
HQ	Hazard quotient
HSWA	Hazardous and Solid Waste Amendments
IR	Infrared spectrophotometer
IRIS	Integrated risk information system
KLH	Keyhole limpet hemocyanin
LaDEQ	Louisiana Department of Environmental Quality
LAWS	Low aromatic white spirits
LBP	Low boiling point
LCA	Louisiana Chemical Assocation
LEV	Low emission vehicles
LFSA	Liquid fuels storage area
LNAPL	Light nonaqueous phase liquid
LOAEL	Low observable adverse effects level
LUST	Leaking underground storage tanks
MCAGCC	Marine Corps Air Ground Combat Center
MCAS	Marine Corps Air Station
MCL	Maximum contaminant level
MDL	Minimum detection limit
MDW	Military District of Washington
Mn	Manganese
MO	Monitoring only
MP	Monitoring points
MS	Mineral spirits
MSVs	Media specific screening values
MTBE	Methyl tert-butyl ether
MW	Monitoring well
N:P	Nitrogen:phosphorous ratio
NA2SO4	Anhydrous sodium sulfate
NAACP	National Association for the Advancement of Colored People
NAPL	Nonaqueous phase liquid
NAS	Naval Air Station
NASL	Naval Air Station, Lemoore
NCEL	Navil Civil Engineering Laboratory
ND	Non detect
NEESA	Naval Energy and Environmental Support Activity
NFA	No further action
NFESC	Naval Facilities Engineering Services Center
NJDEPE	New Jersey Department of Environmental Protection and Energy
NAVFAC	Naval Facilities Engineering Command
NOAEL	No observable adverse effects level
NPL	National Priority List

NYS DEC	New York State Department of Environmental Conservation
OQA	Office of Quality Assurance
OSHA	Occupational Safety and Health Administration
OWS	Oil/water separator
PAH	Polynuclear aromatic hydrocarbons
PAH	Polyaromatic hydrocarbons
PBS	Phosphate buffered saline
PCB	Polychlorinated biphenyls
PCE	Tetrachloroethene
PCS	Petroleum containing soils
PID	Photoionization detector
PLQ	Practical limit of quantification
PNAHs	Polynuclear aromatic hydrocarbons
PRGs	Preliminary remediation goals
PS/DS	Pilot study/Demonstration study
PVC	Polyvinyl chloride
QA/QC	Quality assurance/quality control
QC	Quality control
RA	Risk assessment
RAC	Remedial action contract
RCRA	Resource Conservation and Recovery Act
RF	Radio frequency
RfDs	Reference dosages
RI/FS	Remedial investigations and feasibility studies
RME	Reasonable maximum exposure
ROD	Record of decision
RP	Responsible party
S	Dermal contact rate
S-K	Safety-Kleen Corp.
SA	Surface area of exposed skin
SARA	Superfund Amendments and Reauthorization Act
SCLR	Site clearance report
SCR	Site characterization report
SEM	Standard error of the mean
Si	Silicon
SITE	Superfund Innovative Technology Evaluation
SIVE	Steam injection and vacuum extraction
SOPs	Standard operating procedures
SQL	Sample quantitation limit
SVE	Soil vapor extraction
SVOCs	Semi-volatile organic compounds
SYSCOM	Systems Command
TAC	Time of exchange for air in building
TCAs	Trichloroethane
TCE	Trichloroethylene

TCLP	Toxicity Characterisitic Leachate Procedure
TD	Thermal Desorption
THA	Total hydrocarbon analyzer
Ti	Titanium
TICs	Tentatively identified compounds
TICs	Total ion chromatogram
TPH	Total petroleum hydrocarbons
TPH-GC	Chromatographable hydrocarbons
TPNA	Total polynuclear aromatic hydrocarbon
TRPH	Total recoverable petroleum hydrocarbons
UF	Uncertainty factor
UMass	University of Massachusetts
UST	Underground storage tank
VAR	Ration of building volume to surface area in contact with soil
VOA	Volatile organic analysis
VOCs	Volatile organic compounds
WCFS	Woodward-Clyde Federal Services
WE	Extraction well
WTC	Wastewater Technology Centre

List of Contributors

Mohamed S. Abdel-Rahman, Pharmacology and Toxicology Department, New Jersey Medical School, Newark, NJ

Elizabeth A. Allen, Jacobs Engineering, Sacramento, CA

Mohsen C. Amiran, BioGenesis Enterprises, Inc., Des Plaines, IL.

Pamela E. Bell, Environmental Protection Systems, Charlottesville, VA.

Sheila A. Berglund, Navy Environmental Health Center, Norfolk, VA.

Adolph Bialecki, Naval Civil Engineering Laboratory, Port Hueneme, CA.

John Borovsky, Barr Engineering Co., Minneapolis, MN.

Teresa S. Bowers, Gradient Corporation, Cambridge, MA.

Edward J. Calabrese, School of Public Health, University of Massachusetts, Amherst, MA.

Deh Bin Chan, Naval Civil Engineering Laboratory, Port Hueneme, CA.

Tina Cline-Thomas, Woodward-Clyde Federal Services, Rockville, MD

James O. Crawford, Quantix Systems, Cinnaminson, NJ.

Scott E. Davies, Safety-Kleen Corp., Elgin, IL.

Eric B. Deaver, Environmental Science and Engineering Inc. Herndon, VA.

Richard P. deFilippi, Ariano Technologies, Charlestown, MA.

Margaret Findlay, Bioremediation Consulting, Inc., Newton, MA.

Samuel Fogel, Bioremediation Consulting, Inc., Newton, MA.

Shirley Fu, Gradient Corporation, Boulder, CO.

Ken Gaylord, Tesoro Alaska Petroleum Co., Anchorage, AK.

Scott George, Environmental Science & Engineering, Inc., St. Louis, MO

Edward P. Hagarty, Woodward-Clyde Federal Services, Rockville, MD.

Alexis A. Hartz, formerly of HYDROSYSTEMS, Sterling, VA.

Robert E. Hinchee, Battelle, Columbus, OH.

George C. Hobbib, Quantix Systems, Cinnaminson, NJ.

Ronald E. Hoeppel, Naval Civil Engineering Laboratory, Port Hueneme, CA.

H.T. Hoffman Jr., New Jersey Department of Environmental Protection and Energy, Trenton, NJ.

Raymond S. Kasevich, KAI Technologies, Inc., Woburn, MA.

Bharat B. Kikani, Quantix Systems, Cinnaminson, NJ.

Suresh R. Kikkeri, Woodward-Clyde Federal Services, Rockville, MD.

Jeffrey A. Kittel, Battelle, Columbus, OH.

William A. Kucharski, Louisiana Department of Environmental Quality, Baton Rouge, LA

Phillip N. La Mori, NOVATERRA Inc., Los Angeles, CA.

Susan M. Lasdin, New York State Department of Environmental Conservation, Albany, NY.

Gary A. Long, Safety-Kleen Corp., Elgin, IL.

Ann Lunt, Safety-Kleen Corp., Elgin, IL.

Keith Marcott, Safety-Kleen Corps., Elgin,IL.

Michael C. Marley, VAPEX Environmental Technologies, Inc., Canton, MA.

Nancy B. Matolak, formerly of HYDROSYSTEMS, Charlottesville, VA.

Amy R. Michelson, Gradient Corporation, Cambridge, MA.

M.W. Miller, New Jersey Department of Environmental Protection and Energy, Trenton, NJ.

William Mills, Woodward-Clyde Federal Services, Rockville, MD

Gonzalo J. Mon, Woodward-Clyde, Wayne, NJ

Mark D. Nickelson, HAZWRAP, Martin Marietta Energy Systems, Inc., Oliver Springs, TN

Daniel B. Oakley, HAZWRAP, Science and Technology, Inc., Oak Ridge, TN.

Christopher M. O'Neill, New York State Department of Environmental Conservation, Albany, NY.

William J. Powers, Naval Facilities Engineering Service Center, Port Hueneme, CA.

Stephen L. Price, KAI Technologies, Inc., Woburn, MA.

James H. Rittenburg, Quantix Systems, Cinnaminson, NJ.

Dennis I. Rubin, Woodward-Clyde Consultants, Wayne, NJ

Gretchen A Sauerman, EIT, Gainesville, FL.

Lee R. Shull, EMCON, Sacramento, CA.

Gloria A. Skowronski, Pharmacology and Toxicology Department, New Jersey Medical School, Newark, NJ

Edward J. Stanek, School of Public Health, University of Massachusetts, Amherst, MA.

Mark Stutman, W.L. Gore & Associates, Inc., Elkton, MD.

Alex Tracy, Woodward-Clyde Federal Services, Rockville, MD

Sarah C. Tremaine, Environmental Protection Systems, Charlottesville, VA.

William A. Tucker, Environmental Science and Engineering, Inc., Gainesville, FL.

Rita M. Turkall, Clinical Laboratory Sciences Department, University of Medicine and Dentistry of New Jersey, Newark, NJ

Celeste Twamley, Quantix Systems, Cinnaminson, NJ.

Richard J. Watts, Naval Civil Engineering Laboratory, Pullman, WA.

Jess J. Weiss, Environmental Science and Engineering, Gainesville, FL.

Jimmy L. Wilcher, U.S. Army Corps of Engineers, Baltimore, MD.

Charles L. Wilde, BioGenesis Enterprises, Inc., Springfield, VA.

S. Laura Yeh, Naval Civil Engineering Laboratory, Port Hueneme, CA.

Pedro J. Zavala, Environmental Science and Engineering, Inc., Gainsville, FL.

Thomas C. Zwick, Battelle, Columbus, OH.

INDEX